Atlas of Nuclear Medicine in Musculoskeletal System

Seoung-Oh Yang • So Won Oh
Yun Young Choi • Jin-Sook Ryu
Editors

Atlas of Nuclear Medicine in Musculoskeletal System

Case-Oriented Approach

Springer

Editors
Seoung-Oh Yang
Department of Nuclear Medicine
Dongnam Institute of Radiological and Medical Sciences
Busan, Republic of Korea

So Won Oh
Department of Nuclear Medicine
Seoul National University
Boramae Medical Center
Seoul, Republic of Korea

Yun Young Choi
Department of Nuclear Medicine
Hanyang University College of Medicine
Seoul, Republic of Korea

Jin-Sook Ryu
Department of Nuclear Medicine
Asan Medical Center, University of Ulsan College of Medicine
Seoul, Republic of Korea

ISBN 978-981-19-2676-1 ISBN 978-981-19-2677-8 (eBook)
https://doi.org/10.1007/978-981-19-2677-8

This Springer imprint is published by the registered company Springer Nature Singapore Pte Ltd.
The registered company address is: 152 Beach Road, #21-01/04 Gateway East, Singapore 189721, Singapore

To the patients of all cases presented in this atlas textbook

Preface

Many nuclear medicine textbooks and case studies in forms of atlas have been published so far, but there seems to be no in-depth nuclear medicine imaging atlas focused on diseases of the musculoskeletal system. Since an independent volume focusing on nuclear imaging of musculoskeletal disease has been rare, publication of this book has its significance. In the attempt to cover a specified area of musculoskeletal nuclear medicine, this book includes a large number of correlative clinical images in musculoskeletal disorders. Therefore, the authors wish to write about common cases as well as rare musculoskeletal disorders in which various imaging techniques of nuclear medicine (bone scan, SPECT, SPECT/CT, PET/CT, etc.) are useful based on the author's clinical experience in many different hospitals.

Nuclear medicine imaging in the musculoskeletal system with its ability to assess disease activities has contributed to accurate diagnosis and improved medical and surgical treatment. This book is intended to share the reading experiences of the authors with nuclear medicine and radiology residents and board specialists, and to help other clinicians who manage musculoskeletal disorders such as orthopedic and rheumatology, through various cases of musculoskeletal disorders to support their patient care. We aim to publish an easy-to-read clinical atlas by organizing the proper roles and features of various nuclear medicine imaging technics in musculoskeletal disorders by case-oriented approach.

Please consider that the format of each chapter varies according to the characteristics of each chapter title, and it is challenging to achieve complete integrity by respecting the opinions of the authors of each chapter. The editors wish to thank all contributors who spent much time and efforts in the preparation of their chapters. All the authors who participated in this issue are experts in their field. We are indebted to them for their time and effort.

It is our expectation that the original purpose of publishing cases of musculoskeletal disease including various nuclear medicine images experienced in hospitals in Republic of Korea as a case-oriented textbook has been fulfilled to a certain extent and becomes a helpful book to readers.

Busan, Republic of Korea — Seoung-Oh Yang
Seoul, Republic of Korea — So Won Oh
Seoul, Republic of Korea — Yun Young Choi
Seoul, Republic of Korea — Jin-Sook Ryu

Contents

Contributors

Young-Sil An Department of Nuclear Medicine and Molecular Imaging, Ajou University School of Medicine, Suwon, Republic of Korea

Jang Gyu Cha Department of Radiology, Soonchunhyang University Hospital, Bucheon, Republic of Korea

Jee Won Chai Department of Radiology, Seoul National University Boramae Medical Center, Seoul, Republic of Korea

Young Seok Cho Department of Nuclear Medicine, Samsung Medical Center, Sungkyunkwan University School of Medicine, Seoul, Republic of Korea

Joon Ho Choi Department of Nuclear Medicine, Soonchunhyang University Hospital, Bucheon, Republic of Korea

Yun Young Choi Department of Nuclear Medicine, Hanyang University College of Medicine, Seoul, Republic of Korea

Hye Won Chung Department of Radiology, Asan Medical Center, University of Ulsan College of Medicine, Seoul, Republic of Korea

You Mie Han Department of Nuclear Medicine, Dongtan Sacred Heart Hospital, Hwaseong-si, Gyeonggi-do, Republic of Korea

Jae Pil Hwang Department of Nuclear Medicine, Soonchunhyang University Hospital, Bucheon, Republic of Korea

Tae Joo Jeon Department of Nuclear Medicine, Gangnam Severance Hospital, Yonsei University College of Medicine, Seoul, Republic of Korea

Ji Young Kim Department of Nuclear Medicine, Hanyang University College of Medicine, Seoul, Republic of Korea

Sun Jung Kim Department of Nuclear Medicine, National Health Insurance Service Ilsan Hospital, Goyang, Republic of Korea

Yong-il Kim Department of Nuclear Medicine, Asan Medical Center, University of Ulsan College of Medicine, Seoul, Republic of Korea

Soo Jin Lee Department of Nuclear Medicine, Hanyang University College of Medicine, Seoul, Republic of Korea

Su Jin Lee Department of Nuclear Medicine, Ajou University School of Medicine, Suwon, Republic of Korea

Joo Hyun O Department of Nuclear Medicine, Seoul St. Mary's Hospital, The Catholic University of Korea, College of Medicine, Seoul, Republic of Korea

So Won Oh Department of Nuclear Medicine, Seoul National University Boramae Medical Center, Seoul, Republic of Korea

Jin Chul Paeng Department of Nuclear Medicine, Seoul National University College of Medicine, Seoul, Republic of Korea

Jung Mi Park Department of Nuclear Medicine, Soonchunhyang University Hospital, Bucheon, Republic of Korea

Soon-Ah Park Department of Nuclear Medicine, Wonkwang University School of Medicine, Iksan, Republic of Korea

Jin-Sook Ryu Department of Nuclear Medicine, Asan Medical Center, University of Ulsan College of Medicine, Seoul, Republic of Korea

Ju Won Seok Department of Nuclear Medicine, Chung-Ang University, College of Medicine, Seoul, Republic of Korea

Hye Joo Son Department of Nuclear Medicine, Dankook University College of Medicine, Cheonan, Republic of Korea

Yoo Sung Song Department of Nuclear Medicine, Seoul National University Bundang Hospital, Seongnam-si, Gyeonggi-do, Republic of Korea

Seoung-Oh Yang Department of Nuclear Medicine, Dongnam Institute of Radiological and Medical Sciences, Busan, Republic of Korea

Ie Ryung Yoo Department of Nuclear Medicine, Seoul St. Mary's Hospital, The Catholic University of Korea, College of Medicine, Seoul, Republic of Korea

Joon-Kee Yoon Department of Nuclear Medicine, Ajou University Medical Center, Suwon, Republic of Korea

Yu Sung Yoon Department of Radiology, Soonchunhyang University Hospital, Bucheon, Republic of Korea

Part I

Inflammatory and Infectious Disorders

1 Musculoskeletal Infections

Jung Mi Park, Jae Pil Hwang, Joon Ho Choi,
Jang Gyu Cha, and Yu Sung Yoon

Abstract

Pedal ulcer occurs in approximately 25% of the diabetics. Three-phase bone scan plays a role in the assessment of vascular supply including small arteries and capillary vessels in diabetic foot ulcer. Peri-prosthetic joint infection occurs in 1%–2% of primary and in 4% of revision arthroplasties. Serum CRP may be less specific after post-operative infection and antibiotics therapy; however, combined WBC scan with three-phase bone scan can detect peri-prosthetic infection accurately. Charcot neuropathic osteoarthropathy is a non-inflammatory and progressive destruction of the bone and joint. Bone single-photon emission computed tomography/computed tomography (SPECT/CT) provides an additional anatomical information to distinguish from bone and soft tissue inflammation or infection in evaluating Charcot foot. Typical pyogenic spondylitis affects two adjacent vertebrae and the intervening disc. Differential diagnosis for tuberculous spondylitis could be performed with clinical symptom and imaging findings.

J. M. Park (✉) · J. P. Hwang · J. H. Choi
Department of Nuclear Medicine, Soonchunhyang University Hospital, Bucheon, Republic of Korea
e-mail: jmipark@schmc.ac.kr; zandazanda@schmc.ac.kr; 114780@schmc.ac.kr

J. G. Cha (✉) · Y. S. Yoon
Department of Radiology, Soonchunhyang University Hospital, Bucheon, Republic of Korea
e-mail: mj4907@schmc.ac.kr; yusungy@schcmc.ac.kr

Keywords

Diabetic foot infection · Chronic prosthetic joint infection · Charcot foot · Pyogenic spondylitis

1.1 Diabetic Foot Infection

1.1.1 Clinical Course, Assessment, and Treatment

Development of pedal ulcer can be estimated to occur in 25% of the diabetics. Diabetic foot disorder is the most common cause of lower extremity amputations [1]. Hyperglycemia can cause direct damage to the nerves and blood vessels. Diabetic vascular disease has three components: arteritis and small vessel thrombosis, neuropathy, and large vessel atherosclerosis. Once tissue damage has occurred in ulcer or gangrene, the two main threats are infection and ischemia. Various foot ulcer classifications have been proposed to organize the appropriate treatment plan: the University of Texas diabetic foot ulcer classification is based on ulcer depth and is graded according to the presence or absence of infection and ischemia. Many ulcers where critical ischemia exists fail to heal and lead to irreparable tissue damage and amputation [2].

The 5-year mortality in patients with diabetes and critical limb ischemia is 30%, and the 5-year mortality in patients with diabetic foot infections

S.-O. Yang et al. (eds.), *Atlas of Nuclear Medicine in Musculoskeletal System*,
https://doi.org/10.1007/978-981-19-2677-8_1

who have foot amputations is about 50% [3]. While the neuropathic foot is characterized by warm, dry, bounding pulses as a result of peripheral vasodilation, callosities, painless penetrating ulcers at pressure points, painless necrosis of toes, spreading infection along plantar spaces, and loss of pain and thermal sensation, the ischemic foot is characterized by cold, absent pulses, trophic changes, painful ulcers around heels and toes, and claudication and rest pain. Although these factors may co-exist, it is important to early detect ischemia in the diabetic foot ulcer. Diabetes itself shows a 25% increased risk for peripheral arterial disease [4]. Bone scan can provide a useful assessment of vascular supply including small arteries and capillary vessels [5]. Proper vascular assessment in small vessel disease with associated gangrenous toes can be help to provide a successful treatment with debridement and minor amputation instead of wide amputation. In chronic and progressive diabetes, a conservative surgical approach such as revascularization can be considered. But primary amputation is better than revascularization or percutaneous transluminal angioplasty in the case of bedridden patients and patients with life-threatening sepsis and extensive muscle necrosis.

Case 1.1

A 58-year-old man was referred from an outside hospital; he was treated for necrosis of the left first toe for 3 months. He had a history of having his entire right toes amputated 3 years ago for atherosclerosis obliterans. His left first to third toes were discolored black, and gangrene was progressing. *Enterobacter cloacae* was cultured from his wound; he was treated with antibiotics. His angiography showed multifocal stenosis in both superficial femoral arteries. His plain radiography could not depict any significant bone abnormality on his left toes. However his three-phase bone scan showed perfusion defect in the left first to third toes with complete absence of bone uptake (Fig. 1.1). WBC SPECT/CT demonstrated the strong WBC uptake in the left fourth and fifth toe soft tissue, as well as a cold defect in the left first to third toe gangrene (Fig. 1.2).

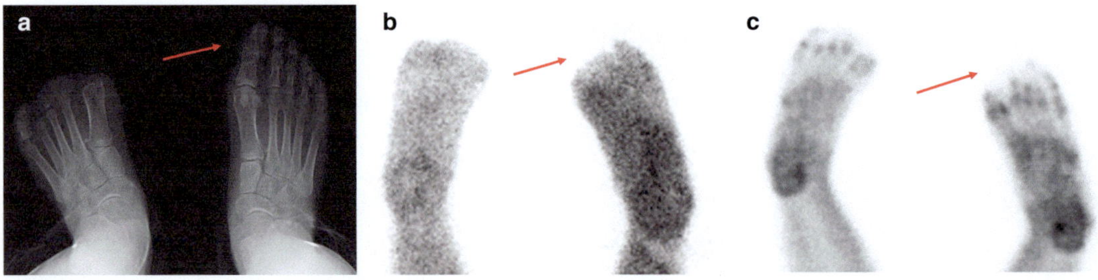

Fig. 1.1 There is no significant abnormal bone lesion in the left foot plain radiography (**a**). Perfusion defects and loss of bone uptake in the left 1st–3rd toes are clearly observed on the blood pool image and bone phase image of the three-phase bone scan (**b**, **c**)

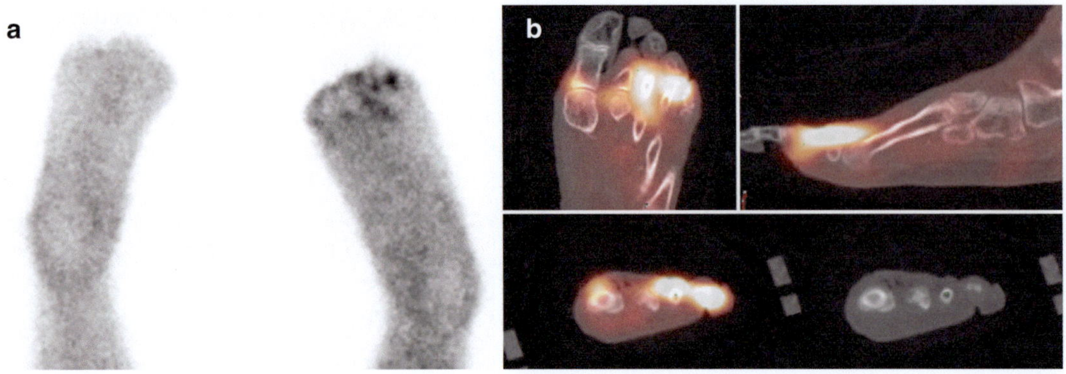

Fig. 1.2 WBC scan and SPECT/CT show cold defects in all of the left toes as well as increased uptake in the soft tissue overlying the 3rd–5th toes (**a**, **b**)

1.2 Chronic Prosthetic Joint Infection

1.2.1 Clinical Course, Assessment, and Treatment

Peri-prosthetic joint infection (PJI) occurs in 1%–2% of primary and in 4% of revision arthroplasties. Management of PJI requires multiple surgical revisions and long-term antimicrobial treatment. About two thirds of PJI results from intra-operative inoculation of microorganisms [6]. However, all prosthetic joints have hematogenous seeding from a distant primary focus, where highly vascular peri-prosthetic tissue is exposed to the highest risk of hematogenous infection in the first years after implantation. The most common primary foci are skin and soft tissue infection, respiratory tract infections, gastrointestinal infections, or urinary tract infections. According to the definition criteria for PJI by the European Bone and Joint Infection Society 2018 in Helsinki, if there is one more criteria, PJI including chronic infection can be diagnosed. It shows better sensitivity for diagnosing PJI [7].

The sensitivity of synovial fluid culture is 45% to 75% with a specificity of 95% [7]. The sensitivity of intra-operative swab is low, and the swab should be avoided. This is because a swab from the wound or sinus tract can mislead by detecting colonizing microorganisms. Generally three to five intra-operative tissue samples should be obtained for the culture. Histopathology of peri-prosthetic tissue should be considered a standard procedure in the diagnosis of PJI.

In PJI caused by low-virulence pathogens, blood tests such as WBC, ESR, and CRP are often normal [8]. CRP can be increased after surgery, due to post-operative inflammation. Serial measurements of CRP are more important for accurate interpretation. In acute post-operative infections (<4 weeks) or acute hematogenous infections, debridement, antibiotics, and implant retention are the best treatment. Local antibiotics can be additionally used during revision surgery. Antibiotic-loaded polymethylmethacrylate (PMMA) beads can become colonized by bacteria due to rapid decrease of local antibiotic concentration, resulting in new biofilm formation [6]. In patients with numerous previous revisions, or when local conditions require time, two-stage exchange with 4- to 6-week antibiotics treatment can be applied. Longer intervals (>8 weeks) of persistent sign of infection, debridement, and antibiotic-loaded spacer cement are used for dead space management with two-stage revision surgery for treatment of golden standard.

Case 1.2

A 78-year-old woman with diabetes visited the hospital for discharge from the right pre-tibial area, which had undergone knee arthroplasty at an outside hospital 7 months ago. She underwent prostheis removal due to septic arthritis and antibiotic bead insertion, and baseline three-phase bone scan showed increased perfusion and joint uptake in the right knee joint and pre-tibial space (arrow) suggesting septic arthritis (Fig. 1.3). Her serum CRP level decreased from 5.2 mg/L to 0.13 mg/L after 2 months of antibiotic IV therapy and antibiotic bead insertion. She underwent a baseline three-phase bone scan (Fig. 1.3) and 2 months later follow up scan (Fig. 1.4). It was to determine an optimal timing of revision of arthroplasty; contrary to expectations, the scan showed severely increased perfusion and bone uptake in the right tibia shaft (Fig. 1.4). WBC scan also showed diffuse WBC uptake along the previously inserted antibiotic beads in the tibia (Fig. 1.4). Rapid decrease of local antibiotic concentration in the inserted antibiotic-coated beads resulted in new biofilm formation. She underwent surgery to remove infectious granulation tissues meticulously in the bone marrow with massive irrigation and new cement insertion with VPMMA for removal of dead space in the tibia. A few months later, she underwent joint replacement surgery. Three-phase bone scan and WBC scan may be useful for accurate diagnosis of infection even when serum CRP returns to normal range after antibiotic treatment.

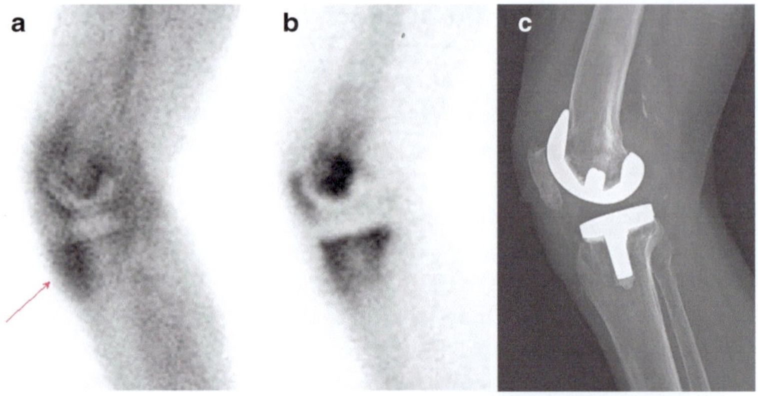

Fig. 1.3 Pretibial soft tissue hyperperfusion (arrow) and diffuse hyperperfusion surrounding the right knee joint are seen on the three-phase bone scan (**a**, **b**). Soft tissue swelling and fluid collection are seen in the patellofemoral compartment of the knee on the plain radiography (**c**)

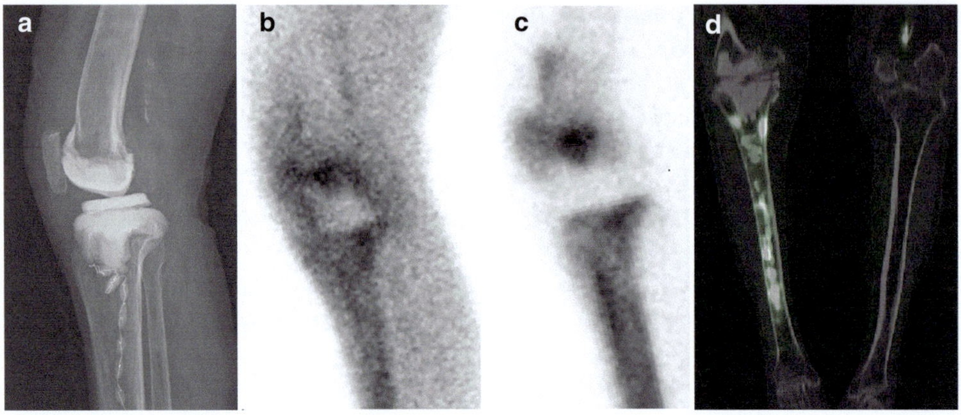

Fig. 1.4 Prosthetic removal and antibiotic bead insertion in the right tibia are seen on the plain radiography (**a**). After 2 months, serum CRP has returned to the normal range. Followed up three-phase bone scan finds the infection widely extends to the tibial shaft (**b**, **c**). WBC SPECT/CT shows strong WBC accumulation in the tibia, consistent with bone marrow infection (**d**)

1.3 Charcot Foot

1.3.1 Etiology and Clinical Significance

Charcot neuropathic osteoarthropathy is a disease spectrum of the bone, joint, and soft tissue and is non-inflammatory and progressive destruction of the bone and joints. Charcot theory is not yet clear for its pathogenesis or mechanism; there is consensus that the cause is multifactorial including polyneuropathy (loss of sensation and proprioception), neurotraumatic, and neurovascular conditions with combined osteoarthropathy [9].

From a clinical perspective, its early phase is characterized by a hot or warm, red, and swelling of foot, often without pain due to polyneuropathy, and by osteopenia with fractures. The disease will progress without proper treatment, and may result in Lisfranc's joint destruction and callopse of the longitudinal arch of the foot. The typical end-stage appearance of a Charcot foot is the rocker bottom deformity. Calcaneal insufficiency fracture is an uncommon, which can be associated with neuroarthropathy or severe osteoporosis, and may be caused by spontaneous condition or repeated microtrauma of the pull of the calcaneal tendon.

1.3.2 Radiographic Imaging

The Charcot foot can be classified using various systems according to anatomical landmarks and clinical symptoms. The most common one is the Sanders and Frykberg classification; this classification identified five zones of disease distribution according to the anatomical location. The most

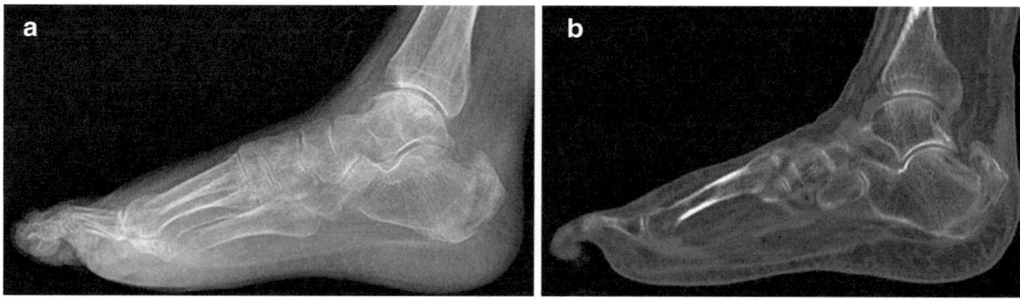

Fig. 1.5 Plain radiography and sagittal image of 3D foot CT show fracture in the calcaneal tuberosity and fluid collections at the posterior aspect of the calcaneus and tibiotalar joints (**a**, **b**)

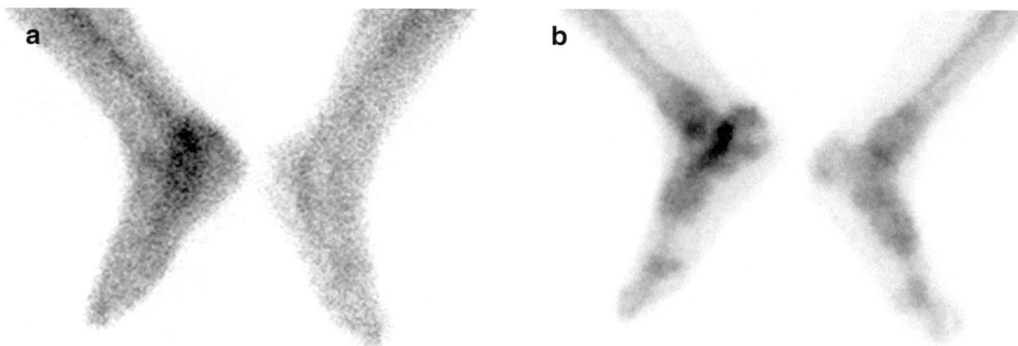

Fig. 1.6 Three-phase bone scan shows decreased radioactivity in the calcaneal fracture site and diffusely and mildly increased perfusion and bone uptake in the talocalcaneal joints (**a**, **b**)

commonly involved areas are about 45% in zone II in about 35% in zone III of cases.

Conventional radiographs of the Charcot foot are traditionally the standard imaging technique to establish the diagnosis, to stage, and to monitor the disease. MRI is a well-known imaging modality to diagnose a suspected early active Charcot disease. Early signs of a Charcot foot in MRI are bone marrow edema, soft tissue edema, joint effusion, and subchondral microfractures. MRI of late-stage Charcot foot shows joint destruction, cortical fractures, joint dislocations, bone marrow edema, superior and lateral dislocation of Lisfranc's joint, prominent well-marginated subchondral cysts, bone proliferation, sclerosis, debris, intraarticular bodies, and dislocation of talus and navicular bones [10].

Three-phase bone scintigraphy is generally used to exclude osteomyelitis in diabetic patients. Increased perfusion and bone uptake are not specific to diagnose osteomyelitis, because they may also occur in chronic soft tissue infections, fractures, and neuropathic joints. Bone SPECT/CT provides an additional anatomical information to distinguish bone and soft tissue inflammation or infection. Bone scintigraphy with radiolabeled leukocytes is more specific for osteomyelitis [11].

Case 1.3

An 82-year-old woman presented to the outpatient clinic due to left heel pain developed 2 days ago. She sprained her foot from walking 3 days ago and had a long time of diabetes history for 25 years. Plain radiography and foot 3D CT revealed right calcaneal tuberosity fracture and fluid collections at posterior aspect of calcaneal fracture site and anterior aspect of tibiotalar joints (Fig. 1.5). ^{99m}Tc-DPD three-phase bone scan and bone SPECT/CT also showed diffusely increased perfusion and bone uptake along the anterior and posterior talocalcaneal joints (Figs. 1.6 and 1.7). These additionally showed decreased perfusion and bone uptake from bony fragmentation at calcaneal avulsion fracture site. Based on the clinical exam including a long his-

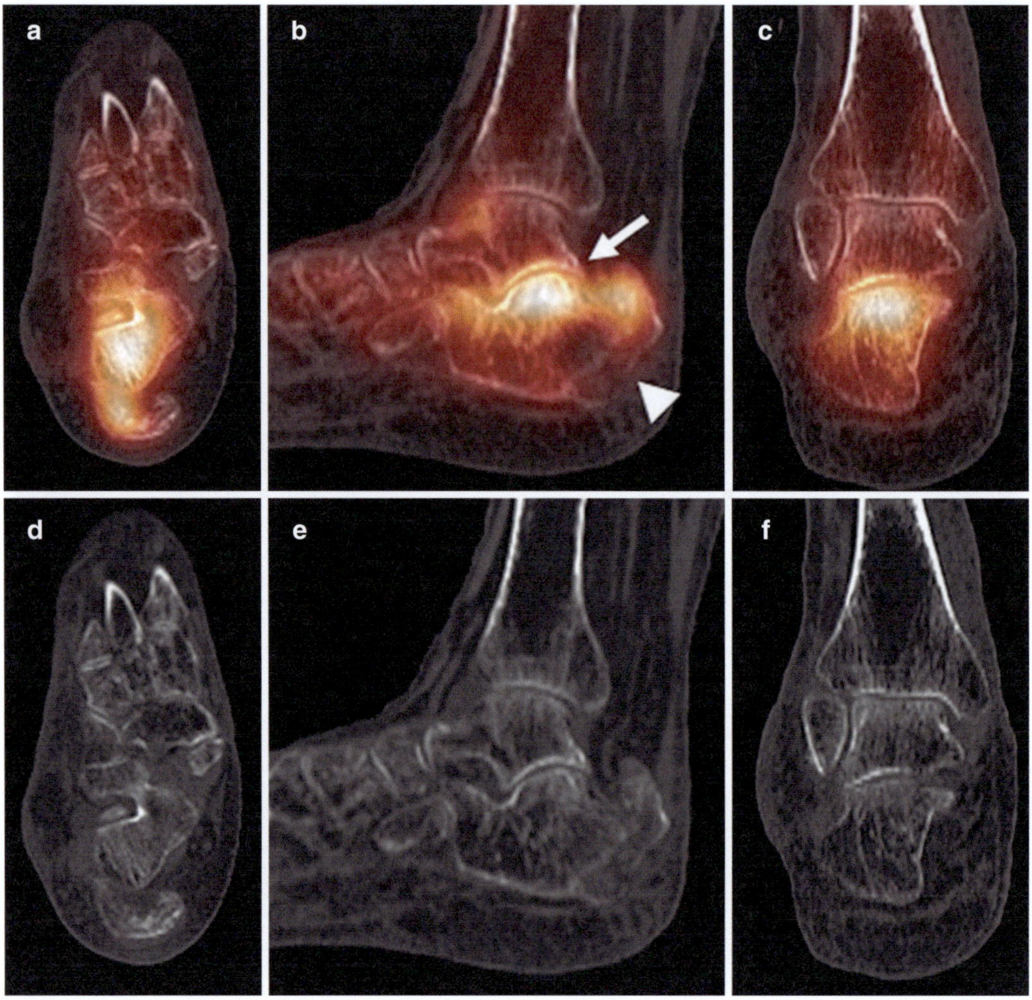

Fig. 1.7 Bone SPECT/CT shows diffuse osteopenia and small bony fragment in the talocalcaneal joint area as well as the avulsion fracture in the calcaneal tuberosity (arrowhead in **b**) on its fusion axial, sagittal, and coronal images (**a**–**c**), axial, sagittal, and coronal CT images (**d**–**f**)

tory of diabetes mellitus, no evidence of tenderness, and imaging work-ups including avulsion fracture and joint activity of common location, early Charcot arthropathy was suggested.

1.4 Malleolar Bursitis

1.4.1 Etiology and Clinical Significance

The bursa is fluid-containing, extra-articular closed sacs that provide cushioning and assist in decreasing friction between skeletal and soft tissue structures, including bone-tendon, bone-skin, and tendon-ligament interfaces. The bursa can be divided into anatomical and adventitious bursae; lateral malleolar bursa is adventitious type. Lateral malleolar bursitis is a rare cause of ankle pain and swelling characterized by bursa wall thickening and excess bursal fluid accumulation. This disease is caused by the inflammation or infection, repetitive irritation, constant pressure, swelling, complication from arthritis, and repeated stress or injury of the lateral malleolar area of the ankle. Treatment includes a lifestyle modification, combination of oral or parenteral antibiotics, and needle aspiration or incisional drainage, and surgical intervention may be necessary in some cases.

1.4.2 Radiographic Imaging

Typical ultrasonographic finding is a fluid-filled anechoic structure with a thickened hyperechoic wall. On MRI, the bursa is seen as a high T2 fluid-filled structure, and CT shows the inflamed bursa as hypodense with an enhancing wall [12]. Three-phase bone scan and perfusion SPECT/CT show hyperemia and focal increased bone uptake. In addition, SPECT/CT can provide higher diagnostic accuracy and anatomical information distinguished bone and soft tissue inflammation or infection due to additional CT imaging technique [11].

Case 1.4

A 52-year-old man presented to the outpatient clinic due to right ankle pain with ulceration (Fig. 1.8). He has had diabetes mellitus for a long time. Radiographs showed no bony abnormality except for soft tissue shadow corresponding the lesion in the right lateral malleolar area (Fig. 1.9). ^{99m}Tc-DPD three-phase bone scan showed increased soft tissue uptake in the right lateral malleolar area on blood pool phase image and mildly increased uptake in the distal fibular area suggesting reactive change on delay bone phase image (Fig. 1.10). Blood pool phase SPECT/CT showed localized increased uptake with diffuse soft tissue swelling centering around the lateral malleolar bursa of right ankle. Otherwise, delay bone phase SPECT/CT showed increased bone uptake suggesting reactive change in the right distal fibula (Fig. 1.11).

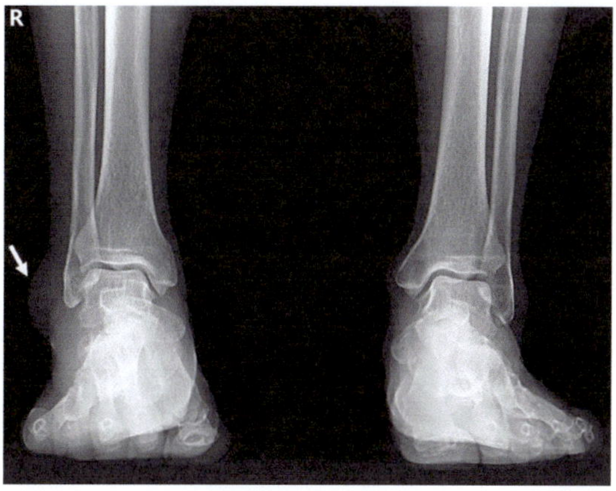

Fig. 1.9 Plain radiography of both feet and ankles

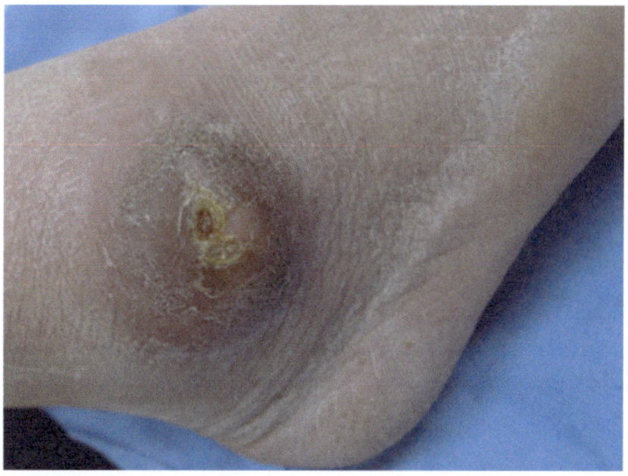

Fig. 1.8 Photograph of lateral malleolar lesion of right ankle at the time of admission

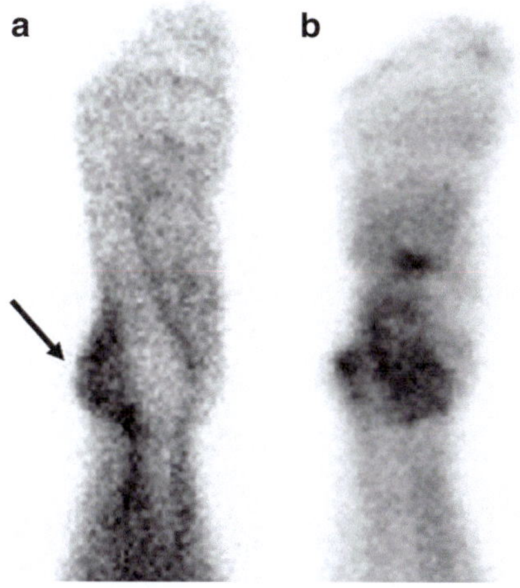

Fig. 1.10 Three-phase bone scan shows increased perfusion in the swelling area of the right lateral malleolus and mildly increased bone uptake in the lateral malleolus (**a**, **b**)

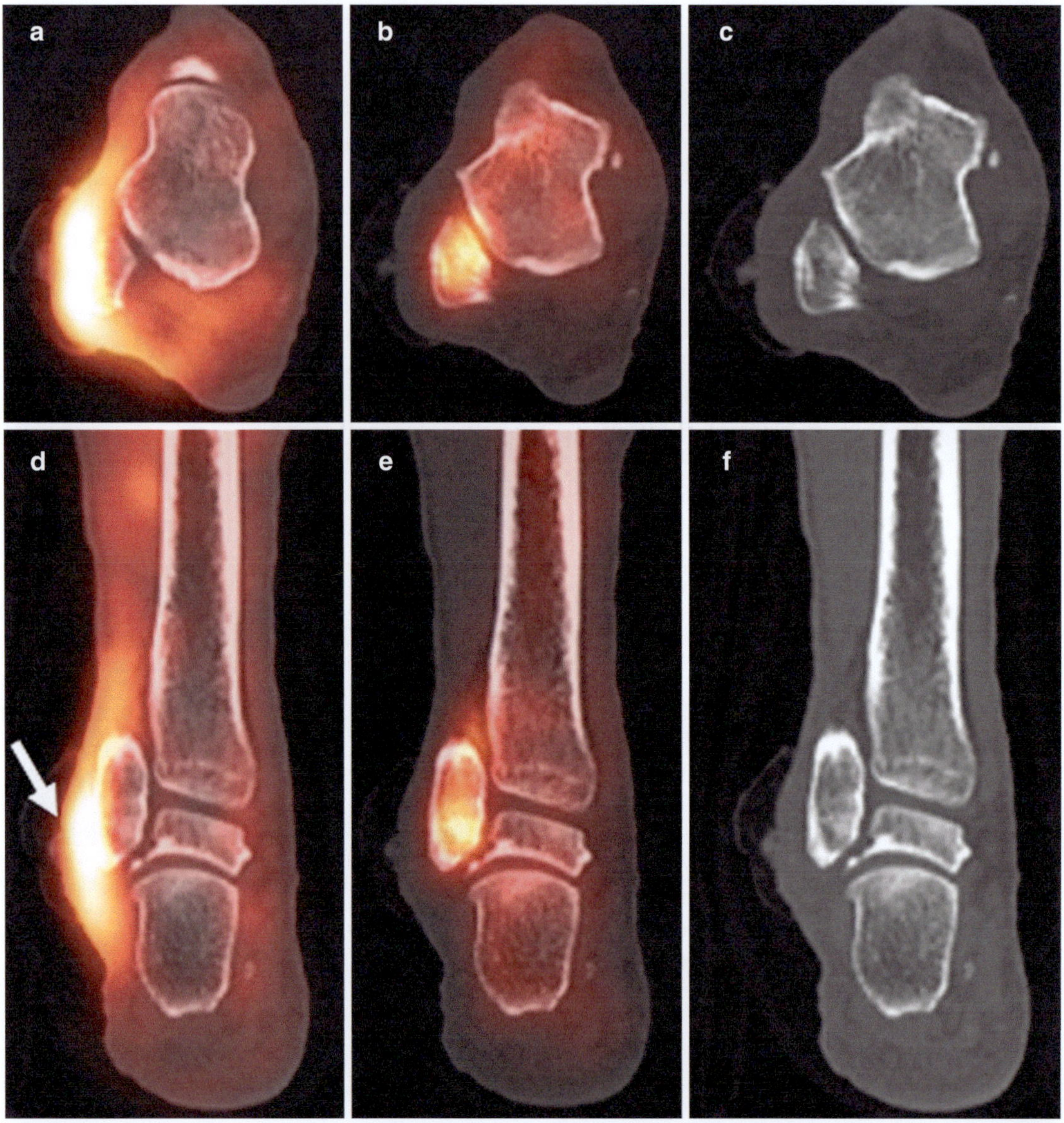

Fig. 1.11 Blood pool and bone SPECT/CT; blood pool phase axial, bone phase axial, bone axial CT images (**a**–**c**), blood pool phase coronal, bone phase coronal, and bone coronal CT (**d**–**f**). SPECT/CT can provide accurate anatomical differentiation between soft tissue and bone, while in a planar three-phase bone scan increased uptake area can be obscure for an exact localization

1.5 Pyogenic Spondylitis

1.5.1 Etiology and Clinical Significance

The term "pyogenic spondylitis" is a broad term which includes pyogenic spondylodiscitis, vertebral osteomyelitis, septic discitis, and epidural abscess. Pyogenic spondylitis usually develops from bacterial origin. The arterial route is more widespread than the venous route, usually from the skin, oral cavity, respiratory tract, and genitourinary tract [13]. The vertebral segmental artery provides an intervening disc as well as the upper and lower portion of vertebrae. Thus, typical pyogenic spondylitis affects two adjacent vertebrae and the intervening disc. The spines infections could involve all levels of the spines. The result shows the lumbar spine (45–50%) is the most common site, and the rest of the level is the thoracic (35%), cervical (3–20%), and sacral regions [14].

1.5.2 Radiographic Imaging

Radionuclide studies showed more sensitive results than radiograph images in early stages. Bone scans reveal little anatomical details and can be positive in osteoporotic fractures and neoplastic disease. Magnetic resonance imaging (MRI) is known as the gold standard for detecting pyogenic spondylitis. The infection commonly begins at the anterolateral vertebral body near the endplate [15]. Associated edema is declared and includes much of the vertebral body and intervertebral disc. MRI is also a dependable method for evaluating and assessing the spinal canal, especially the epidural space and spinal cord. Epidural abscess with neurological deficit is a surgical emergency [13].

1.5.3 Differential Diagnosis with Pyogenic Spondylitis Versus Tuberculous Spondylitis

Infective spondylitis may result from hematogenous spread, direct external inoculation, or contiguous tissues. The hematogenous arterial route is predominant in pyogenic spondylitis, starting infection from various sites to the vertebral column. Contrary to pyogenic infections, tuberculous infection usually spread from the venous system such as Batson's venous plexus. In the case of tuberculous spondylitis, there are few clinical symptoms such as fever, pain, and swelling due to infection, and the disease progresses gradually. However, infective spondylitis is highly likely to be accompanied by severe pain and high fever [16].

The most characteristic features of tuberculosis spondylitis are (a) predominantly pattern of bone destruction, (b) relatively preserved disc due to a lack of proteolytic enzymes in mycobacteria [17], (c) enhanced focal and heterogeneous contrast of vertebral bodies, (d) well-defined perivertebral regions of abnormal signal intensity, and (e) rim enhancement of vertebral intraosseous lesion in the sagittal plane. On the other hand, the common findings of pyogenic spondylitis are (a) mainly the appearance of intervertebral disc disease, (b) mild to moderately peridiscal bone involvement, (c) relatively diffuse and homogeneous enhancement of the vertebral body, (d) ill-defined abnormal signal intensity paraspinal region, and (e) intervertebral rim enhancement findings. If three or more of the five criteria are found, it is strongly suggestive of tuberculosis or pyogenic spondylitis [17].

Case 1.5
An 87-year-old woman visited an outpatient clinic with her back pain for 4 months, and tenderness was elicited at left lower back area. The laboratory findings showed elevated ESR and CRP. MR showed enhancement of bone marrow and disc in L4–L5 with bilateral paravertebral abscess and phlegmon (Fig. 1.12a). Three-phase bone scan with bone SPECT/CT showed diffuse increased perfusion and bone uptake in the L4 and L5 vertebare (Fig. 1.12c–f). Pyogenic spondylitis was diagnosed by bone biopsy.

Case 1.6
A 64-year-old man visited an outpatient clinic for back pain and left leg numbness sensation with fever. Laboratory results showed positive for the blood TB-specific antigen. MR revealed well-defined paravertebral soft tissue abscess formation (Fig. 1.13), combined with edematous bone change and heterogenous cortical loss but relatively preserved disc. Three-phase bone scan and following SPECT/CT showed increased perfusion and bone uptake in the L3–L4 bodies with increased perfusion in the paravertebral soft tissues at the L3–L5 level (Fig. 1.13c).

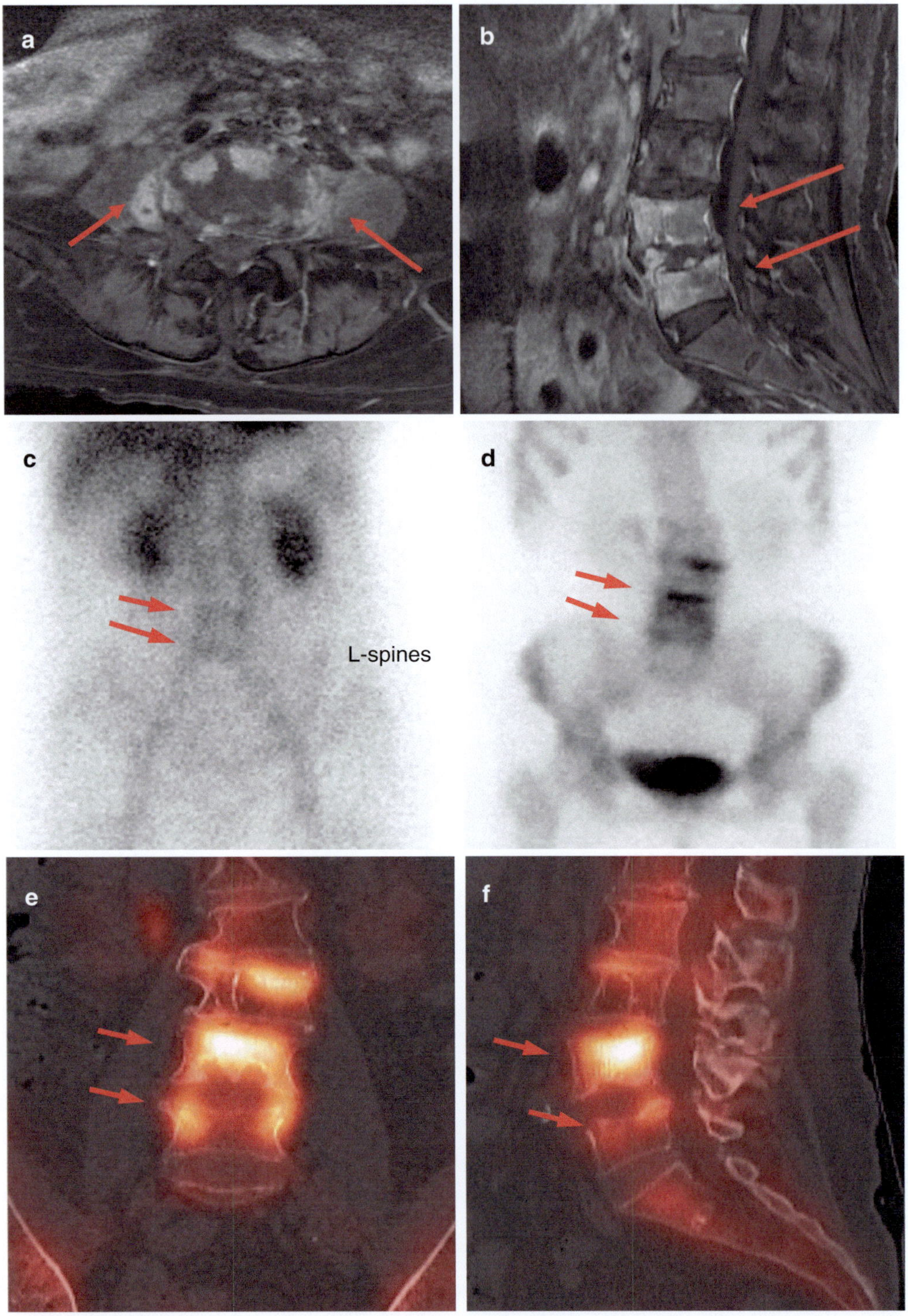

Fig. 1.12 Contrast-enhanced MR images of L-spines show enhancement of the bilateral paravertebral abscesses (arrows in **a**) and two adjacent vertebrae with the intervening disc (arrows in **b**). Three-phase bone scan (**c**, **d**) and bone SPECT/CT (**e**, **f**) show increased perfusion and bone uptake in the L4 and L5 spines

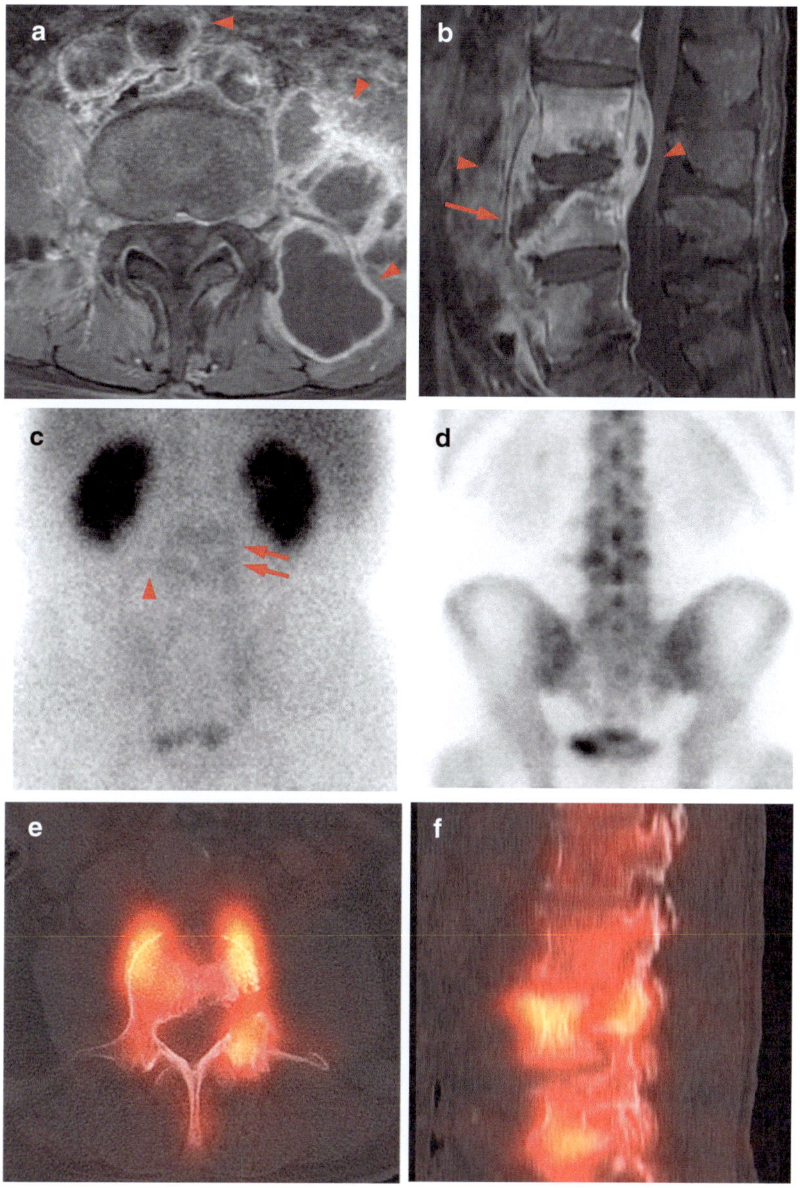

Fig. 1.13 Contrast-enhanced MR images of L-spines show multiple paravertebral abscesses (arrowheads in **a**, **b**) and bone loss in the L3 (arrow in **b**). Posterior view of three phase bone scan shows subtle increased soft tissue perfusion in the left paravertebral area (arrowhead in **c**), mildly increased perfusion in the L3 and L4 (arrows in **c**), and relatively subtle increased bone uptake in the L3 and L4 (**c**, **d**). Bone SPECT/CT shows bone defect with mildly increased bone uptake in the L4 body (**e**, **f**)

Case 1.7

A 58-year-old man visited an outpatient clinic due to back pain after receiving interbody fusion 4 months ago. He was treated with antibiotics intensively, however his clinical symtpoms were not improved. MR showed hyperenhancement on L2 and L3 bodies and paravertebral soft tissue (Fig. 1.14a, b). Prosthetic loosening and associated edema were also revealed. Three-phase bone scan showed increased perfusion and bone uptake in the left side of screw of L3 body (Fig. 1.14c, d). White blood cell scan with SPECT/CT demonstrated cold defect in L2 and L3 spines (Fig. 1.14e, f) suggesting osteomyelitis. In chronic sponydlitis, the presence of necrotic bones can reduce the effectiveness of antibiotic treatment by preventing the antibiotics from entering the tissue, which in turn may produce a new inflammation or thrombosis and result in more severe necrosis.

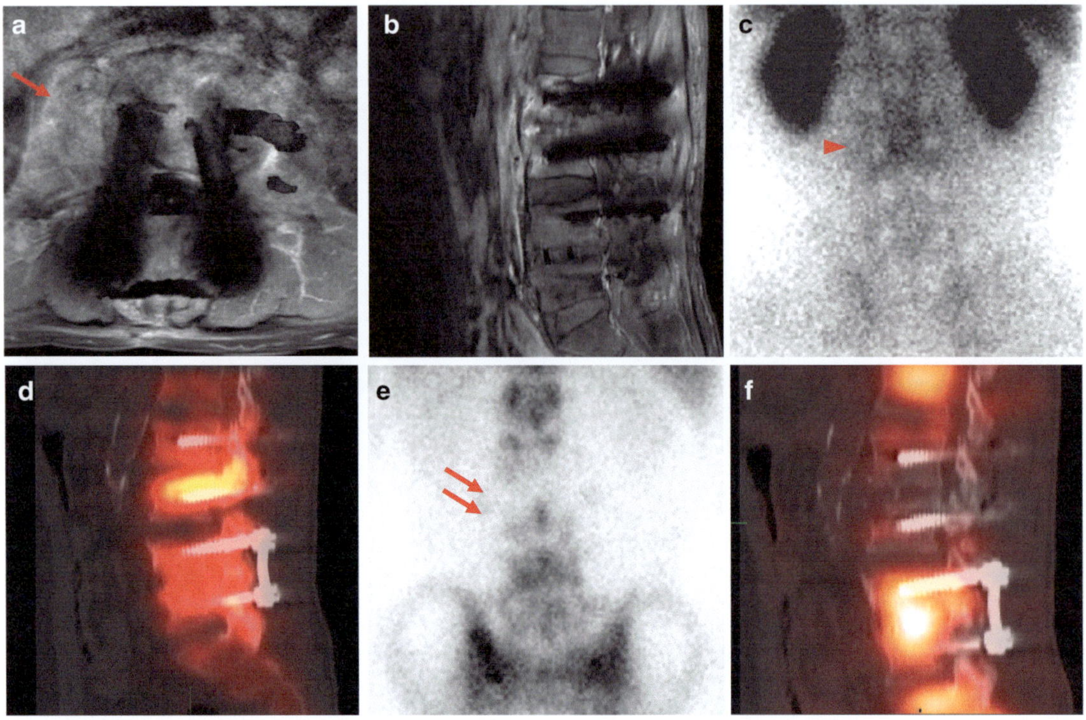

Fig. 1.14 Contrast-enhanced MR images of L-spines show enhancement of paravertebral soft tissue at the level of L2–L3 (**a**, **b**). Bone scan and SPECT/CT show increased perfusion and bone uptake in the level of L2-L3 (**c**, **d**). WBC scan and SPECT/CT show cold defects in the L2 and L3 bodies in comparison to the uptake in other lumbar spines suggesting osteomyelitis (**e**, **f**)

Case 1.8

A 78-year-old man presented to the outpatient clinic with neck pain and fever. Laboratory study showed elevation of ESR and CRP. MR demonstrated decreased intervertebral space and paravertebral abscess at C6–C7 level with anterior epidural abscess formation (Fig. 1.15a). Three-phase bone scan revealed mildly increased perfusion and bone uptake in the lower C spines at anterior and oblique views (Fig. 1.15c–e). Empirical antibiotic treatment was applied for pyogenic spondylitis. Bone scan for cervical spondylitis should be carefully reviewed, because it has a relatively low incidence and bone uptake of C spine lesion is easily obscured in comparison to the thoraco-lumbar spines.

Teaching Points

- Bone scan can provide a useful assessment of vascular supply including small arteries and capillary vessels in diabetic foot.
- Even CRP can be less specific after post-operative infection and antibiotics therapy, combining WBC scan with three-phase bone scan can be useful for detecting peri-prosthetic infection accurately.
- Early detection and proper treatment of Charcot foot are important for prevention of disease progression and prediction of disease prognosis.

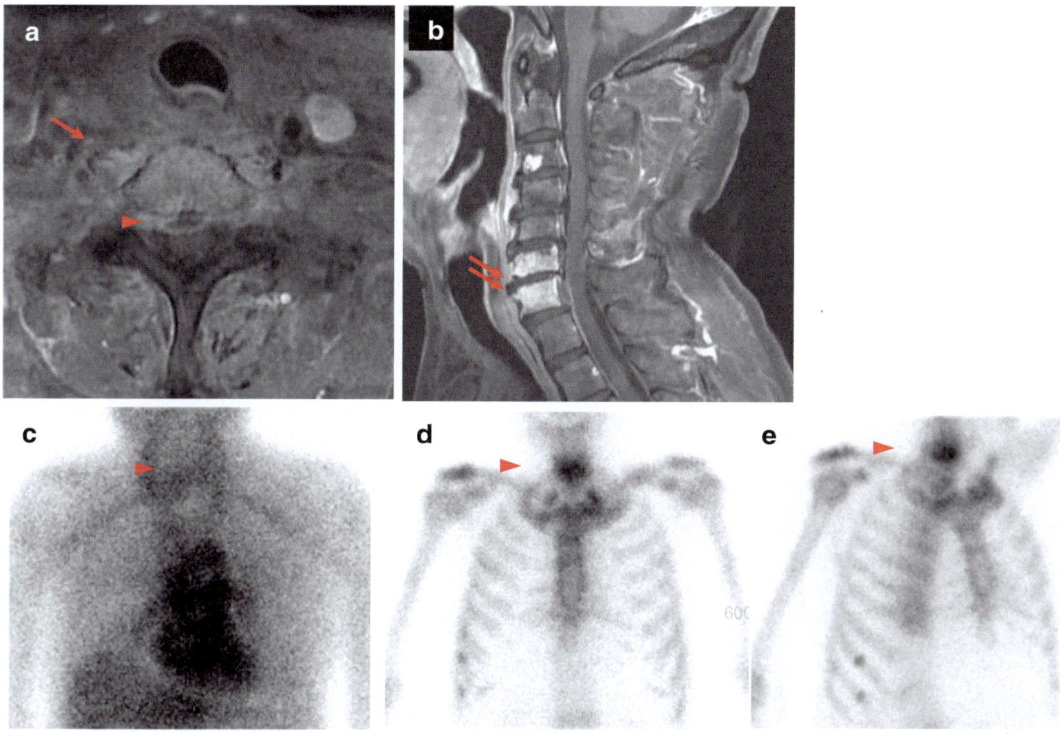

Fig. 1.15 Contrast-enhanced MR images of C-spines show paravertebral abscess at the level of C4–C7 (arrow, double arrows in **a, b**) and anterior epidural abscess at the C6–C7 level (arrowheads in **a**). Suspicious mildly increased perfusion in the lower C spine area and increased bone uptake in the lower C spines on the three-phase bone scan (arrowheads in **c**–**e**)

- SPECT/CT allows accurate anatomical correlation with CT to functional information with SPECT; it can improve the diagnostic accuracy for inflammation or infection, traumatic injury, and degenerative change of the foot and ankle.
- WBC SPECT/CT can help increase diagnostic accuracy for infections in violated bone lesions compared to relatively low sensitivity of three-phase bone scan.
- Malleolar bursitis is a rare inflammatory disease involving the soft tissue of the ankle and foot.
- Blood pool and delay bone phase SPECT/CT can help discriminate the involvement of bony inflammation or infection.
- Pyogenic spondylitis involves various clinical entities such as pyogenic spondylodiscitis, septic discitis, vertebral osteomyelitis, and epidural abscess.
- Pyogenic spondylitis affects two adjacent vertebrae and intervening disc and infectious spondylitis can show cold defect in WBC scan.
- Differential diagnosis between pyogenic spondylitis and tuberculous spondylitis can be made by clinical symptom and imaging findings.

References

1. Palestro CJ, Love C. Nuclear medicine and diabetic foot infections. Semin Nucl Med. 2009;39:52–65.
2. Lipsky BA, Berendt AR, Deery HG, Embil JM, Joseph WS, Karchmer AW, LeFrock JL, Lew DP, Mader JT, Norden C, Tan JS. Diagnosis and treatment of diabetic foot infections. Clin Infect Dis. 2004;39:885–910.
3. Lipsky BA, Berendt AR, Cornia PB, Pile JC, Peters EJ, Armstrong DG, Deery HG, Embil JM, Joseph WS, Karchmer AW, Pinzur MS, Senneville E. Infectious diseases society of America. Clinical practice guidelines for the diagnosis and treatment of diabetic foot infections. Clin Infect Dis. 2012;54:132–73.
4. Selvin E, Marinopoulos S, Berkenblit G, et al. Meta-analysis: glycosylated hemoglobin and cardiovascular disease in diabetes mellitus. Ann Intern Med. 2004;141:421–31.
5. Masaoka S. Evaluation of arterial obstructive leg and foot disease by three-phase bone scintigraphy. Ann Nucl Med. 2001;15:281–9.
6. Zimmerli W, Trampuz A, Ochsner PE. Prosthetic-joint infections. N Engl J Med. 2004;351:1645–54.
7. Izakovicova P, Borens O, Trampuz A. Periprosthetic joint infection: current concepts and outlook. Efort Open Rev. 2019;4:482–94.
8. Perez-Prieto D, Portillo ME, Puig-Verdie L, et al. C-reactive protein may misdiagnose prosthetic joint infections, particularly chronic and low-grade infections. Int Orthop. 2017;41:1315–9.
9. Jones E, Manaster B, May D, Disler D. Neuropathic osteoarthropathy: diagnostic dilemmas and differential diagnosis. Radiographics. 2000; https://doi.org/10.1148/radiographics.20.suppl1.g00oc22s279.
10. Rosskipf A, Loupatatzis C, Pfirrmann C, Boni T, Berli M. The Charcot foot: a pictorial review. Insight Imaging. 2019;10:77.
11. Yoo IR. Bone SPECT/CT of the foot and ankle: potential clinical application for chronic foot pain. Nucl Med Mol Imaging. 2020;54:1–8.
12. Hirji Z, Hunjun J, Choudur H. Imaging of the Bursae. J Clin Imaging Sci. 2011; https://doi.org/10.4103/2156-7514.80374.
13. Cheung WY, Luk KD. Pyogenic spondylitis. Int Orthop. 2012;36(2):397–404.
14. Jaramillo-de la Torre JJ, Bohinski RJ, Kuntz C. Vertebral osteomyelitis. Neurosurg Clin N Am. 2006;17(3):339–51. vii
15. Modic MT, Feiglin DH, Piraino DW, Boumphrey F, Weinstein MA, Duchesneau PM, et al. Vertebral osteomyelitis: assessment using MR. Radiology. 1985;157(1):157–66.
16. Tsiodras S, Falagas ME. Clinical assessment and medical treatment of spine infections. Clin Orthop Relat Res. 2006;444:38–50.
17. Chang MC, Wu HT, Lee CH, Liu CL, Chen TH. Tuberculous spondylitis and pyogenic spondylitis: comparative magnetic resonance imaging features. Spine (Phila Pa 1976). 2006;31(7):782–8.

2 Septic Arthritis

You Mie Han

Abstract

Septic arthritis is a painful infection in a joint induced by an infectious agent. Release of proteolytic enzyme from bacteria and inflammatory cells may cause articular cartilage damage within hours. So, prompt diagnosis and treatment are essential to prevent significant morbidity and mortality. Although arthrocentesis is commonly used to make an accurate diagnosis of septic arthritis, imaging modalities are helpful to evaluate the disease. Whole-body or three-phase bone scintigraphy has been widely used in diagnosis of septic arthritis. Although its findings are nonspecific, it is a sensitive study to diagnose septic arthritis and detect associated bone erosion or osteomyelitis under suspicion of infectious condition. A total of six cases of septic arthritis are presented in this chapter: four bacteria-confirmed and one bacteria-suspected infections and one tuberculous infection. Each case contains a closely correlated combination of images of three-phase bone scintigraphy, simple radiography, MRI, and/or PET/CT.

Y. M. Han (✉)
Department of Nuclear Medicine, Dongtan Sacred Heart Hospital,
Hwaseong-si, Gyeonggi-do, Republic of Korea
e-mail: youme@hallym.or.kr

Keywords

Septic · Infectious · Arthritis · Tuberculous Bone · Scintigraphy

2.1 Etiology and Pathophysiology

Septic arthritis is also known as infectious arthritis or pyogenic arthritis, a painful infection in a joint induced by an infectious agent. It can be caused by bacterial, viral, mycobacteria, or fungal infections. The most common causative organism is *S. aureus* (*Staphylococcus aureus*). An organism can enter the joint by the blood stream from another infected body focus, by contiguous spread from infected periarticular tissue, or by direct inoculation via penetrating injury, surgery, or injection. Knees and hips are commonly affected joints, but septic arthritis can affect other joints including both large and small joints. Symptoms and signs of septic arthritis are acute pain, swelling, redness, and heating sensation on the affected joint with discomfort and limited range of motion. Active bacterial proliferation resulted from invasion of the highly vascular synovium. Release of proteolytic enzyme from bacteria and inflammatory cells may cause articular cartilage damage within hours. Furthermore, increased intra-articular pressure from accumulation of the purulent fluid results in

S.-O. Yang et al. (eds.), *Atlas of Nuclear Medicine in Musculoskeletal System*,
https://doi.org/10.1007/978-981-19-2677-8_2

necrosis of the synovium, cartilage, and bone. Revascularization, synovial proliferation, granulation tissue, and finally bony ankylosis can also develop according to progression of arthritis. Septic arthritis is potentially serious, because it can cause rapid joint destruction leading to permanent deformities and irreversible loss of joint function in 25–50% [1].

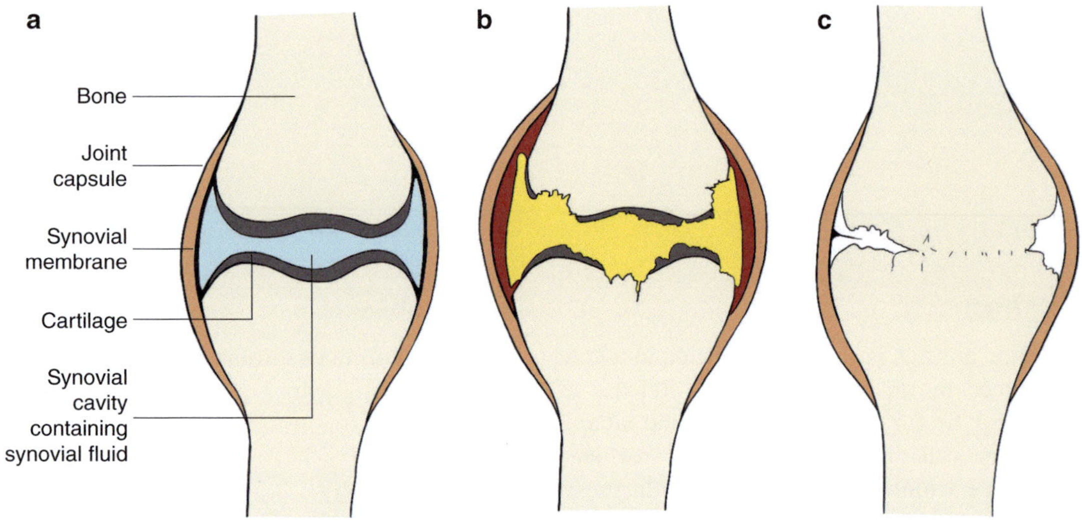

Septic arthritis – pathophysiology Normal (a). In the acute stage (b), there is an acute synovial inflammation with a purulent joint effusion. Soon articular cartilage is damaged by proteolytic enzyme secreted from bacteria and cells. If the infection is not controlled, the cartilage may be completely destroyed and subcortical bone is eroded. Healing may occur with irregular joint space narrowing and bony ankylosis (c)

2.2 Diagnosis

Diagnosis of septic arthritis is generally based on the patient's history, clinical examination, and laboratory and imaging findings. Imaging modalities such as radiography, CT (computed tomography), MRI (magnetic resonance image), ultrasound, or bone scintigraphy can help determine areas of inflammation but cannot confirm the infection. Arthrocentesis is used to make an accurate diagnosis of septic arthritis. However, false-negative gram stains and cultures of synovial fluid can occur. The infection can damage rapidly and severely the cartilage and bone within the joints, so urgent treatment is needed. Prompt diagnosis is essential for the better outcome, and MRI is the initial imaging study of choice for the septic arthritis. Septic arthritis should be differentiated from acute osteomyelitis because the treatment strategies are not identical. Sometimes, septic arthritis and acute osteomyelitis can co-exist.

Scintigraphy with ^{99m}Tc-labeled phosphonates is helpful for a supportive study in the septic arthritis and is sensitive, though not specific, to detect destructive bone change or associated osteomyelitis which shows increased bone turnover. In three-phase bone scintigraphy, because of hyperemia in synovial vessels to the affected joint, all three phases (flow, blood pool, delayed) show increased radionuclide uptake [2, 3]. Flow and blood pool images show diffusely increased activity at the suspected periarticular area. Delayed bone images obtained at 2–4 h after injection of radiopharmaceuticals may demonstrate diffuse mild bone marrow uptake in the articular confinement and continued intense bone uptake with process of destructive cortical bone change. Periarticular bone marrow uptakes also possibly represent so-called reactive bone marrow edema on MRI [4, 5]. In addition, other factors (e.g., trauma, osteoarthritis) could also cause a false-positive scan.

^{18}F-FDG PET (fluorine-18 fluorodeoxyglucose positron emission tomography)/CT has an incremental value in detection of infectious disease due to its excellent sensitivity and specificity. In pyogenic arthritis, FDG uptake is increased at synovium which has abundant neutrophils. However, increased FDG uptake is a usual feature in various types of arthritis, because of the increased cellularity of the synovial membrane in synovitis and synovial hypertrophy. Therefore, it is difficult to distinguish the septic arthritis from other types of arthritis with PET/CT images only. The advantages of PET/CT are high spatial resolution and the ability of detecting tissue metabolic state, which reflect well the extent and severity of the disease [6].

2.3 Tuberculous Arthritis

Tuberculous arthritis is a slowly progressive, chronic monoarticular infection and is almost always combined with tuberculous osteomyelitis. Joint invasion may be a result from hematogenous synovial infection or, more commonly, from epiphyseal or metaphyseal bone infection that erodes into the joint space. Hip is the second most common site followed by vertebra; it accounts for about 15% of all cases of musculoskeletal tuberculosis [7]. As synovial inflammation is started, granulomatous tissue develops and expands over the bone at the synovial reflections, with subsequent cartilage destruction and bone erosions. However, joint destruction occurs in the late phases of disease, because the lack of proteolytic enzymes in tuberculosis preserves the cartilage for a considerable length of time [8, 9].

Case 2.1
A 46-year-old man was admitted to the hospital under suspicion of acute osteomyelitis. He complained of pain and swelling of the right knee with heating sensation that had been developed on the same day after a slip down. He had a history of debridement and skin grafting over the right knee due to the burn injury 5 months ago. Purulent discharge (*S. aureus*) was coming from a small external wound on the right knee.

Postcontrast FS (fat-saturated) T1-weighted (W) sagittal and axial MRI showed enhanced thick synovial membrane and grafted tissue (*), a large joint effusion, and mildly enhanced bone marrow in the periarticular bones. ^{99m}Tc-HDP (hydroxymethylene diphosphonate) three-phase bone scintigraphy was performed on the third day after the MRI. Images of flow and blood pool phases showed diffusely increased soft tissue uptake about right knee joint, suggesting synovial hyperemia and inflammation. Delayed bone phase image showed asymmetric diffuse and mildly increased periarticular bone uptake at the right knee probably due to regional hyperemia (Fig. 2.1).

Case 2.2
A 56-year-old woman presented with continuous pain in the right shoulder. She had a history of surgical drainage of pus (*S. aureus*) and antibiotic therapy for the right shoulder joint and muscle infection, which had been developed after injections at a local clinic, 2 months ago.

Three-phase bone scintigraphy showed no significantly increased blood flow activity at the right shoulder. Asymmetric, uneven hot uptake was noted at the right shoulder on blood pool image. There was diffuse mild periarticular increased bone uptake with two focal areas of intense hot uptake at the right humerus head on delayed bone image. There were intra-articular erosive bone changes at the right humeral head. Plain radiography showed focal radiolucencies at the anatomical neck of the right humerus. These areas were corresponding to the areas with focal hot uptake on the delayed bone image of three-phase bone scintigraphy. Postcontrast FS T1W coronal MRI showed focal cortical defects at the same areas of the humerus as shown on plain radiography and bone scintigraphy. There was thick synovial enhancement with small joint effusion, enhancement of surrounding muscles and tendons, and reactive bone marrow edema in the humerus head. During arthroscopic surgery, pus from the scapular area and synovial proliferation were noted. Pathologic report was chronic active inflammation, revealing chronic infectious arthritis (Figs. 2.2 and 2.3).

Case 2.3
A 47-year-old woman was hospitalized under the impression of septic arthritis of the right hip. She

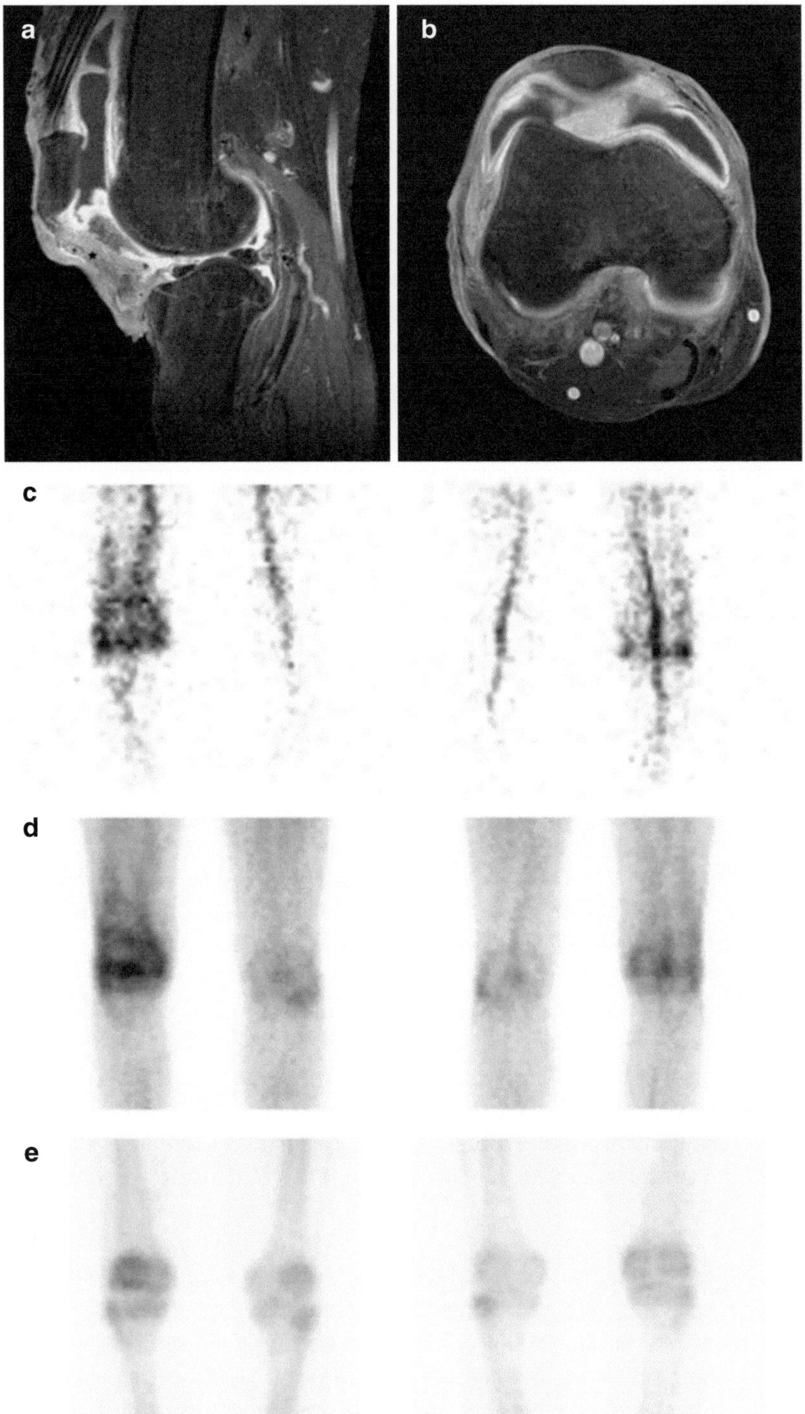

Fig. 2.1 (**a**, **b**) Postcontrast FS T1W MRI: synovial inflammation and reactive bone marrow edema in the periarticular bones, grafted tissue (asterisk). Three-phase bone scintigraphy 3 days later: (**c**, **d**) periarticular hot uptake at right knee on flow and blood pool phases, associated with septic arthritis. (**e**) Asymmetric diffuse mild periarticular increased bone uptake at right knee, suggestive of periarticular bone edema

complained right hip pain, which had developed 2 months ago and aggravated recently, extending to inguinal and buttock areas. The result of aspiration biopsy was chronic active inflammation. No microorganisms were found in the bacterial culture.

Precontrast T1W and postcontrast FS T1W axial MRI showed right hip joint inflammation

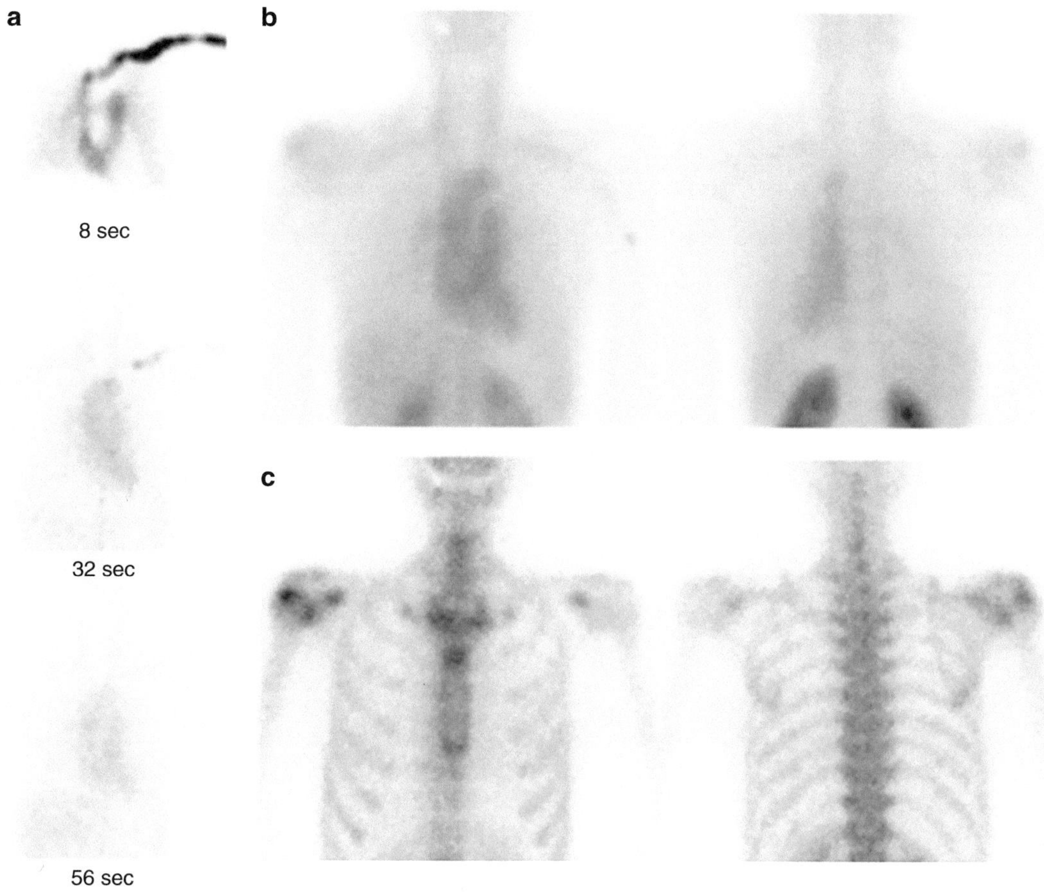

Fig. 2.2 Three-phase bone scintigraphy: (**a**) no significant hyperemia at the right shoulder on flow image. (**b**) Asymmetric uneven hot uptake at the right shoulder on blood pool image. (**c**) Diffuse mild periarticular increased bone uptake with two focal areas of intense hot uptake at the right humerus head on delayed image

with enhanced thick synovial membrane and enhanced periarticular soft tissue. Heterogeneous T1 low signal intensities and contrast enhancements were in the right femoral head and neck and in the acetabulum. Non-enhanced T1 low signal intensity area was at the posterior aspect of the right femoral head, suggesting osteonecrosis. ^{99m}Tc-HDP three-phase bone scintigraphy showed asymmetric hot uptake at the right hip on flow and blood pool images. Delayed image showed asymmetric increased bone uptake in the right hip joint. There was no significant bony lesion on the initial plain radiography. Plain radiography taken 7 months later showed uneven narrowing of the right hip joint space with bone erosions and sclerosis in the femoral head and the acetabulum (Fig. 2.4).

Case 2.4

A 67-year-old woman was admitted due to spontaneous painful swelling in the left wrist for 2 weeks. There was purulent discharge (*Streptococcus agalactiae*) from the left wrist.

Plain radiography of the left wrist showed soft tissue swelling, uneven joint space narrowing, and periarticular bone erosion and sclerosis. FS T2W coronal MRI showed high signal intensity of synovial and parasynovial inflammation in the left wrist joint with uneven joint space narrowing, subchondral bone erosions,

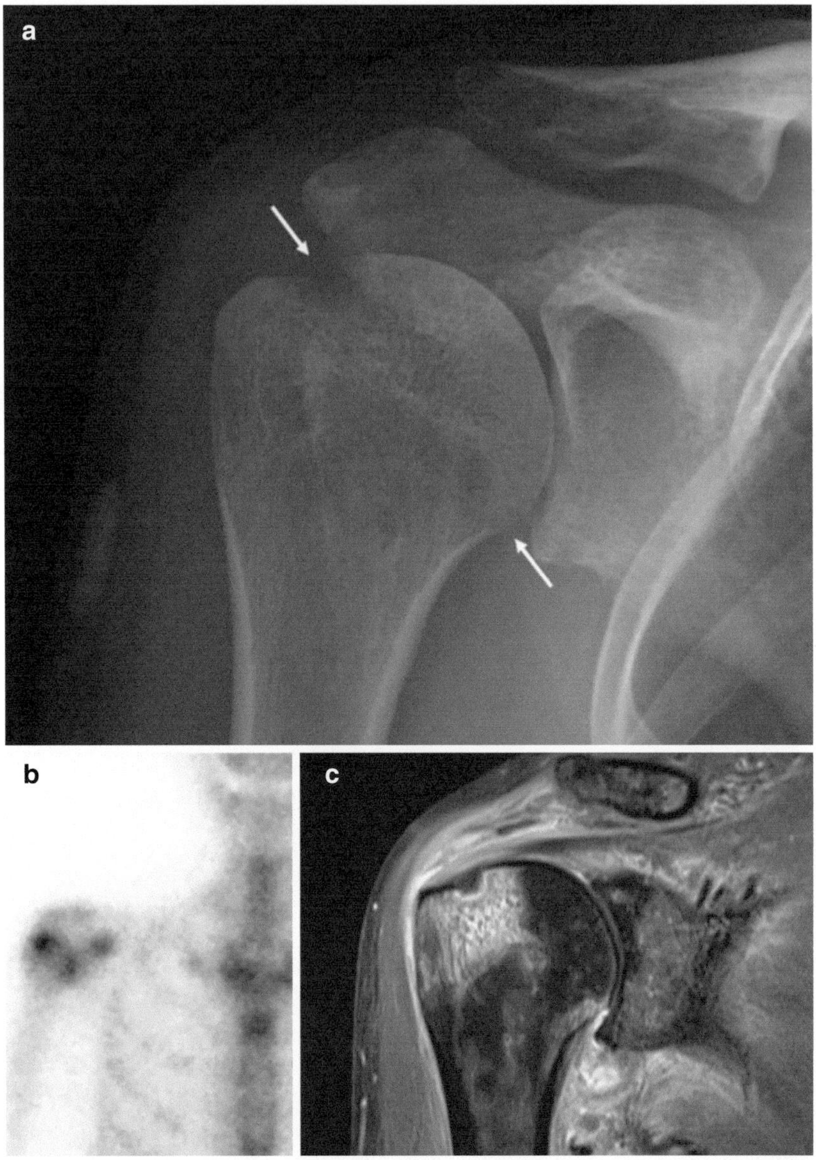

Fig. 2.3 (**a**) Plain radiography: focal bone erosions (arrows) at the anatomical neck of the right humerus. (**b**) Bone scintigraphy: focal hot uptakes at right humerus head corresponding to bone erosions. (**c**) Postcontrast FS T1W MRI: bone erosions with reactive bone marrow edema in the humerus head and synovial and adjacent soft tissue inflammation

and patchy bone marrow edema. Mid-carpal joint space was relatively preserved. ^{99m}Tc-HDP three-phase bone scintigraphy showed diffuse hot uptake throughout the left wrist on both perfusion and blood pool images, indicating articular hyperemia and inflammation. Delayed scan shows diffuse periarticular increased bone uptake with intense radiotracer uptakes at proximal and distal carpal (especially second to fourth carpometacarpal) joint areas (Fig. 2.5).

Case 2.5

A 64-year-old man was admitted to the hospital due to incidentally detected gastric cancer during health screening. He complained pain and swelling on both knees. He had a clinical history of intra-articular injection at a local clinic 5 days ago. He underwent arthroscopic pus (*S. aureus*) drainage and irrigation.

Initial plain radiography of the right knee shows distension of suprapatellar bursa without evidence of bone lesion. ^{18}F-FDG PET/CT was taken 1 day

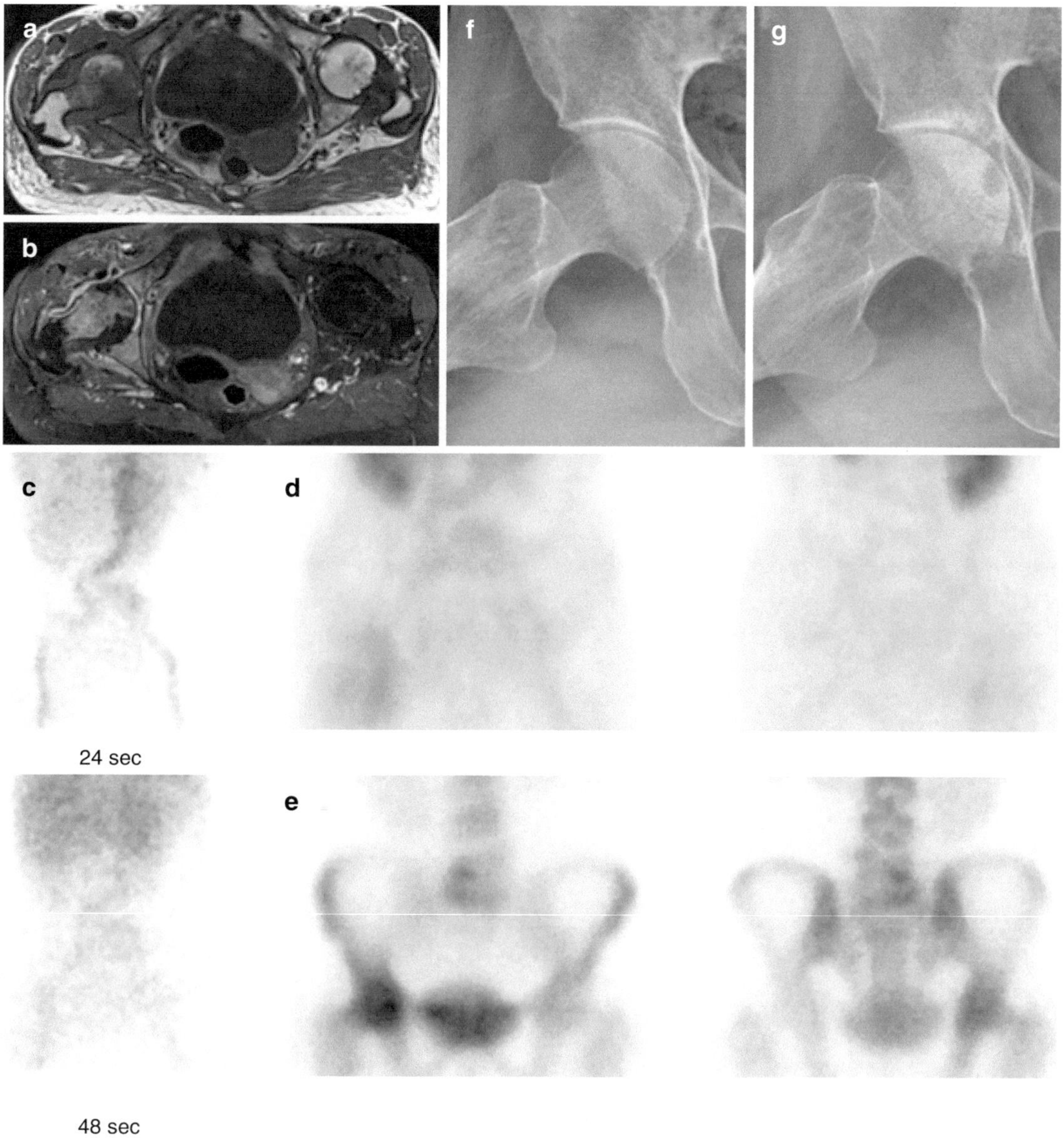

Fig. 2.4 (**a**) Precontrast T1W and (**b**) postcontrast FS T1W MRI: right hip joint and adjacent soft tissue inflammation with bone marrow change in femoral head and neck and in acetabulum. Three-phase bone scintigraphy: (**c**) asymmetric mild hyperemia, (**d**) hot uptake at right hip on blood pool image, (**e**) periarticular increased bone uptake in right femoral head and neck and in acetabulum. (**f**) Initial plain radiography: no significant bone lesion. (**g**) Plain radiography taken 7 months later: uneven joint space narrowing with bone erosions and sclerosis in femoral head and acetabulum

after surgical pus drainage and irrigation. Maximum intensity projection (MIP) image shows intense FDG uptake at the right knee. Coronal and sagittal PET/CT images showed intense FDG uptake in the right knee joint along the synovial lining without evidence of bone involvement (Fig. 2.6).

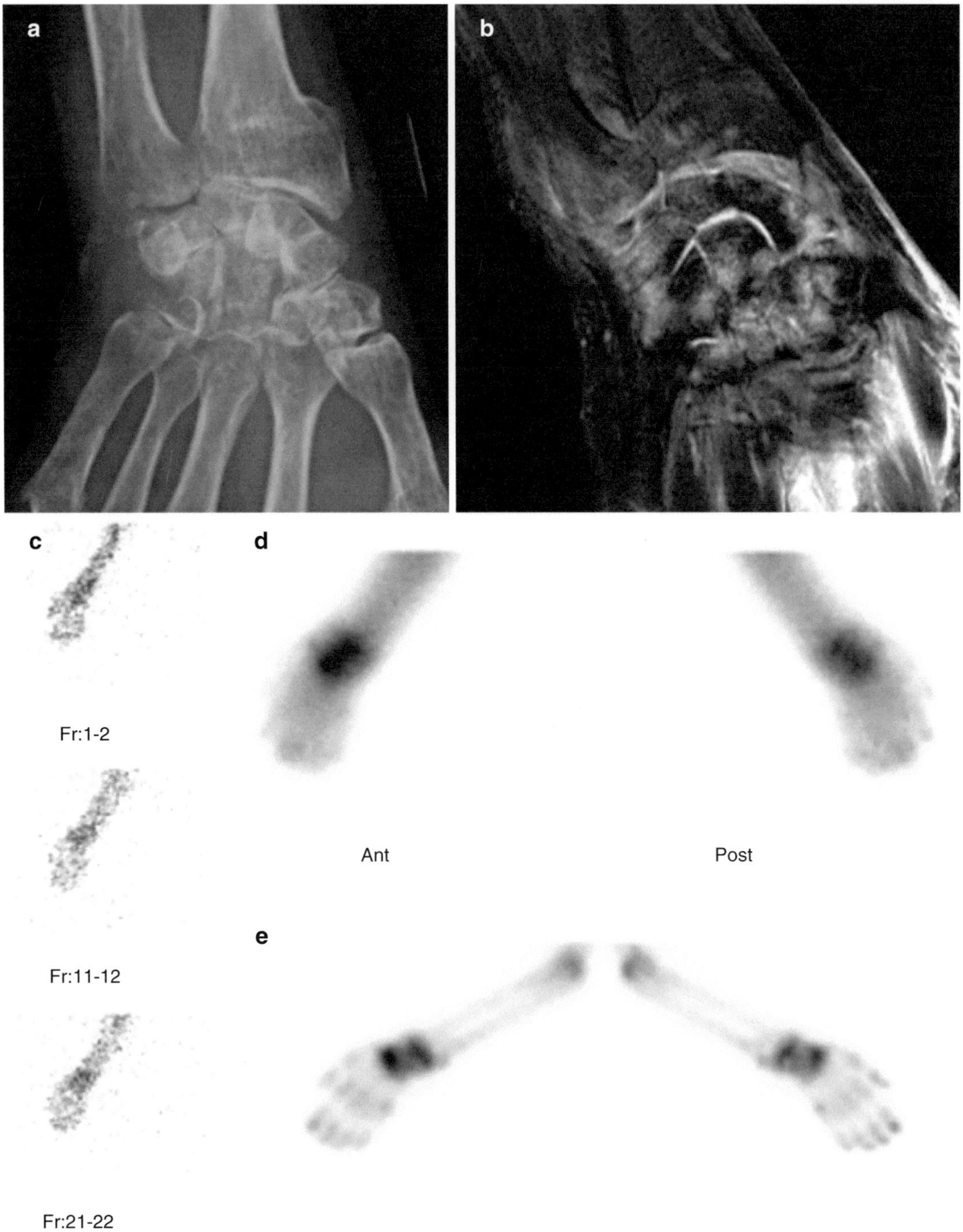

Fig. 2.5 (**a**) Plain radiography: soft tissue swelling, uneven joint space narrowing, and periarticular bone erosion and sclerosis. (**b**) FS T2W MRI: high signal intensity of synovial and parasynovial inflammation with uneven joint space narrowing, subchondral bone erosions, and patchy bone marrow edema. Three-phase bone scintigraphy: (**c**, **d**) diffuse hot uptake throughout left wrist on both perfusion and blood pool images and (**e**) periarticular hot uptakes at carpal bones on delayed scan

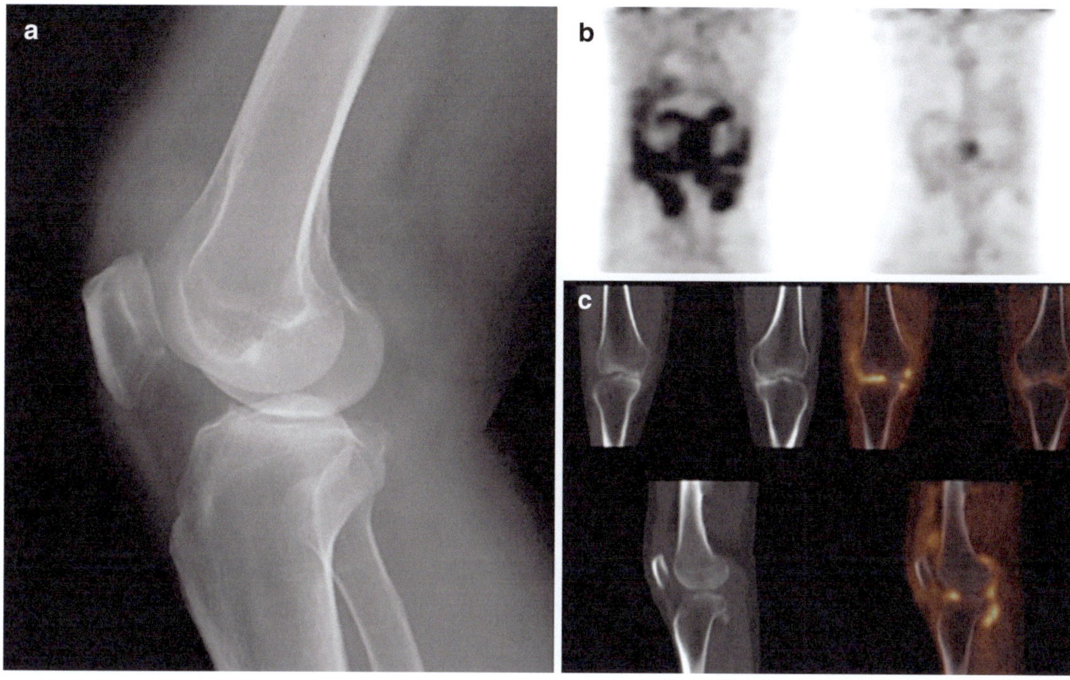

Fig. 2.6 (**a**) Plain radiography: distended suprapatellar bursa without evidence of bone lesion. FDG PET/CT after surgical pus drainage and irrigation: (**b**) intense FDG uptake at right knee on MIP image. (**c**) Intense FDG uptake in right knee joint along synovial lining without evidence of bone involvement on CT and PET/CT images

Case 2.6

A 79-year-old woman spontaneously developed left hip pain a week ago. Operative findings were necrosis of the greater trochanter of the left femur, multiple abscess pockets around the greater trochanter, and granuloma and inflammatory tissue around abscess. The pathologic report of hip joint biopsy was active granulomatous inflammation with caseous necrosis. MTB-PCR result was positive.

Plain radiography of the left hip showed periarticular radiolucencies in the acetabulum, the femoral head, and the proximal femur. Mixed erosive and sclerotic bone lesions were in the greater trochanter. FS T2W coronal MRI showed heterogeneous intermediate to high signal intensity of bone marrow changes in the acetabulum and in the head and intertrochanteric area of the left femur. Fluid accumulation (cold abscesses) of mixed high and low signal intensity was in the left hip joint space and in the femur, suggesting tuberculous arthritis combined with tuberculous osteomyelitis. Fluid accumulations were also noted in para-articular soft tissues and in the trochanteric bursa. Bone erosions were at the femoral head and the greater trochanter of the left femur. ^{99m}Tc-HDP bone scintigraphy showed periarticular increased bone uptakes in the left acetabulum, left femoral head, and trochanteric area. A round photopenia was in the intertrochanteric area, which is corresponding to intramedullary abscess in the femur on MRI (Fig. 2.7).

Teaching Points

- Three-phase bone scintigraphy is a good modality showing active tissue inflammation and bone change. However, it is nonspecific to detect a infection and is only representing tissue hyperemia and bone turnover. So, similar findings can be demonstrated in aseptic other joint disease.
- Mild periarticular increased bone uptake may be a finding of reactive bone change resulted from synovial hyperemia or reactive bone marrow edema.
- Associated cortical bone destructions in the course of the disease can be represented as focal intense bone uptakes.

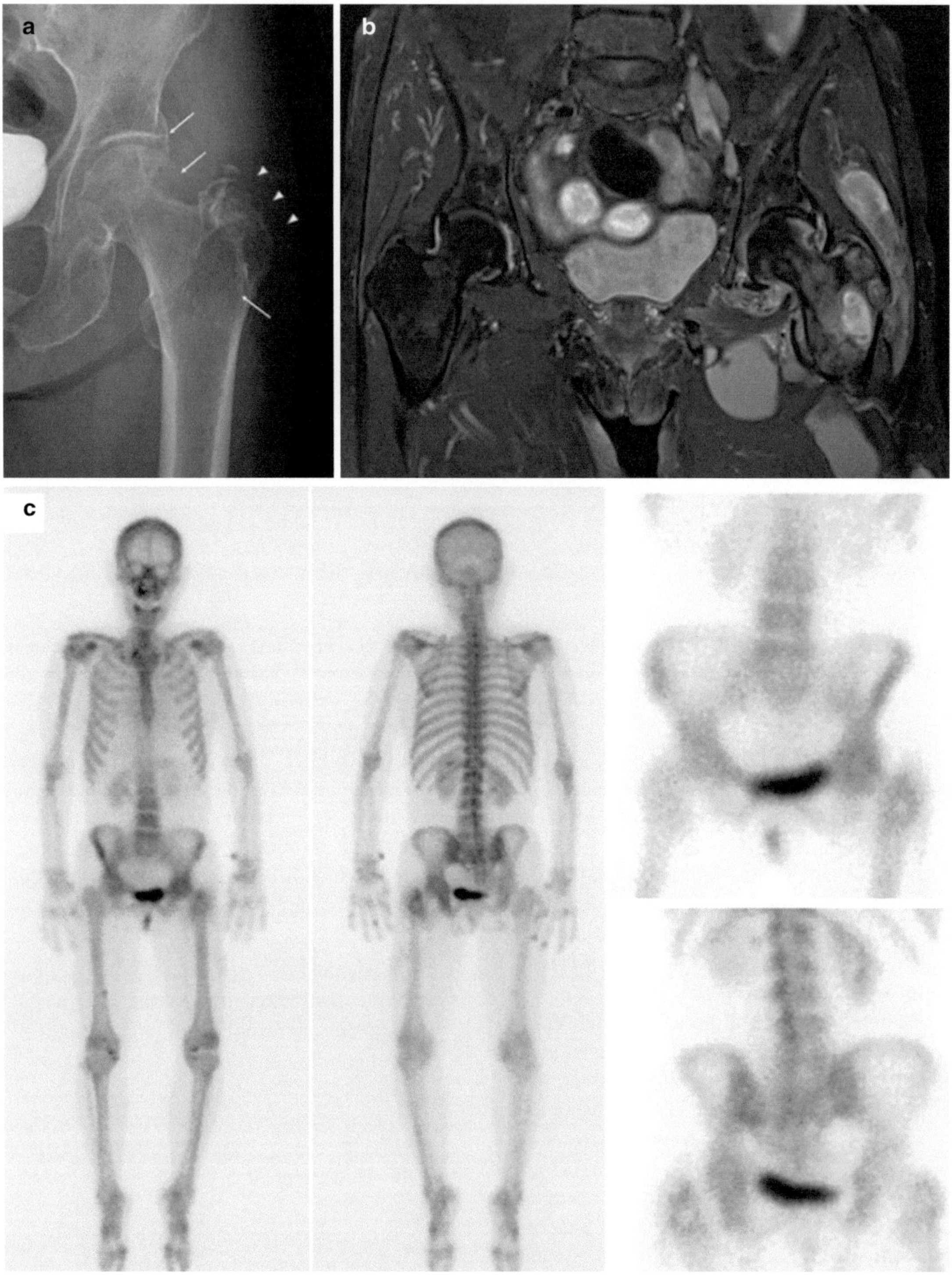

Fig. 2.7 (**a**) Plain radiography: periarticular radiolucencies (arrows) in acetabulum, femoral head, and proximal femur. Mixed erosive and sclerotic bone lesions (arrowheads) in greater trochanter. (**b**) FS T2W MRI: bone marrow changes in acetabulum and proximal femur with bone erosions. High signal intensities of cold abscesses in joint space, proximal femur, trochanteric bursa, and para-articular soft tissues. (**c**) Bone scintigraphy: periarticular increased bone uptake at left hip with small round photopenia in proximal femur, corresponding to intramedullary abscess

References

1. Mathews CJ, Weston VC, Jones A, Field M, Coakley G. Bacterial septic arthritis in adults. Lancet. 2010;375:846–55.
2. Gilday DL, Paul DJ, Paterson J. Diagnosis of osteomyelitis in children by combined blood pool and bone imaging. Radiology. 1975;117:331–5.
3. Maurer AH, Chen DC, Camargo EE, et al. Utility of three-phase skeletal scintigraphy in suspected osteomyelitis: concise communication. J Nucl Med. 1981;22:941–9.
4. Starr AM, Wessely MA, Albastaki U, Pierre-Jerome C, Kettner NW. Bone marrow edema: pathophysiology, differential diagnosis, and imaging. Acta Radiol. 2008;49:771–86.
5. Eriksen EF, Ringe JD. Bone marrow lesions: a universal bone response to injury? Rheumatol Int. 2012;32:575–84.
6. Hotta M, Minamimoto R, Kaneko H, Yamashita H. Fluorodeoxyglucose PET/CT of arthritis in rheumatic diseases: a pictorial review. Radiographics. 2020;40:223–40.
7. Tuli SM. Tuberculosis of the skeletal system (bones, joints, spine and bursal sheaths), vol. 4. 4th ed. New Delhi: Jaypee Brothers Medical Publishers Pvt, Ltd; 2010. p. 69–110.
8. De Vuyst D, Vanhoenacker F, Gielen J, Bernaerts A, De Schepper AM. Imaging features of musculoskeletal tuberculosis. Eur Radiol. 2003;13:1809–19.
9. Davidson PT, Horowitz I. Skeletal tuberculosis. A review with patient presentations and discussion. Am J Med. 1970;48:77–84.

3 Inflammatory Arthritis

Ju Won Seok

Abstract

Inflammatory arthritis is a joint inflammation caused by an overactive immune system. It usually affects many joints throughout the body at the same time. Inflammatory arthritis is much less common than osteoarthritis, which affects most people in their later stages of life. The major types of inflammatory arthritis including rheumatoid arthritis, seronegative spondyloarthropathies (ankylosing spondylitis), and crystal-induced arthritis (gout and pseudogout) will be presented in this chapter.

Clinical symptoms, physical examination, blood tests, and imaging techniques, including plain radiography, ultrasonography of joints, CT, and MRI, are essential to make an accurate diagnosis. Bone scintigraphy is frequently used in the workup of patients with inflammatory arthritis, because it is not specific, but sensitive in the detection of inflammatory joint diseases.

Keywords

Rheumatoid arthritis · Ankylosing spondylitis Gout · Synovial hyperplasia · Joint effusion Bone erosions · Tenosynovitis

3.1 Ankylosing Spondylitis

3.1.1 Etiology and Clinical Significance

Ankylosing spondylitis (AS) is a chronic inflammatory disease that affects the sacroiliac (SI) joints and/or spine in particular. AS is often more common in men and becomes symptomatic in the second or third decades as lower back pain and spinal immobility [1]. In addition, approximately 90% of AS patients are HLA-B27 positive.

Though the pathogenesis of AS has not yet been fully understood, it is now clear that spinal bone formation in AS is a post-inflammatory tissue remodeling reaction. Enthesitis is an important pathologic feature of AS and believed to represent the primary pathogenic process in such a group of disease [2]. Studies have shown predisposing factors such as genetic background, microbial infection, endocrine abnormalities, and immune responses associated with the occurrence of AS [3–5].

J. W. Seok (✉)
Department of Nuclear Medicine, Chung-Ang University, College of Medicine, Seoul, Republic of Korea
e-mail: joneseok@cau.ac.kr

S.-O. Yang et al. (eds.), *Atlas of Nuclear Medicine in Musculoskeletal System*,
https://doi.org/10.1007/978-981-19-2677-8_3

3.1.2 Radiographic Imaging

Symmetrical and bilateral sacroiliitis is usually the first manifestation. The sacroiliac joints were first widened, and subchondral erosions, sclerosis, and proliferation on the iliac side of the SI joints were detected. Early spondylitis, along with reactive sclerosis, is characterized by small erosions at the corners of vertebral bodies. AS is the most common cause of vertebral body squaring. It usually includes several steps and generally begins in the lumbar spines and precedes the bamboo spine.

Chronic structural changes such as erosions, subchondral sclerosis, and bony ankylosis are better observed in CT. MRI may play a role in early diagnosis of sacroiliitis. MRI is more sensitive in detecting inflammatory changes such as bone marrow edema, synovitis, and capsulitis. Bone scan may be helpful in selected patients with normal or equivocal findings on sacroiliac joint, and quantitative analysis by uptake ratio of SI joint to sacrum may be useful.

Teaching Points
- Bone scan may be helpful with ambiguous findings on SI joint in conventional imaging methods.
- Qualitative evaluation of radionuclide accumulation in SI joints can be difficult due to normal uptake at this location. Therefore, quantitative analysis may be more useful.

Case 3.1
A 16-year-old man with left wrist and right hip pain that started several months ago. Bone scan shows markedly increased uptake in the left wrist and right sacroiliac joint. MRI shows bone marrow edema around the right sacroiliac joint, representing osteitis with erosions, synovitis, and capsulitis, suggesting right active sacroiliitis. He was clinically diagnosed with ankylosing spondylitis (Fig. 3.1).

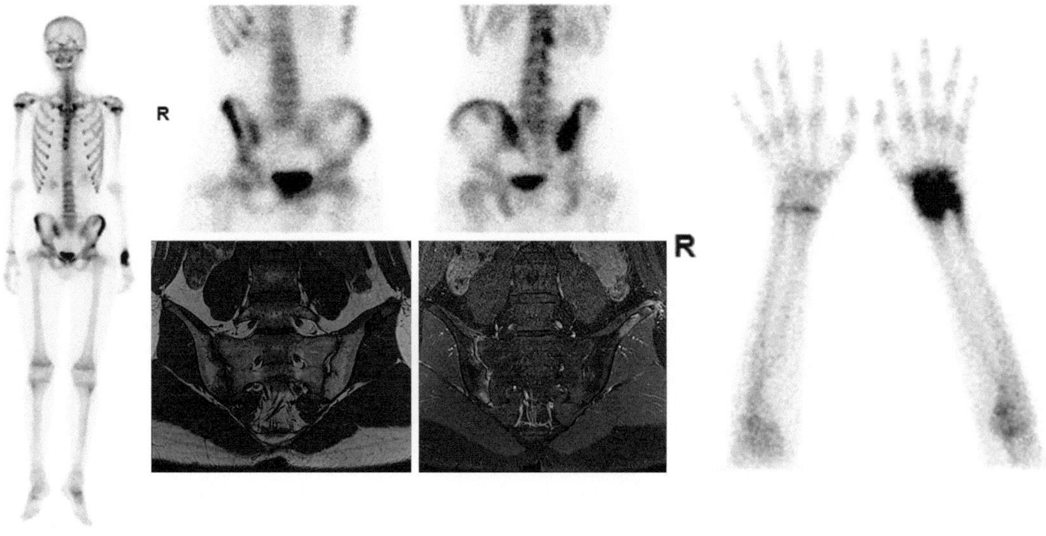

Fig. 3.1 Bone scan images show increased uptake of left wrist and right sacroiliac joint, and MRI also shows findings suggesting sacroiliitis

Case 3.2

A 17-year-old man with persistent bilateral hip and back pain. Radiologic imaging shows bilateral sacroiliitis. Bone scan shows increased uptake in both SI joints. The uptake ratio of sacroiliac joint to sacrum was measured high 2.46 on the right and 2.86 on the left (normal value, within 1.2), meaning that uptake of SI joints increased due to sacroiliitis (Fig. 3.2).

Case 3.3

A 35-year-old man with ankylosing spondylitis has had stiffness and pain in his back since he was 20 years old. He had never been treated, and the pain has worsened recently. Radiographic imaging shows bilateral sacroiliitis. Bone scan shows increased uptake in both sternoclavicular junctions and both SI joints. He was clinically diagnosed with SAPHO syndrome accompanied by ankylosing spondylitis (Fig. 3.3).

3.2 Rheumatoid Arthritis

3.2.1 Etiology and Clinical Significance

Rheumatoid arthritis (RA) is a systemic autoimmune disease characterized by inflammatory arthritis and extra-articular involvement [6]. Although the cause of RA is unknown, a genetic predisposition and an environmental trigger were generally considered to have led autoimmune resactions [7]. Activation and accumulation of CD4 T cells in the synovium cause a continuation of inflammatory reactions [8]. An inflammatory reaction induces pannus formation. Pannus gradually erodes at the bare area at first, followed by the articular cartilage, and it causes fibrous ankylosis which becomes an ossfication [9].

The most common clinical manifestation of RA is the polyarthritis of the small joints of the

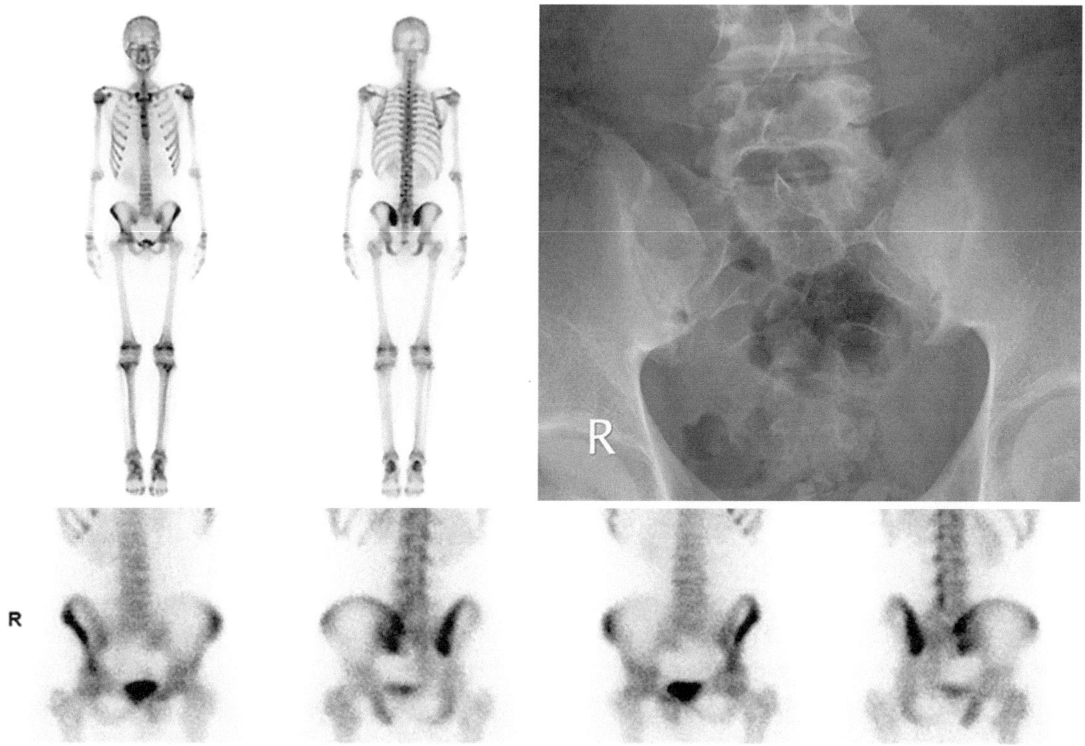

Fig. 3.2 Sacroiliitis is observed in both sacroiliac joints on X-ray images, and increased uptake of both sacroiliac joints is also observed on bone scan images

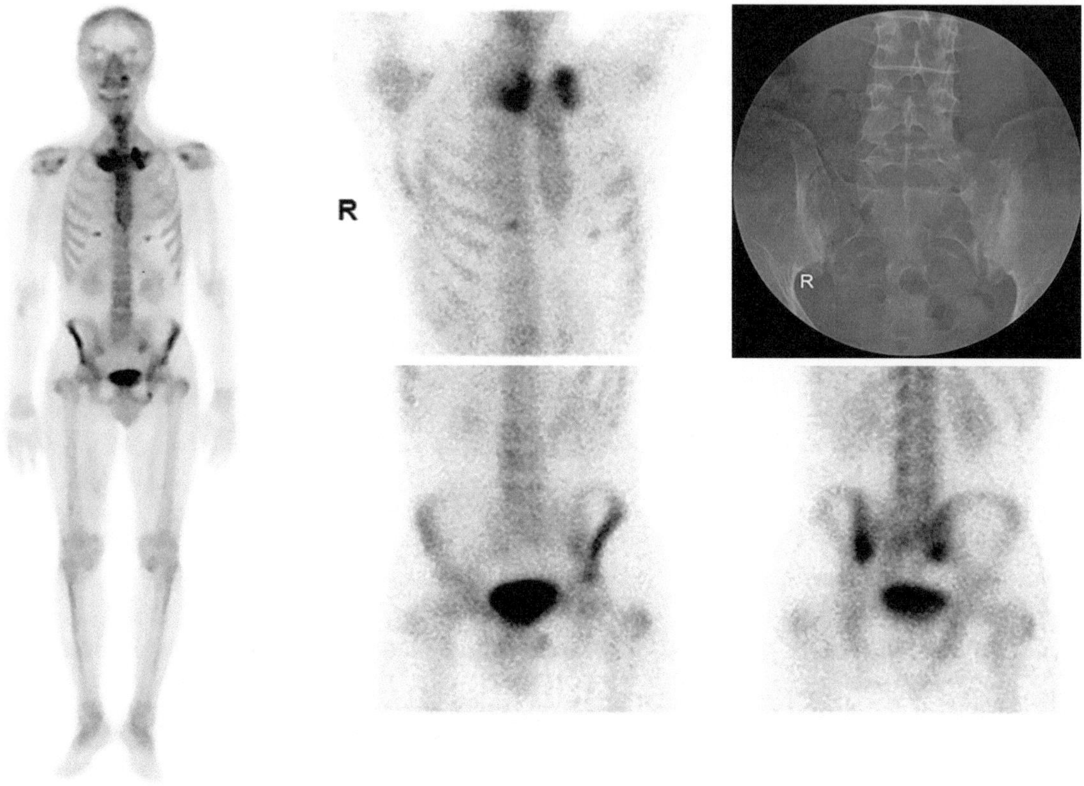

Fig. 3.3 Bone scan images show increased uptake in both sacroiliac joints. Characteristically, increased uptake in both sternoclavicular junctions is observed in bone scan images

hands: proximal interphalangeal (PIP), metacarpophalangeal (MCP) joints, and wrist. Other joints that are generally affected include wrists, elbows, shoulders, hips, knees, ankles, and metatarsophalangeal (MTP) joints. The arthropathy has a typical inflammatory phenotype with joint stiffness, reduced range of motion, and decreased function.

3.2.2 Radiographic Imaging

Radiographic features of RA are marginal erosions, soft tissue swelling, osteoporosis, and narrowing of joint space. Diagnosis and follow-up of patients with RA generally include images of hands and wrist. The disease tends to affect the proximal joints in a bilaterally symmetrical distribution. The acquired changes of RA are subchondral cyst formation, hitchhiker's thumb deformity, scapholunate dissociation, and ankylosis. The feet are the same as the hands, and PIP and MTP joints are preferred.

Ultrasonography can evaluate soft tissue manifestations such as synovial proliferation and inflammation of the superficial joints, tenosynovitis, and bursitis [10]. MRI is particularly sensitive to the initial and subtle characteristics of RA. Characteristics of RA, which are best demonstrated by MRI, include synovial hyperemia, synovial hyperplasia, pannus formation, reduction in the thickness of cartilage, subchondral cysts and erosion, juxta-articular bone marrow edema, and joint effusions [11].

Teaching Points

- Bone scan appeared to be a more sensitive method for detecting inflammatory joint disease than conventional imaging methods and more sensitive than clinical evaluation in diagnosis of joint inflammation.
- The occurrence of erosion of RA can be predicted through bone scan.
- When the high activity persists, erosions were most likely to occur in joints showing high radionuclide uptake.

Case 3.4

A 52-year-old woman presented with pain in all finger joints and wrists lasting more than 10 years. She had pain, swelling, and stiffness in the knuckles in the morning, which lasted for more than 1 h. Plain radiograph of both hands shows degenerative change and erosions on metacarpophalangeal joints of both hands. Bone scan shows increased uptake in both hands, wrists, elbows, both knees, ankles, and both feet, suggestive of polyarthritis (Fig. 3.4).

Case 3.5

A 50-year-old woman presented with pain in the wrist and knee joints. Radiologic imaging of both feet showed bone erosions at left first interphalangeal joint, both third and fourth metatarsophalangeal joint, and left fifth metatarsophalangeal joint, subluxation of right third and left fourth metatarsophalangeal joint, and soft tissue swelling around left fifth metatarsophalangeal joint. It suggested rheumatoid arthritis. There was no significant bony abnormality on both knees and both hands, except for joint effusion of the left knee. Bone scan shows increased uptake in both wrists; both knees; right first, second, and third metatarsophalangeal joints; and left third, fourth, and fifth metatarsophalangeal joints (Fig. 3.5).

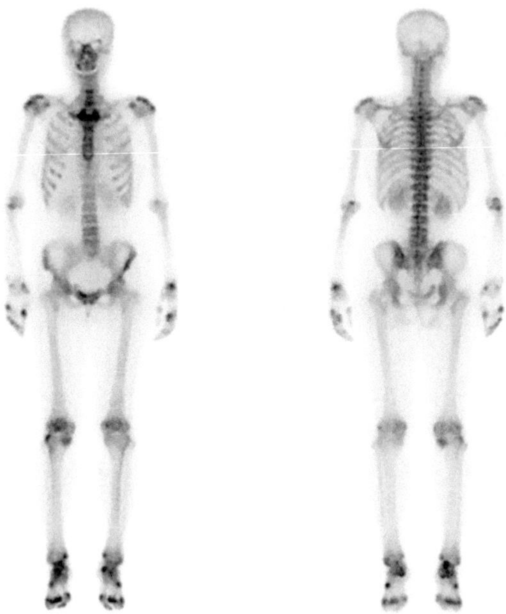

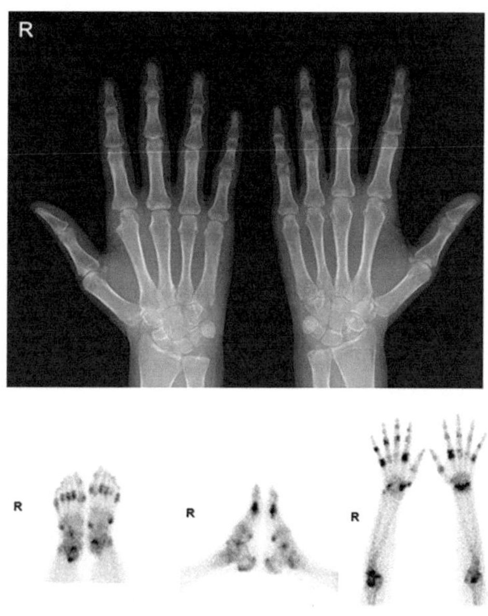

Fig. 3.4 Increased uptake of both wrists; the second and fifth metacarpophalangeal joints; the third, fourth, and fifth proximal interphalangeal joints; and the second and third distal interphalangeal joints of the right hand; the first, second, and third metacarpophalangeal joints and the second, third, and fourth proximal interphalangeal joints of the left hand; both ankles; the first, second, third, fourth, and fifth metatarsophalangeal joints of the right foot; and the first, second, third, and fifth metatarsophalangeal joints of the left foot are observed in bone scan images

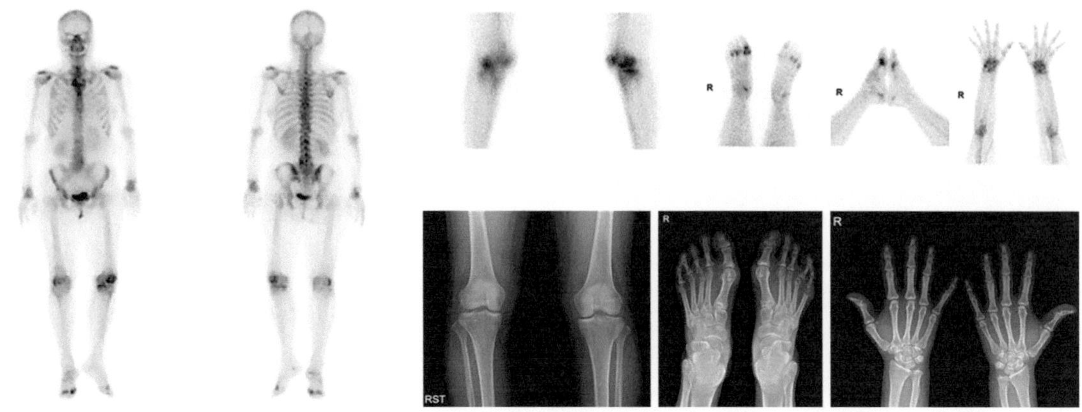

Fig. 3.5 Bone scan images show increased uptake of multiple metatarsophalangeal joints of both feet, and X-ray images also show bone erosion of multiple metatarsophalangeal joints of both feet

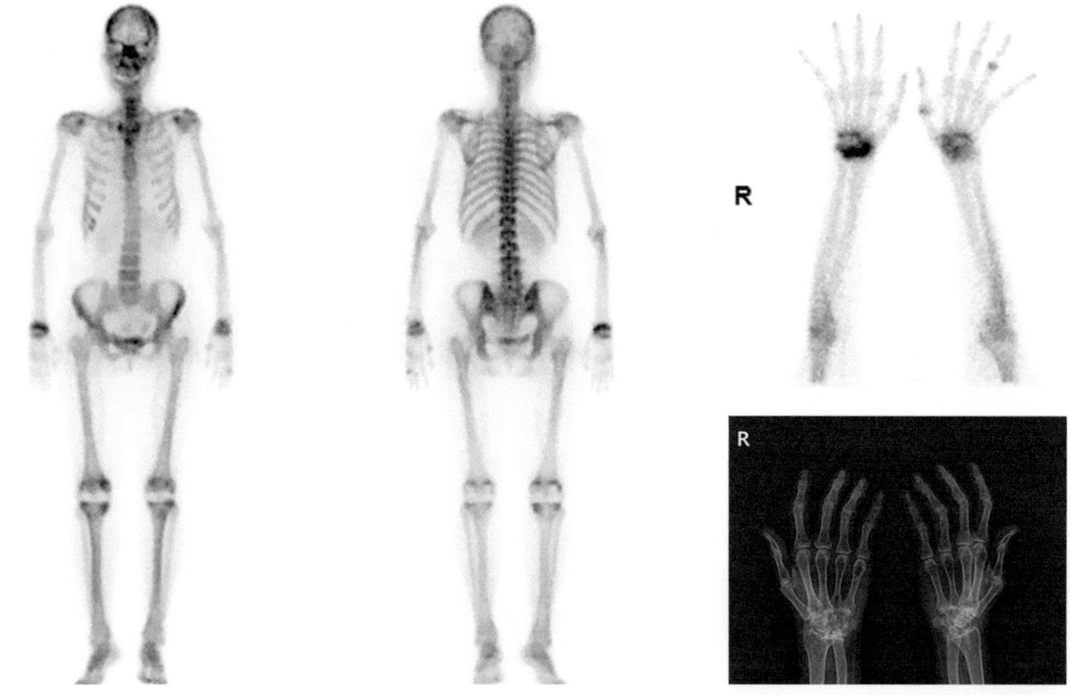

Fig. 3.6 Severe deformity is also observed in X-ray imaging in both wrist joints where increased uptake is observed in bone scan imaging

Case 3.6
A 61-year-old woman was diagnosed with rheumatoid arthritis 10 years ago due to multiple joint pains and was treated at another hospital, but did not improve, and was admitted to the outpatient hospital. Radiologic imaging shows severe deformity on both wrist joints. Bone scan shows increased uptake in both wrists, left first metacarpophalangeal joint, and fourth proximal interphalangeal joint of the left hand (Fig. 3.6).

Case 3.7
A 47-year-old woman was admitted with wrist pain lasting more than 1 year. Radiologic imag-

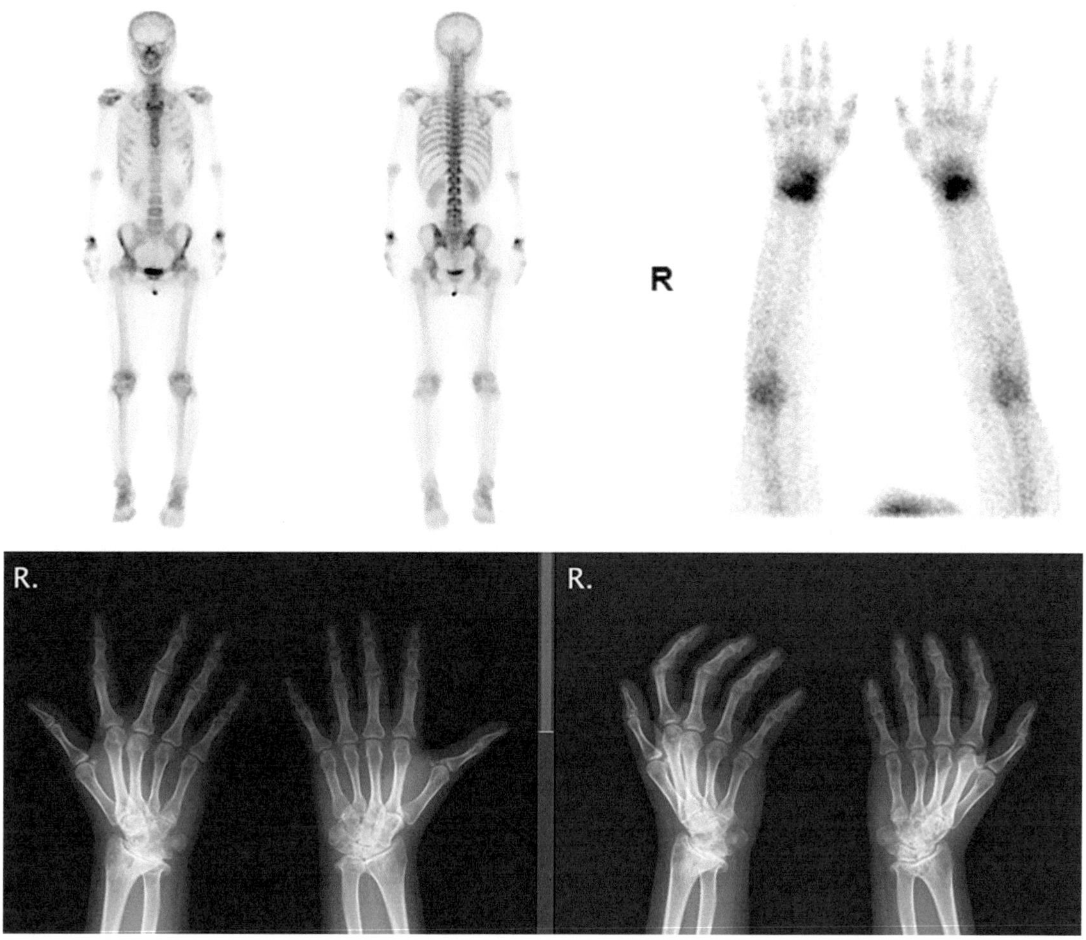

Fig. 3.7 In both wrist joints, bone scan images show increased uptake, and severe deformity was observed in X-ray images

ing suggested advanced rheumatoid arthritis on both wrists. Bone scan shows markedly increased uptake in both wrist joints (Fig. 3.7).

3.3 Gout

3.3.1 Etiology and Clinical Significance

Gout is a metabolic disorder [12]. However, since clinical presentations are very similar to arthritis, gout is also classified as a form of crystal-induced arthritis [13]. Acute gout arthritis represents a monoarticular redness, inflammation, and swollen joints, typically in the lower limb, and classically affects the first metatarsophalangeal joint. Gout accumulated monosodium crystals in tissues; it causes arthritis, soft tissue mass, nephrolithiasis, and urate nephropathy [14].

The main risk factor is hyperuricemia, which can leave uric acid crystals such as needles inside joints [15]. The main symptom is joint pain that appears often first on the big toe. Other joints that may be affected include ankles, feet, knees, and, in severe cases, wrists, elbows, and fingers [16]. A similar condition, known as pseudogout, has similar symptoms. In both conditions, white blood cells surround chemical crystals that cause inflammation. In pseudogout, the associated crystals are formed from calcium pyrophosphate dihydrate, rather than uric acid as in gout, and knee joints are primarily affected.

3.3.2 Radiographic Imaging

Although not all patients progress to this stage, characteristic radiologic changes occur in the chronic stage. Small joints of the hands and feet are preferred. The earliest change is the swelling of soft tissue. At a later stage, erosions occur that may be far from the articular cortex. These erosions are well defined, often sclerotic and with edges, often protruding edges. It is because there are urate sediments in the bone. These sediments are so large that they can cause extensive bone destruction. Usually, there is no osteoporosis. Due to the collection of sodium urate known as tophi, localized soft tissue lumps may occur in the periarticular tissues. The swellings may be large and sometimes calcification may be shown [17].

Although there may be changes in appearance, the tophi are hyperechoic and heterogeneous and tend to be poorly defined contours in ultrasound. CT and MRI can distinguish between urate mineralization and calcification and can be useful if clinical and biochemical presentations are atypical.

Teaching Points

- Bone scan has high sensitivity to osseous abnormality detection, but the scintigraphic findings in gout are often non-specific.
- Asymmetrical, bilateral, and multifocal joint involvement tends to be associated with severe abnormal uptake area.
- The intense uptake usually extends beyond the associated joints, because of the swelling of soft tissue.

Case 3.8

A 34-year-old man was admitted with a 1-month history of pain in the ankle joints followed by involvement of both first metatarsophalangeal joints. Radiographs show erosive changes on the right medial hallux sesamoid bone and small erosion on the left first proximal phalangeal base. Bone scan shows increased uptake in both first metatarsophalangeal joints. Ultrasound image shows synovial thickening and joint effusion with echogenic nodular lesions of medial capsule of bilateral metatarsophalangeal joints. It suggested gout arthritis (Fig. 3.8).

Case 3.9

A 48-year-old man presented with sudden right foot pain. Radiographic imaging shows degenerative change and soft tissue swelling on the right first metatarsophalangeal joint. Bone scan shows increased uptake in the right first metatarsophalangeal joint. Ultrasound image shows echogenic foci and capsular thickening on right first metatarsophalangeal joint; it suggested gout arthritis (Fig. 3.9).

Case 3.10

A 41-year-old man was diagnosed with gout at an outside hospital and was admitted. He complained of pain in both knee and ankle joints. Radiographic imaging shows moderate osteoarthritis on both knee joints, but no abnormal findings were found in both ankles. Bone scan shows increased uptake in the right knee and right ankle joints. Ultrasound image shows echogenic tophi on medial aspect of both ankles and right knee (Fig. 3.10).

Case 3.11

A 47-year-old woman was admitted with pain in both feet lasting for 1 year. Radiographic imaging showed diffuse osteopenia and osteoarthritis on both feet. Bone scan shows increased bone uptake in both cuboid bones of both feet and joint uptake in the first metatarsophalangeal joint and proximal interphalangeal joints of the right foot. Ultrasound image shows mild synovitis and echogenic change on both first metatarsophalan-

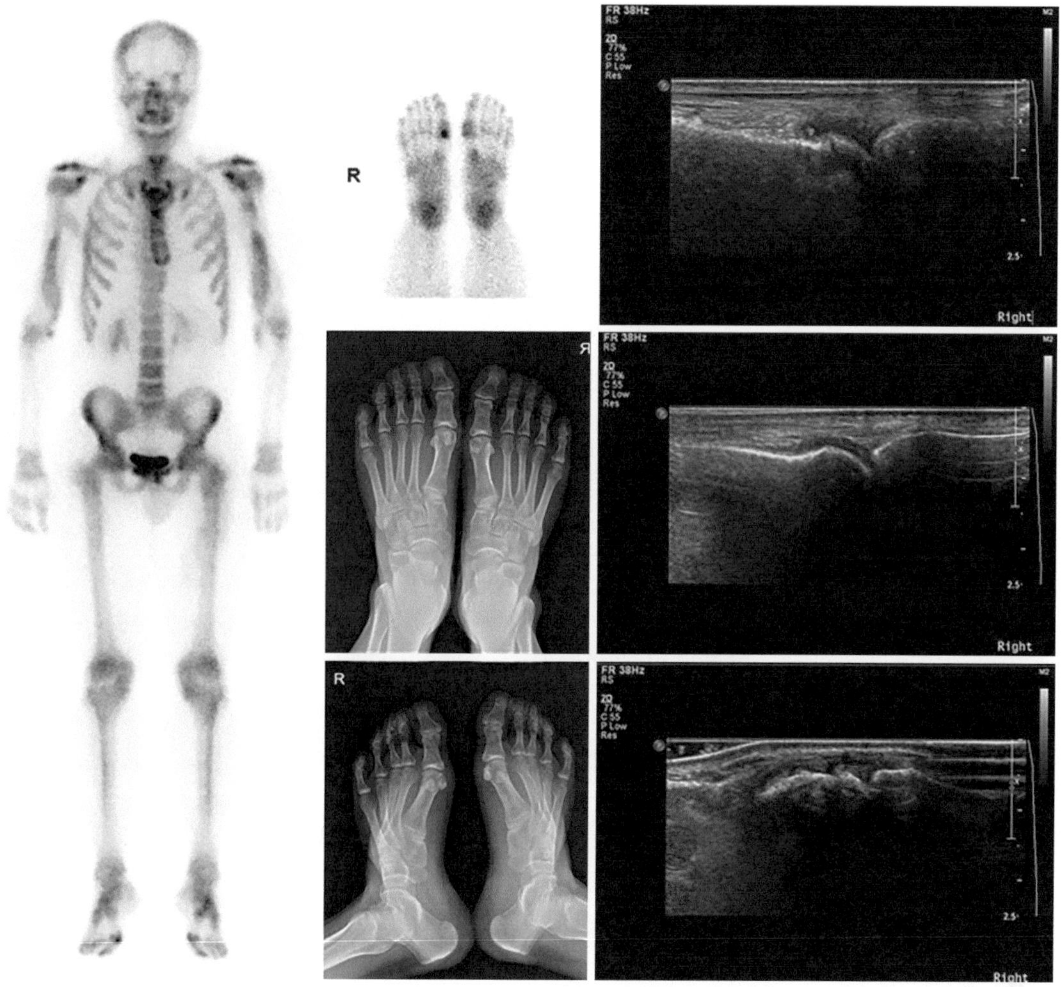

Fig. 3.8 In both first metatarsophalangeal joints, increased uptake is observed in bone scan images, bone erosion is observed in X-ray images, and synovial thickening was observed in ultrasound images

geal joints and synovial thickening and erosive change with joint effusion on tarsometatarsal joints of both feet. The patient was clinically diagnosed with gout (Fig. 3.11).

Case 3.12

A 42-year-old man presented with unbearable pain in the right first toe. Radiographic imaging showed no abnormality on both feet. Bone scan shows increased uptake in the right first metatarsophalangeal joint, both knee joints, and both ankle joints. Ultrasound image shows large echogenic foci with bony erosion and synovial thickening and small joint effusion. CT image with uric acid spectral CT shows gout tophi on the right first toe (Fig. 3.12).

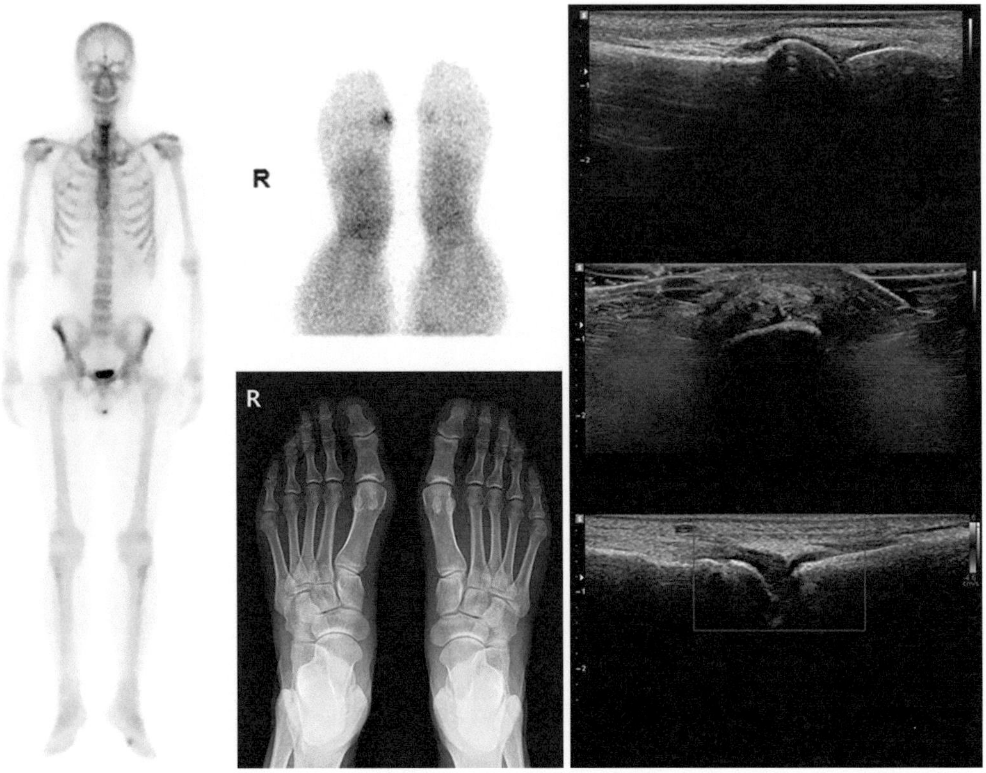

Fig. 3.9 Increased uptake is observed in the first metatarsophalangeal joint on the right foot, and echogenic foci is observed in ultrasound images

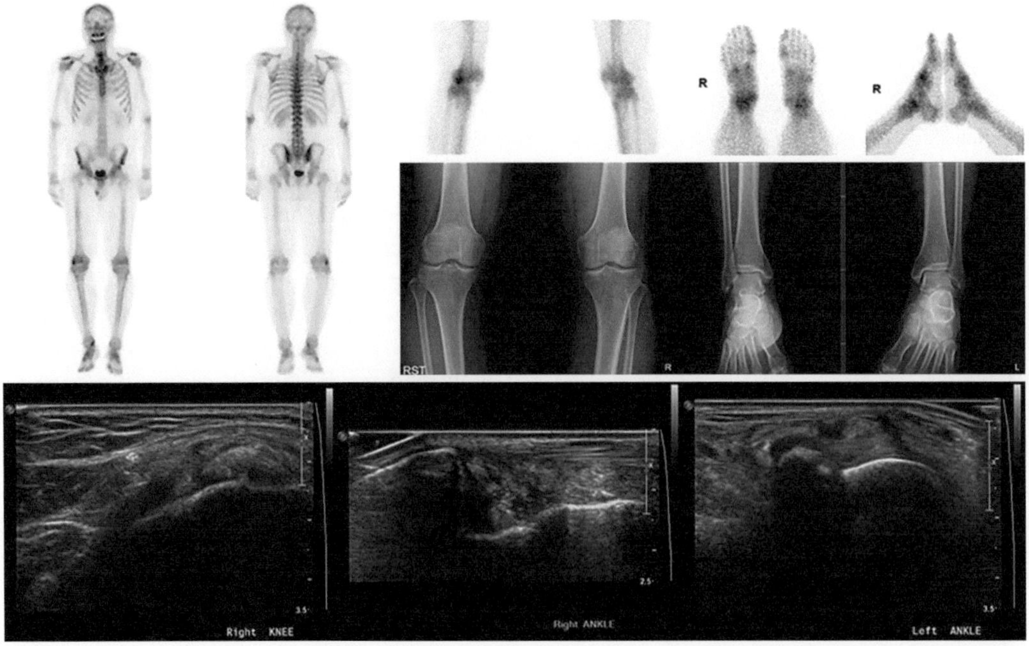

Fig. 3.10 Increased uptake is observed in the right knee and right ankle joints in bone scan images, and tophi is observed in the ultrasound images of the same area

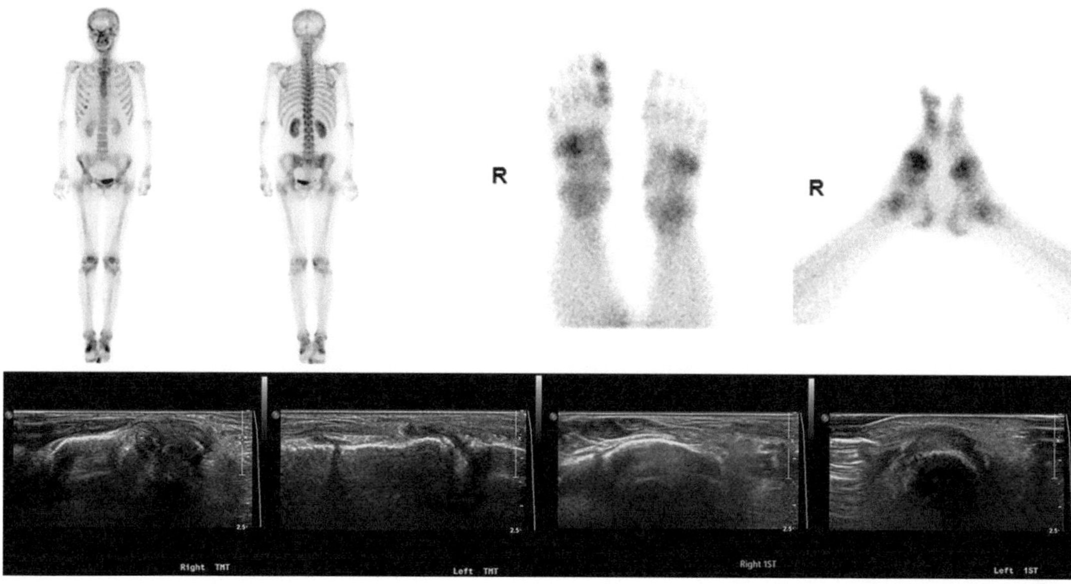

Fig. 3.11 Bone scan images shows increased uptake in the first metatarsophalangeal joint and the first proximal interphalangeal joint of the right foot

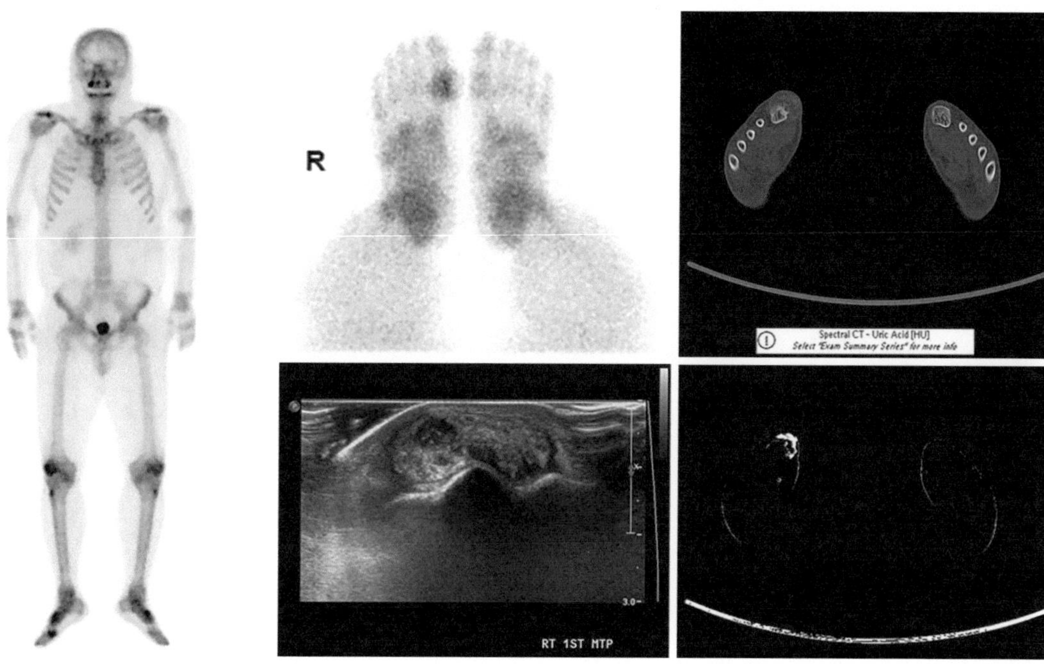

Fig. 3.12 In the bone scan images, the increased uptake of the first metatarsophalangeal joint of the right foot is observed, and the tophi is observed in the uric acid spectral CT image in the same area

References

1. Proft F, Poddubnyy D. Ankylosing spondylitis and axial spondyloarthritis: recent insights and impact of new classification criteria. Ther Adv Musculoskelet Dis. 2018;10(5-6):129–39.
2. Bridgewood C, Watad A, Cuthbert RJ, McGonagle D. Spondyloarthritis: new insights into clinical aspects, translational immunology and therapeutics. Curr Opin Rheumatol. 2018;30(5):526–32.
3. Wang R, Ward MM. Epidemiology of axial spondyloarthritis: an update. Curr Opin Rheumatol. 2018;30(2):137–43.
4. van den Berg R, Jongbloed EM, de Schepper EIT, Bierma-Zeinstra SMA, Koes BW, Luijsterburg PAJ. The association between pro-inflammatory biomarkers and nonspecific low back pain: a systematic review. Spine J. 2018;18(11):2140–51.
5. Kucybała I, Urbanik A, Wojciechowski W. Radiologic approach to axial spondyloarthritis: where are we now and where are we heading? Rheumatol Int. 2018;38(10):1753–62.
6. Carbone F, Bonaventura A, Liberale L, Paolino S, Torre F, Dallegri F, Montecucco F, Cutolo M. Atherosclerosis in rheumatoid arthritis: promoters and opponents. Clin Rev Allergy Immunol. 2020;58(1):1–14.
7. du Teil EM, Gabarrini G, Harmsen HJM, Westra J, van Winkelhoff AJ, van Dijl JM. Talk to your gut: the oral-gut microbiome axis and its immunomodulatory role in the etiology of rheumatoid arthritis. FEMS Microbiol Rev. 2019;43(1):1–18.
8. Bao YK, Weide LG, Ganesan VC, Jakhar I, McGill JB, Sahil S, Cheng AL, Gaddis M, Drees BM. High prevalence of comorbid autoimmune diseases in adults with type 1 diabetes from the HealthFacts database. J Diabetes. 2019;11(4):273–9.
9. López-Mejías R, Carmona FD, Genre F, Remuzgo-Martínez S, González-Juanatey C, Corrales A, Vicente EF, Pulito-Cueto V, Miranda-Filloy JA, Ramírez Huaranga MA, Blanco R, Robustillo-Villarino M, Rodríguez-Carrio J, Alperi-López M, Alegre-Sancho JJ, Mijares V, Lera-Gómez L, Pérez-Pampín E, González A, Ortega-Castro R, López-Pedrera C, García Vivar ML, Gómez-Arango C, Raya E, Narvaez J, Balsa A, López-Longo FJ, Carreira P, González-Álvaro I, Rodríguez-Rodríguez L, Fernández-Gutiérrez B, Ferraz-Amaro I, Gualillo O, Castañeda S, Martín J, Llorca J, González-Gay MA. Identification of a 3'-untranslated genetic variant of Rarb associated with carotid intima-media thickness in rheumatoid arthritis: a genome-wide association study. Arthritis Rheumatol. 2019;71(3):351–60.
10. Baffour FI, McKenzie GA, Bekele DI, Glazebrook KN. Sonography of active rheumatoid arthritis during pregnancy: a case report and literature review. Radiol Case Rep. 2018;13(6):1233–7.
11. Mochizuki T, Ikari K, Yano K, Okazaki K. Evaluation of factors associated with locomotive syndrome in Japanese elderly and younger patients with rheumatoid arthritis. Mod Rheumatol. 2019;29(5):733–6.
12. Neogi T. Gout. Ann Intern Med. 2016;165(1):ITC1–ITC16.
13. Dalbeth N, Merriman TR, Stamp LK. Gout Lancet. 2016;388(10055):2039–52.
14. Abhishek A, Roddy E, Doherty M. Gout - a guide for the general and acute physicians. Clin Med (Lond). 2017;17(1):54–9.
15. Merriman TR, Choi HK, Dalbeth N. The genetic basis of gout. Rheum Dis Clin N Am. 2014;40(2):279–90.
16. Towiwat P, Chhana A, Dalbeth N. The anatomical pathology of gout: a systematic literature review. BMC Musculoskelet Disord. 2019;20(1):140.
17. Hughes GR, Barnes CG, Mason RM. Bony ankylosis in gout. Ann Rheum Dis. 1968;27(1):67–70.

Non-inflammatory Arthritis: Osteoarthritis

4

Young-Sil An

Abstract

Osteoarthritis is the most common form of non-inflammatory arthritis. Osteoarthritis mainly involves the knee, hip, and hand joints, and obesity or repetitive joint damage is known risk factors. Diagnosis of osteoarthritis is based on clinical and/or radiological features; nuclear medicine imaging studies can be helpful when the diagnosis is ambiguous or when evaluating disease severity. Bone scans are traditional imaging studies used in the field of nuclear medicine for evaluating osteoarthritis, and bone single-photon emission computed tomography (SPECT) or SPECT/computed tomography is also clinically used to compensate for the limitations of bone scans. Here, we will elucidate cases where nuclear medicine imaging studies has provided valuable information in diagnosing and evaluating osteoarthritis.

Keywords

Non-inflammatory arthritis · Osteoarthritis
Bone scan · Bone SPECT · Bone SPECT/CT

Y.-S. An (✉)
Department of Nuclear Medicine and Molecular Imaging, Ajou University School of Medicine, Suwon, Republic of Korea

4.1 Etiology and Pathophysiology

Non-inflammatory arthritis is so named because it does not show inflammatory features such as warmth or swelling in the joint area and is mostly known to be associated with osteoarthritis (OA) [1, 2]. Therefore, this chapter will mainly focus on OA.

OA usually occurs frequently in people over the age of 50, and aging and being overweight are known risk factors. In addition, OA can occur due to joint injury and repetitive joint damage due to daily activities, such as occupation-related activities or hobbies. OA commonly involves weight-bearing large joints (such as the knee and hip joints) and small joints (such as the hands) [2, 3]. Patients with OA usually complain of joint pain, stiffness, and restriction without systemic involvement of other organs [1].

OA can cause breakdown of cartilage and periarticular bones [3]. This leads to alteration of osteoclast and osteoblast activity and changes in bone material properties and architecture, leading to the formation of osteophytes [4]. In addition, hyperplasia of the joint synovium may appear in OA, which can be observed in imaging findings such as magnetic resonance imaging (MRI) and ultrasonography, and could be correlated with joint symptoms of OA [3, 5].

S.-O. Yang et al. (eds.), *Atlas of Nuclear Medicine in Musculoskeletal System*,
https://doi.org/10.1007/978-981-19-2677-8_4

4.2 Diagnosis

Most patients with OA visit the hospital mainly because of symptoms such as joint pain or discomfort. Diagnosis of OA is mainly conducted by evaluating patients' symptoms; however, the primary aim is to differentiate OA from other arthritis such as rheumatoid arthritis, ankylosing spondylitis, gouty arthritis, septic arthritis, and psoriatic arthritis. This can help rule out other diseases by assessing the rheumatoid factor, erythrocyte sedimentation rate, and C-reactive protein levels through blood tests.

Imaging studies can assist when the clinical diagnosis of OA is unclear or when evaluating disease severity. Typical findings of simple X-ray imaging in OA include joint space narrowing, osteophyte formation, and subchondral sclerosis. However, in early OA, these findings may not be clear, and MRI may be useful in these cases. A bone scan is the most commonly used nuclear medicine imaging study to evaluate OA. This imaging tool can be used to deposit bone-seeking radiopharmaceuticals in areas where osteoblastic activity and perfusion are increased in OA lesions [6]. However, bone scan has a limitation in evaluation of OA, because a bone scan can provide only planar images and it can be supplemented by using bone single-photon emission computed tomography (SPECT) or SPECT/CT. Because SPECT can provide a three-dimensional image of the joint area, the localization of the lesion can be more clearly evaluated. In particular, it is possible to obtain a fusion image of SPECT and CT images from SPECT/CT; therefore, its clinical utility in arthritis is expected to increase [7, 8].

Teaching Points

- When a bone scan is performed to evaluate OA, a regional view can be helpful in finding more detailed lesions.
- SPECT/CT may be more useful than planar bone scan in evaluating OA.
- In a bone scan, the whole body can be covered with a single examination, so it is possible to detect OA in areas the patient is not aware of.

Case 4.1

A 69-year-old man presented with bilateral knee pain that began 3 years prior. The patient manifested with a bilateral sore pain in his knees, necessitating him to rest after a 20-min walk due to pain. In the simple radiograph performed at our hospital, joint space narrowing was observed in both knees, suggesting arthritis (Fig. 4.1a). The patient underwent a bone scan in our department for further evaluation of OA in both knees.

On the anterior and posterior view images of the bone scan, hot uptakes were observed in the medial compartments and patellar region of both knees (Fig. 4.1b). However, localization of the lesion is limited due to the nature of the views; therefore, medial and lateral images were additionally obtained after flexion of the patient's knee using a staircase tool. During the evaluation of the additional images, the hot uptakes were located in the right medial tibial condyle, the posterior portion of the medial femoral condyle, and patella, and the patellofemoral joint was also accompanied by a hot uptake in the right knee (Fig. 4.1c). Additional regional view images of the left knee showed a hot uptake in the medial tibial condyle and patellofemoral joint (Fig. 4.1d). According to this case, it is clearly shown that a more detailed lesion location that was not known in simple anterior and posterior view images can be confirmed in an additional view obtained by flexing the joint.

Case 4.2

A 77-year-old woman visited our hospital complaining of pain in the right knee, which started 5 months prior. The patient's pain worsened during a squatting position and when she stands up from a sitting position. The patient underwent a simple radiograph to evaluate pain in both knees, and the findings showed joint space narrowing in both knees, which was suggestive of arthritis (Fig. 4.2a). The patient further underwent a bone scan and bone SPECT/CT of both knees in our department for further evaluation.

On planar bone scan, intense hot uptakes were observed in the medial, lateral, and patellar regions of the right knee (Fig. 4.2b). Although there was no pain in the patient's left knee joint, mild radiopharmaceutical deposition was also

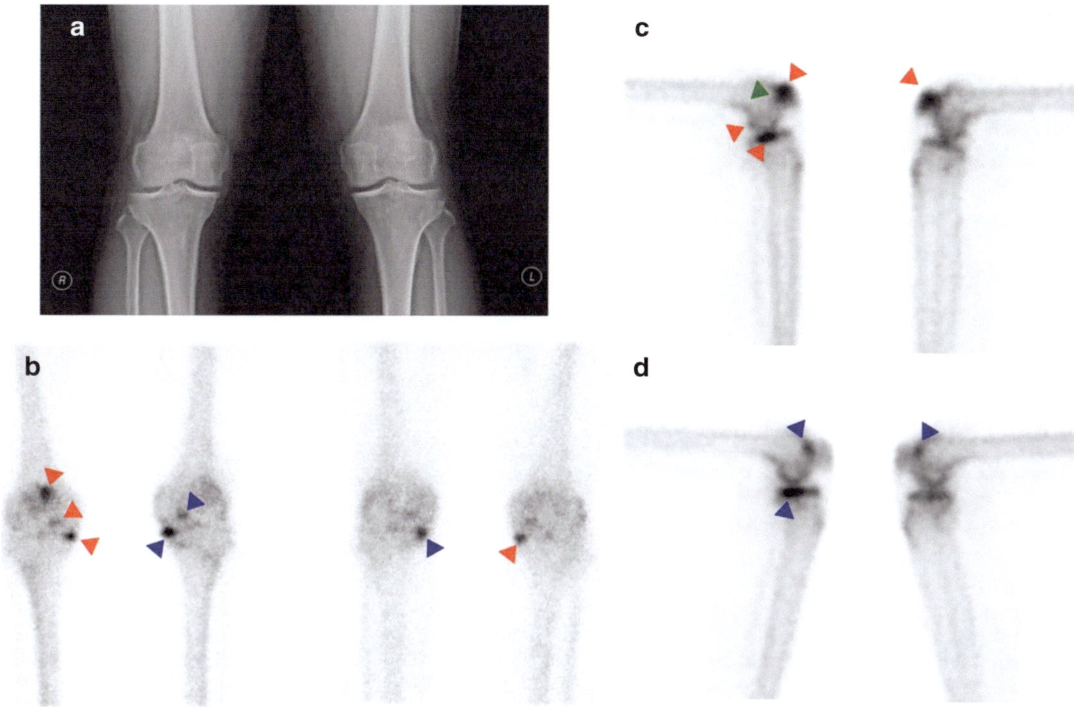

Fig. 4.1 (**a**) A simple radiograph showed narrowing of the bilateral knee joint spaces. (**b**) Hot uptakes were observed in the medial compartments and patellar region of both knees on bone scan (red arrowheads for the right knee and blue arrowheads for the left knee). (**c**) Additionally, hot uptakes were confirmed in the right medial tibial condyle, the posterior portion of the medial femoral condyle, and patella in the flexion view of the right knee (red arrowheads), which was also accompanied by hot uptakes in the patellofemoral joint (green arrowhead). (**d**) In the regional view of the left knee, hot uptakes were noted in the medial tibial condyle and patellofemoral joint (blue arrowheads)

observed in the medial compartment and patellar region of the left knee (Fig. 4.2b). However, there is a limit to clearly distinguishing anatomical regions of hot uptake in knees with only a planar bone scan image. On additional bone SPECT/CT, intense hot uptake lesions were observed in the medial and lateral femoral condylar region, patella, and patellofemoral joint of the right knee. It was confirmed that mild hot uptakes of the left knee were lesions of the left medial femoral condylar area and left patellofemoral joint (Fig. 4.2c, d, f and g). In the CT image, it was additionally observed that the space of the bilateral patellofemoral joints was narrowed (Fig. 4.2e). The patient was diagnosed with bilateral knee joint OA (more active on the right side). In this case, it shows that bone SPECT/CT provides a clearer anatomical information about OA lesions than bone scan.

Case 4.3

A 49-year-old man visited our hospital complaining of persistent pain in both ankles for 8 months. Pain is mainly evident during a squatting position. A simple radiograph showed arthritis in both ankle joints (Fig. 4.3a). The patient was referred to our department for a bone scan and bone SPECT/CT examination for a more detailed evaluation of arthritis.

Hot uptake was observed in both ankle joints on a bone scan (Fig. 4.3b). These hot uptake lesions were more clearly confirmed to be lesions of both tibiotalar and fibulotalar joints on SPECT/CT images (Fig. 4.3c–f). The patient was finally diagnosed with OA of both ankle joints. As seen in this case, the hot uptake seen in the bone scan shows a clearer localization through bone SPECT/CT.

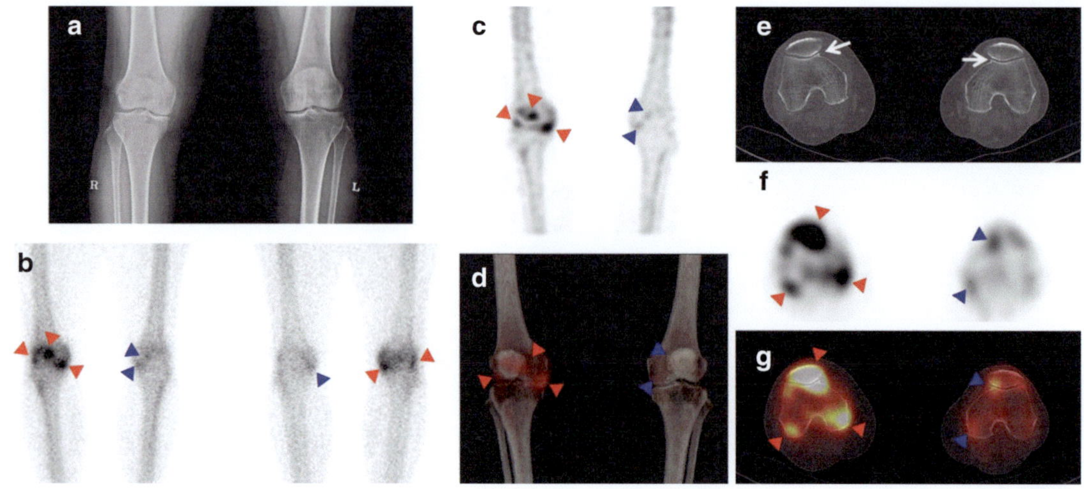

Fig. 4.2 (**a**) On a simple radiograph, joint space narrowing was observed in both knees. (**b**) Intense hot uptakes were noted in the medial, lateral, and patellar regions of the right knee (red arrowheads), and mild hot uptakes were also noted in the medial region of the left knee on bone scan (blue arrowheads). (**c–g**) Intense hot uptakes in the right medial, lateral femoral condyle, patella, and patellofemoral joints (red arrowheads in **c** [maximum intensity projection (MIP) image], **d** [MIP image of fusion with CT], f [SPECT image], and g [SPECT fusion with CT]) and mild hot uptakes in the left medial femoral condyle and patellofemoral joint (blue arrowheads in **c**, **d**, **f**, and **g**) were confirmed by SPECT/CT. Also, it was found that both patellofemoral joint spaces were narrowed on CT image (arrows in **e**)

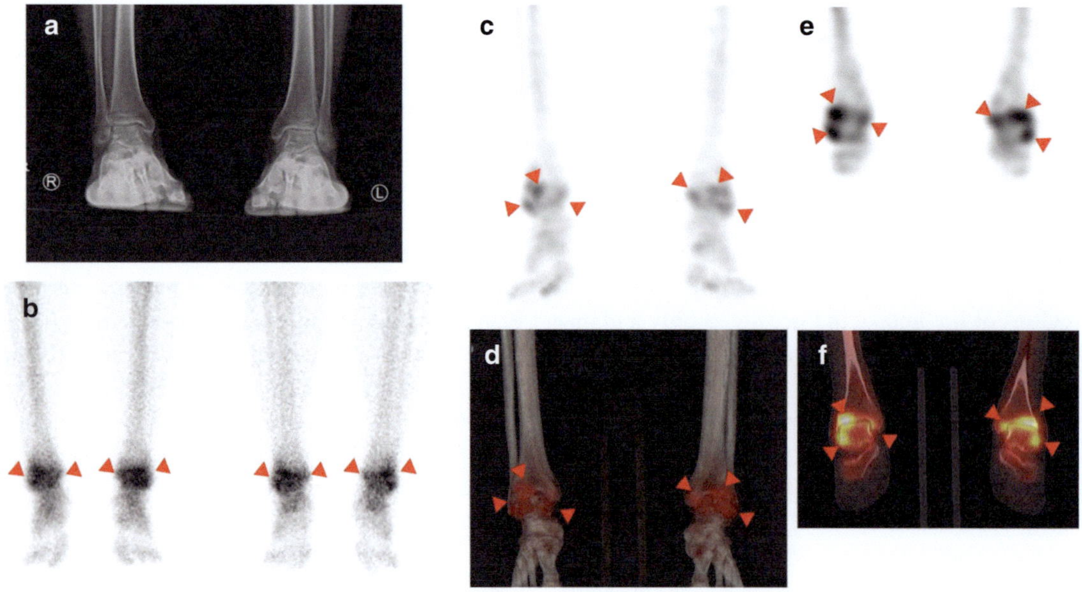

Fig. 4.3 (**a**) A simple radiograph showed that the spaces between the ankle joints were narrowed. (**b**) Hot uptakes were observed in both ankle joints on a bone scan (arrowheads). (**c–f**) SPECT/CT images showed hot uptake lesions in both tibiotalar and fibulotalar joints (arrowheads in **c** [MIP image], **d** [MIP image of fusion with CT], **e** [coronal SPECT image], and **f** [coronal SPECT fusion with CT])

Case 4.4

A 34-year-old man presented with left foot pain. The patient had a fracture of the left calcaneus due to a fall 2 years prior and underwent surgery. Subsequently, pain in the left foot area persisted during the recovery process. X-ray of his left foot region was performed and showed no specific findings other than a metallic prosthesis from the left calcaneus surgery (Fig. 4.4a). Bone scan and bone SPECT/CT were performed in our department for further evaluation of foot pain.

In the bone scan, hot uptake with a diffuse mild pattern was observed in the left foot region (Fig. 4.4b). Bone SPECT/CT showed a mildly hot uptake with a postoperative change pattern in the left calcaneus area (Fig. 4.4c, d, f and g), and the inserted pins were also confirmed on the CT image (Fig. 4.4e). Another hot uptake lesion was observed in the left talocalcaneal joint above the surgical site (Fig. 4.4c, d, h and i), and this area coincided with the patient's main pain area; therefore, OA was confirmed. There were no specific symptoms in the patient's right foot, but a hot uptake was incidentally observed in the right intercuneiform joint on bone SPECT/CT (Fig. 4.4c, d, f and g). Moreover, a possible arthritic change in this area was considered. In this case, bone SPECT/CT was advantageous, detecting lesions that were not visible on bone scans in posttraumatic OA.

Case 4.5

A 55-year-old woman who was diagnosed with left breast cancer 4 years previously underwent a bone scan and ^{18}F-fluorodeoxyglucose (^{18}F-FDG) positron emission tomography (PET)/CT for follow-up examination. The patient's bone scan showed no suspicious hot uptake indicative of a metastasis, and a mild radiopharmaceutical accumulation at the right shoulder joint was observed (Fig. 4.5a). ^{18}F-FDG PET/CT showed no recurrent malignancy or metastasis, but hot uptake was observed in the right shoulder joint, which was more active than that in the bone scan (Fig. 4.5b–d). The patient mainly used her right arm due to surgery on the left breast and was diagnosed with OA of the right shoulder joint. In this case, we show an OA caused by the excessive use of the contralateral joint due to the deterioration of the unilateral joint due to surgery or trauma.

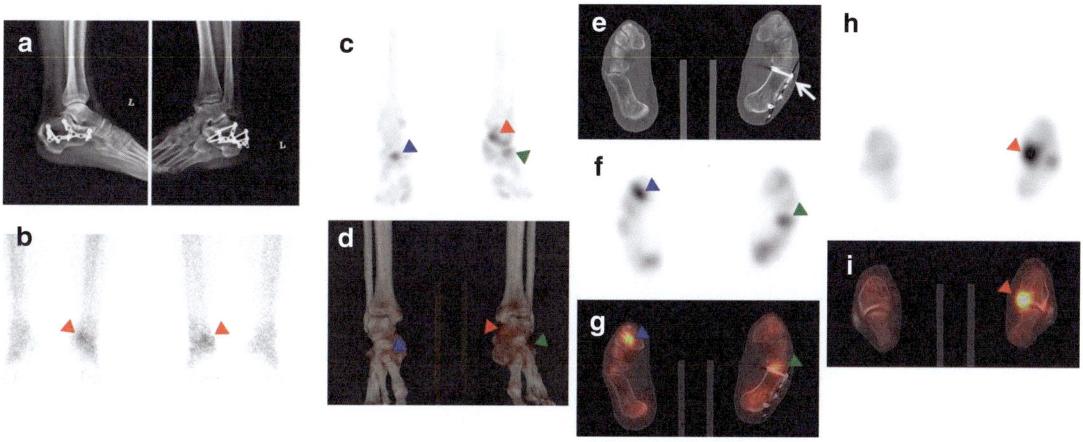

Fig. 4.4 (**a**) On a simple radiograph of the patient's left foot, there were no specific findings except for the metallic prosthesis from surgery. (**b**) Hot uptake with mild diffuse pattern is shown in the left foot area on the bone scan. (**c**–**i**) On SPECT/CT images, there was mildly hot uptake lesion in the left calcaneus area with a postoperative change pattern (green arrowheads in **c** [MIP image], **d** [MIP image of fusion with CT], **f** [SPECT image], and **g** [SPECT fusion with CT]). In the CT image, the pins inserted into the left calcaneus can also be confirmed (arrow in **e**). Another hot uptake lesion was seen in the left talocalcaneal joint, which coincided with the patient's pain area (red arrowheads in **c**, **d**, **h** [SPECT image], and **i** [SPECT fusion with CT]). Also, hot uptake in the right intercuneiform joint is an incidental lesion found only in SPECT/CT (blue arrowheads in **c**, **d**, **f**, and **g**)

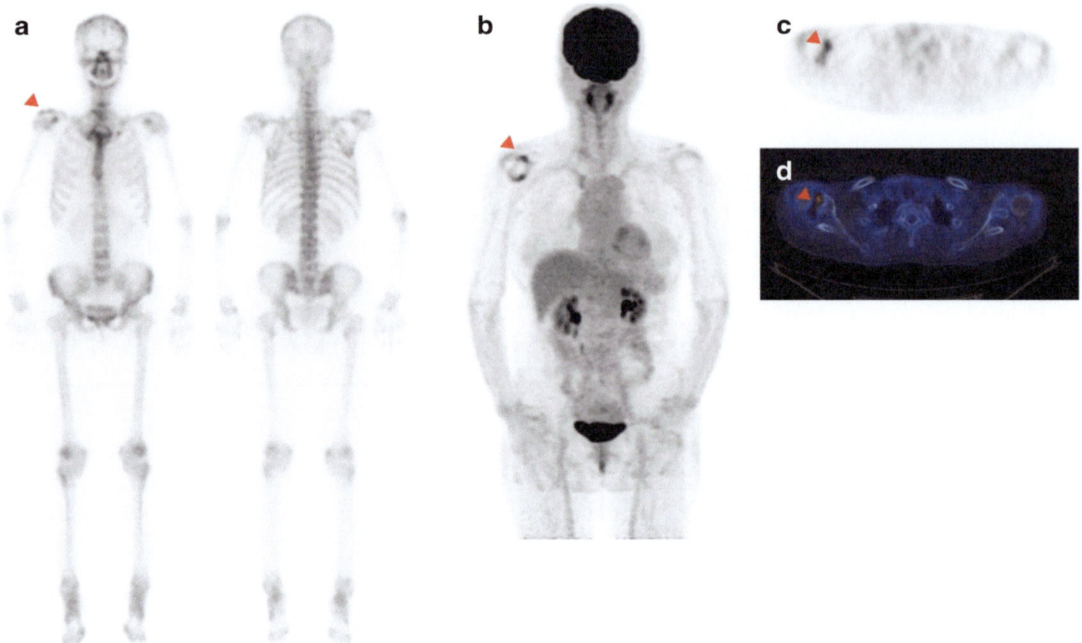

Fig. 4.5 (**a**) Mildly hot uptake lesion was noted in right shoulder joint on bone scan (arrowhead). (**b–d**) More active hot uptake lesion of right shoulder joint was observed on ^{18}F-FDG PET/CT (arrowheads in **b** [MIP] image], **c** [PET image], and d [PET fusion with CT])

Case 4.6
A 55-year-old man visited our hospital complaining of bilateral knee and elbow pain. The patient has been working on a construction site for 15 years and has had persistent pain in the knee and elbow since about 8 years prior, and the pain worsened while working. A simple radiograph of both knees was performed, and both knee joint spaces were narrowed, suggesting arthritis (Fig. 4.6a). He performed a bone scan in our department for a more detailed evaluation of pain in the joints.

In the bone scan, hot uptake was observed in both elbows and bilateral knee joints (Fig. 4.6b), which were associated with OA. As in this case, a patient may complain of joint pain in several areas instead of one location, and this case showed that a bone scan encompassing the whole body with one examination can be useful for evaluating multiple OA.

Case 4.7
A 73-year-old man visited our hospital with left hip joint pain that had begun 2 years previously. The patient had no specific past history other than a history of lumbar disc surgery 3 years previously. A simple X-ray was performed to evaluate the presence of arthritis. As a result, severe joint space narrowing was observed in the left hip joint (Fig. 4.7a), which was highly suggestive of OA. The patient underwent a bone scan in our department for a more detailed evaluation.

On bone scan, a significantly large intense hot uptake lesion was observed in the left hip joint, suggesting severe advanced OA (Fig. 4.7b). In addition, hot uptakes of both shoulder joints and small joints of both hands were also seen in the bone scan, confirming OA in this area as well (Fig. 4.7b). As seen in this case, the hip and hand joints are areas where OA can easily occur, and bone scans show that the uptake level of radiopharmaceuticals can reflect the severity of the disease.

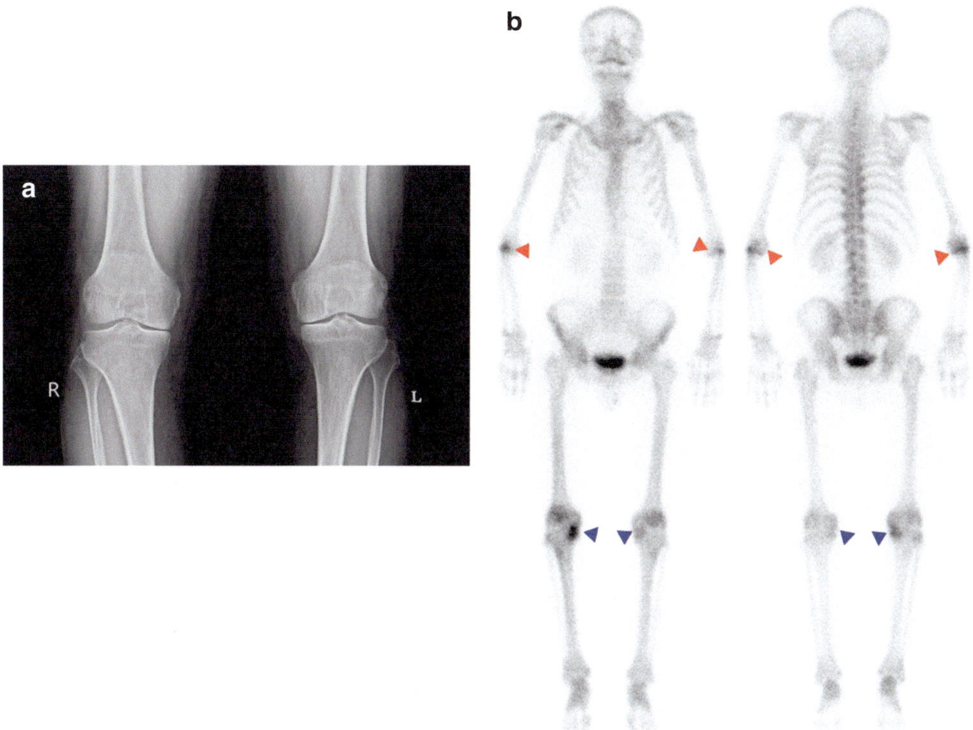

Fig. 4.6 (**a**) On a simple radiograph, joint space narrowing of both knees was observed. (**b**) Hot uptakes in both elbows (red arrowheads) and bilateral knee joints (blue arrowheads) were noted on bone scan

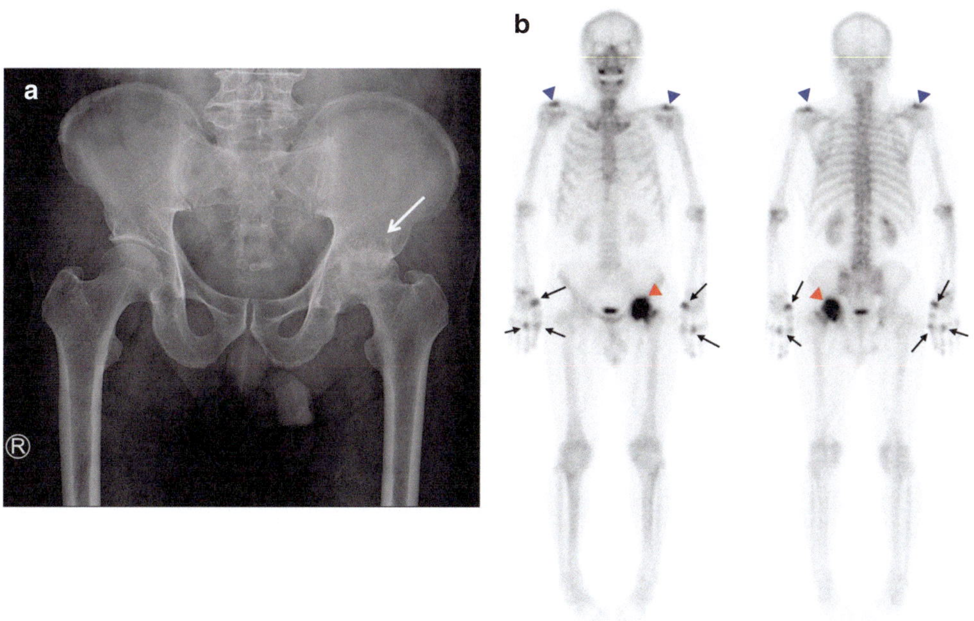

Fig. 4.7 (**a**) A simple radiograph showed the left hip joint space was severely narrowed (arrow). (**b**) Intense hot uptake lesion was observed in left hip joint on bone scan (red arrowheads). Additionally, hot uptakes in both shoulders (blue arrowheads) and small joints of both hands (arrows) were noted in the bone scan

References

1. Pujalte GG, Albano-Aluquin SA. Differential diagnosis of polyarticular arthritis. Am Fam Physician. 2015;92(1):35–41.
2. Mies Richie A, Francis ML. Diagnostic approach to polyarticular joint pain. Am Fam Physician. 2003;68(6):1151–60.
3. Martel-Pelletier J, Barr AJ, Cicuttini FM, Conaghan PG, Cooper C, Goldring MB, et al. Osteoarthritis. Nat Rev Dis Primers. 2016;2:16072. https://doi.org/10.1038/nrdp.2016.72.
4. Burr DB, Gallant MA. Bone remodelling in osteoarthritis. Nat Rev Rheumatol. 2012;8(11):665–73. https://doi.org/10.1038/nrrheum.2012.130.
5. Pelletier JP, Raynauld JP, Abram F, Haraoui B, Choquette D, Martel-Pelletier J. A new non-invasive method to assess synovitis severity in relation to symptoms and cartilage volume loss in knee osteoarthritis patients using MRI. Osteoarthr Cartil. 2008;16(Suppl 3):S8–13. https://doi.org/10.1016/j.joca.2008.06.007.
6. Park DY, Jin LH, Min BH, Kwack KS, An YS, Kim YJ. Subchondral bone scan uptake correlates with articular cartilage degeneration in osteoarthritic knees. Int J Rheum Dis. 2017;20(10):1393–402. https://doi.org/10.1111/1756-185X.12909.
7. An YS, Park DY, Min BH, Lee SJ, Yoon JK. Comparison of bone single-photon emission computed tomography (SPECT)/CT and bone scintigraphy in assessing knee joints. BMC Med Imaging. 2021;21(1):60. https://doi.org/10.1186/s12880-021-00590-8.
8. Kim J, Lee HH, Kang Y, Kim TK, Lee SW, So Y, et al. Maximum standardised uptake value of quantitative bone SPECT/CT in patients with medial compartment osteoarthritis of the knee. Clin Radiol. 2017;72(7):580–9. https://doi.org/10.1016/j.crad.2017.03.009.

Hypertrophic Osteoarthropathy

5

Young Seok Cho

Abstract

Hypertrophic osteoarthropathy (HOA) is a syndrome characterized by abnormal skin proliferation at the distal parts of the extremities as well as periosteal proliferation of the long bones. Bone scintigraphy, usually with ^{99m}Tc methylene diphosphonate (MDP), is usually more sensitive for the detection and characterization of the extent of HOA than radiography alone. Typically, there is symmetrically increased tracer uptake at the periosteum in a linear fashion along the cortical margins of the diaphysis and metaphysis of the long tubular bones, termed "the tram line" or "double stripe sign."

Keywords

Hypertrophic osteoarthropathy · HOA
Hypertrophic pulmonary osteoarthropathy
HPO · Clubbing · Periosteal reaction

Y. S. Cho (✉)
Department of Nuclear Medicine, Samsung Medical Center, Sungkyunkwan University School of Medicine, Seoul, Republic of Korea
e-mail: ysnm.cho@samsung.com

5.1 Etiology and Clinical Significance

Hypertrophic osteoarthropathy (HOA) is a syndrome defined by abnormal skin proliferation at the distal parts of the extremities as well as periosteal generation of the long bones. HOA can be a primary disease entity, known as pachydermoperiostosis, or can be secondary to extraskeletal conditions, with different prognoses and management implications for each. There is a high association between secondary HOA and thoracic malignancy, especially non-small cell lung cancer. In such cases, it can be considered a form of paraneoplastic syndrome. The most prevalent secondary causes of HOA are pulmonary in origin, which is why this condition was formerly referred to as hypertrophic pulmonary osteoarthropathy (HPO). HOA can also be associated with pleural, mediastinal, and cardiovascular causes, as well as extrathoracic conditions such as gastrointestinal tumors and infections, cirrhosis, and inflammatory bowel disease [1]. The main clinical features are a peculiar bulbous deformity of the tips of the fingers conventionally described as *clubbing*, periosteal reaction of the tubular bones, and synovial effusions. In HOA, there is a spectrum of symptoms. At one extreme, patients may be asymptomatic and unaware of the deformity of their fingers and toes. Other patients, in particular those with lung cancers, may notice a burning sensation of the fingertips

S.-O. Yang et al. (eds.), *Atlas of Nuclear Medicine in Musculoskeletal System*,
https://doi.org/10.1007/978-981-19-2677-8_5

and may also experience incapacitating bone and joint pain. Characteristically, this pain is deep-seated, more prominent in the lower extremities, and aggravated by dependency of the limbs [2].

5.2 Imaging

Plain X-ray images of the extremities are often the first imaging modality used to evaluate the pain and may demonstrate abnormalities even in asymptomatic patients. Periosteal reaction is the imaging hallmark of HOA and manifests along the shafts of tubular bones and usually spares the epiphyses in the earliest phases. Symmetric and widely distributed bone involvement is a typical finding in primary and generalized secondary HOA. The tibia, fibula, radius, and ulna are the most commonly affected bones, followed by the phalanges of the fingers. The patterns of periosteal reaction may be solid, linear, dense, or layered [1, 3].

Periosteal reaction at MR imaging typically exhibits low-to-intermediate signal intensity on T1-weighted images and low signal intensity on T2-weighted images. Its appearance at MR imaging usually correlates with the radiographic findings and can manifest as simple periosteal elevation or laminated or onion-skin periosteal reaction [1, 4].

Bone scintigraphy, usually with ^{99m}Tc methylene diphosphonate (MDP), is usually more sensitive for the detection and characterization of the extent of HOA than radiography alone [5]. Typically, there is symmetrically increased tracer uptake at the periosteum in a linear fashion along the cortical margins of the diaphysis and metaphysis of the long tubular bones, termed *the tram line* or *double stripe sign* [6, 7]. Prominent tracer uptake in the digits is reflective of digital clubbing [8]. Case reports of PET/CT with ^{18}F-fluorodeoxyglucose (FDG) and sodium fluoride ([^{18}F]NaF) have reported uptakes corresponding to the periosteal thickening seen on the corresponding CT image [9, 10].

Case 5.1

A 59-year-old man who was diagnosed with a 4-cm-sized pulmonary adenocarcinoma of the right lung lower lobe with ipsilateral hilar lymph node metastasis had a ^{99m}Tc-MDP whole body bone scan to check for bone metastasis. Heterogeneous cortical uptakes with relatively symmetrical distribution can be seen in the cortex of the metaphysis and diaphysis of both femurs (Fig. 5.1).

Case 5.2

A 63-year-old man who underwent right lung upper lobectomy and mediastinal lymph node dissection for adenocarcinoma of the right lung upper lobe 7 years prior had periodic ^{99m}Tc-MDP whole-body bone scan to screen bone metastasis. At the time of bone scan, multiple pulmonary nodules suggesting lung-to-lung metastasis were seen on chest CT. Symmetric cortical uptakes with diffuse pattern are seen in the whole appendicular skeletons (Fig. 5.2a). Periosteal reactions were observed on X-ray images of bilateral humeri (Fig. 5.2b) and CT images of bilateral femurs (Fig. 5.2c).

Case 5.3

A 35-year-old man was hospitalized for hemoptysis as chief compliant. His chest CT showed multiple thin-walled cystic lesions containing soft tissue with nodular growth pattern in both lungs suggesting benign lung disease such as tuberculosis or aspergillosis. Bronchoscopy with transbronchial lung biopsy was performed for differential diagnosis. The biopsy specimen showed acute inflammation with many eosinophils suggesting pulmonary aspergillosis. In ^{99m}Tc-MDP whole-body bone scan, the cortical bone uptakes of bilateral upper and lower extremities were diffusely increased (Fig. 5.3a, b). X-ray showed periosteal thickening along the outer cortices (Fig. 5.3c, d).

Case 5.4

A 67-year-old man who was recently diagnosed with poorly differentiated adenocarcinoma of right lung upper lobe performed a whole-body bone scan for staging. His clinical stage was T2aN0M0. The patient had complained arthralgia of both hands and knees and clubbing of fingers for 3 years. On ^{99m}Tc-MDP bone scintigraphy, heterogeneous patterns of uptakes were observed

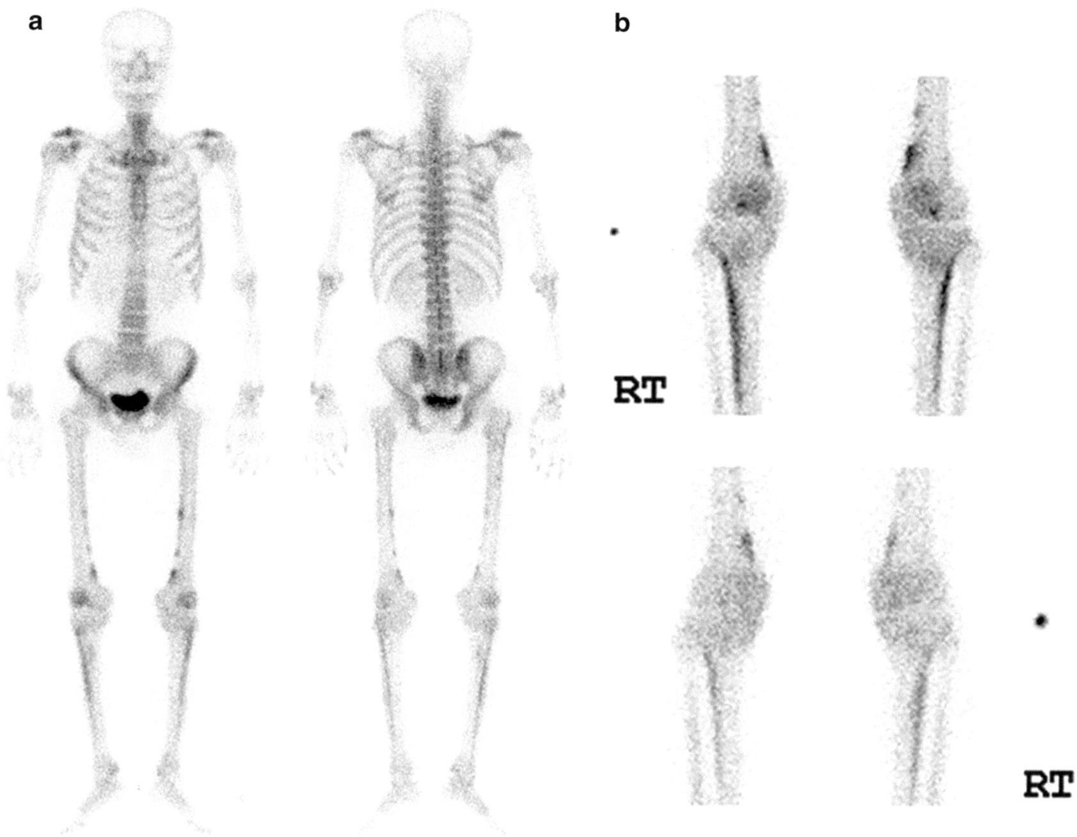

Fig. 5.1 Symmetrical cortical uptakes with heterogeneous pattern were observed in the cortex of the metaphysis and diaphysis of both femurs on whole-body images obtained by continuous acquisition (**a**) and additional planar spot view images (**b**)

along the appendicular skeleton of the whole body (Fig. 5.4a). In particular, increases in radiouptake were prominent in the bilateral distal femurs and the bones of both hands, but the periosteal reactions in these areas were not clearly seen on X-rays of both hands and both knees (Fig. 5.4b, c). On ^{18}F-FDG PET/CT scan, mild periosteal reactions and faint FDG uptake were seen along the medial aspect of the proximal femurs (Fig. 5.4d).

Case 5.5
A 66-year-old man with a neuroendocrine tumor located in the central portion of the right lung with extensive malignant lymphadenopathy in right pulmonary hilum and subcarinal area and hepatic metastasis performed a ^{99m}Tc-MDP whole-body bone scan for staging. The whole-body bone scan taken at the time of initial diagnosis showed only mild degenerative changes, and there was no demonstrable abnormal radiouptake suggesting bone metastasis or hypertrophic osteoarthropathy (Fig. 5.5a). But, in whole-body bone scan taken 9 months later, newly developed bone metastasis was shown, and the cortical uptakes of both tibiae were increased in diffuse manner (Fig. 5.5b). Comparing CT images, the subcarinal lymphadenopathy worsened in the intervening period (Fig. 5.5c, d).

Case 5.6
A 57-year-old man with a 7-cm-sized adenocarcinoma in the upper lobe of the left lung and ipsilateral mediastinal lymph node metastasis underwent a ^{99m}Tc-MDP whole-body bone scan

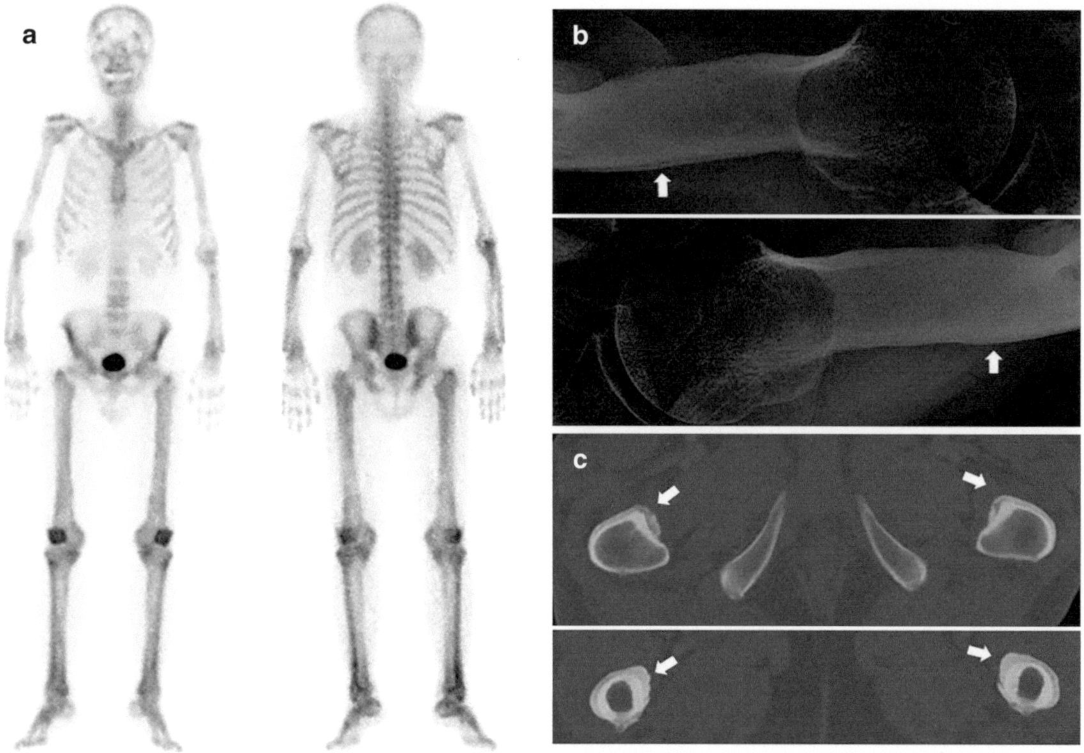

Fig. 5.2 Symmetric cortical radiouptakes with diffuse pattern were observed in the cortex of both humeri, both radii, both ulnae, both femurs, and both tibiae on whole-body bone scan images (**a**). Periosteal reactions (arrows) were observed in the cortex of bilateral distal humeri on shoulder X-ray images (**b**) and the cortex of bilateral proximal femurs on abdomen and pelvis CT images (**c**)

for screening of bone metastasis. The cortical uptake of the whole appendicular skeletons was increased in a diffuse manner, which is typical of hypertrophic osteopathy. But, the X-ray images of both wrists and both ankles did not show a clear sign of periosteal reaction (Fig. 5.6).

Case 5.7

A 53-year-old man with thymic carcinoma and pulmonary metastasis who had extended total thymectomy and adjuvant chemoradiation therapy 2 years prior underwent a ^{99m}Tc-MDP whole-body bone scan for annual follow-up. In the bone scan images, the cortical uptakes of both femurs and tibiae were significantly increased in a heterogeneous pattern (Fig. 5.7a). On the follow-up bone scan performed 4 years later, the cortical uptakes of both femurs and tibiae decreased, but the intense uptakes of multiple bone metastases were newly observed (Fig. 5.7b). During the interval period, the sizes of mediastinal metastatic lymph nodes and pulmonary metastatic nodules were significantly decreased on chest CT images (images not shown).

Case 5.8

A 68-year-old woman who underwent mastectomy for right breast cancer 15 years prior and total thyroidectomy for papillary thyroid cancer 5 years prior had a ^{99m}Tc-MDP whole-body bone scan for annual follow-up. On this scan, the linear radiouptakes consistent with the typical *tram line* or *double stripe sign* were shown along the cortical margins of the diaphysis of both femurs and tibiae (Fig. 5.8a). X-ray images of both knees showed no demonstrable finding of periosteal

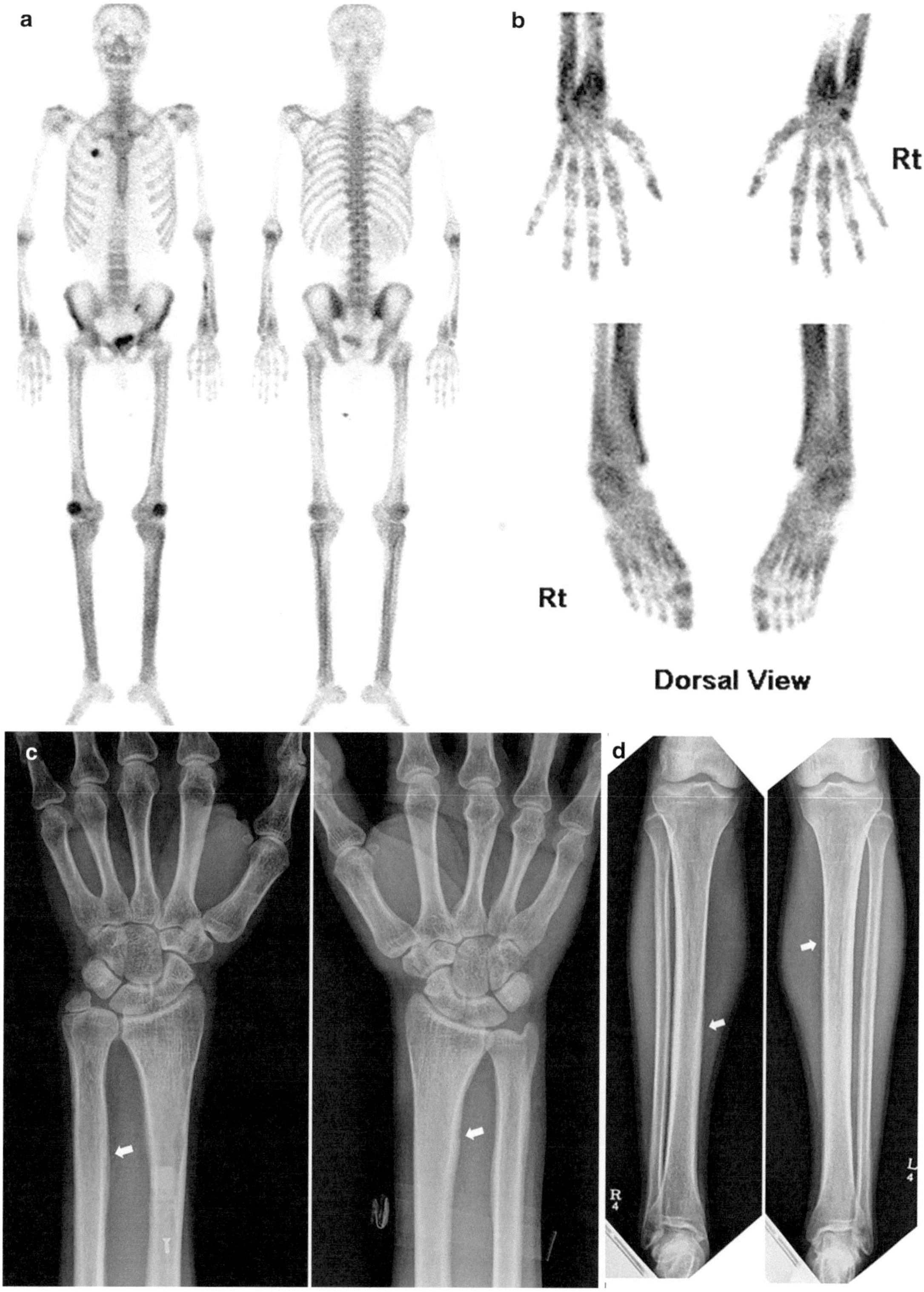

Fig. 5.3 Diffuse increases of radiouptake were seen in the cortex of both radii, both ulnae, both femurs, both tibiae, and small bones of both hands and feet on whole-body bone scan images (**a**) and planar spot images of both hands and feet (**b**). X-ray images of both hands (**c**) and both lower legs (**d**) demonstrated periosteal thickening along the outer cortices of bilateral distal ulnae, radii, tibiae, and fibulae (arrows)

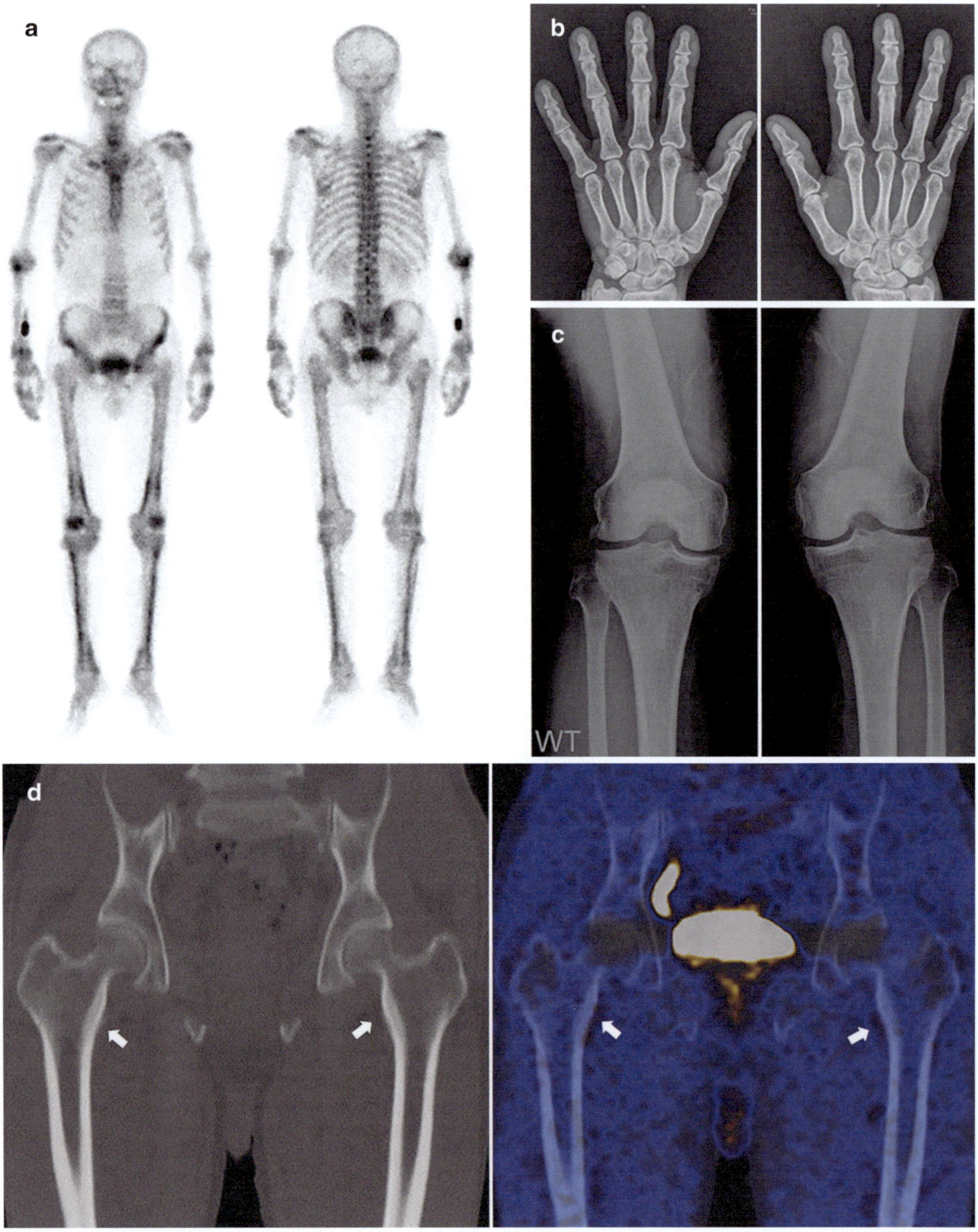

Fig. 5.4 Heterogeneous cortical radiouptakes were observed in bilateral upper and lower extremities on whole-body bone scan (**a**). Particularly, the uptakes were increased in the distal portion of both femurs and tibiae and the small bones of both hands. X-ray images of both hands (**b**) and both knees (**c**) demonstrated no significant cortical thickening suggesting periosteal reaction. The fusion PET/CT images (right) and CT images (left) of torso FDG PET/CT showed faint FDG uptakes (SUV_{max} = 1.3) and mild irregular cortical thickenings (arrows) of both proximal femurs (**d**)

reaction (Fig. 5.8b). Chest CT performed at that time did not show any abnormal finding suggestive of primary lung cancer, pulmonary metastasis, or mediastinal malignant lymphadenopathy (image not shown).

Case 5.9

A 23-year-old man who had chemoradiotherapy for nasopharyngeal 4 years prior underwent a ^{99m}Tc-MDP whole-body bone scan for screening of bone metastasis. The cortical bone uptakes in bilateral upper and lower extremities were increased in a heterogeneous pattern (Fig. 5.9a). The chest CT images at the time of bone scan showed multiple nodules due to pulmonary metastases and enlarged lymph nodes suggesting mediastinal lymph node metastasis (Fig. 5.9b).

Teaching Points

- Bone scintigraphy is more sensitive for the detection and characterization of hypertrophic osteoarthropathy than radiography alone.
- Typical finding of hypertrophic osteoarthropathy is symmetrical radiouptake at the periosteum along the cortical margins of the long tubular bones, termed "the tram line" or "double stripe sign".

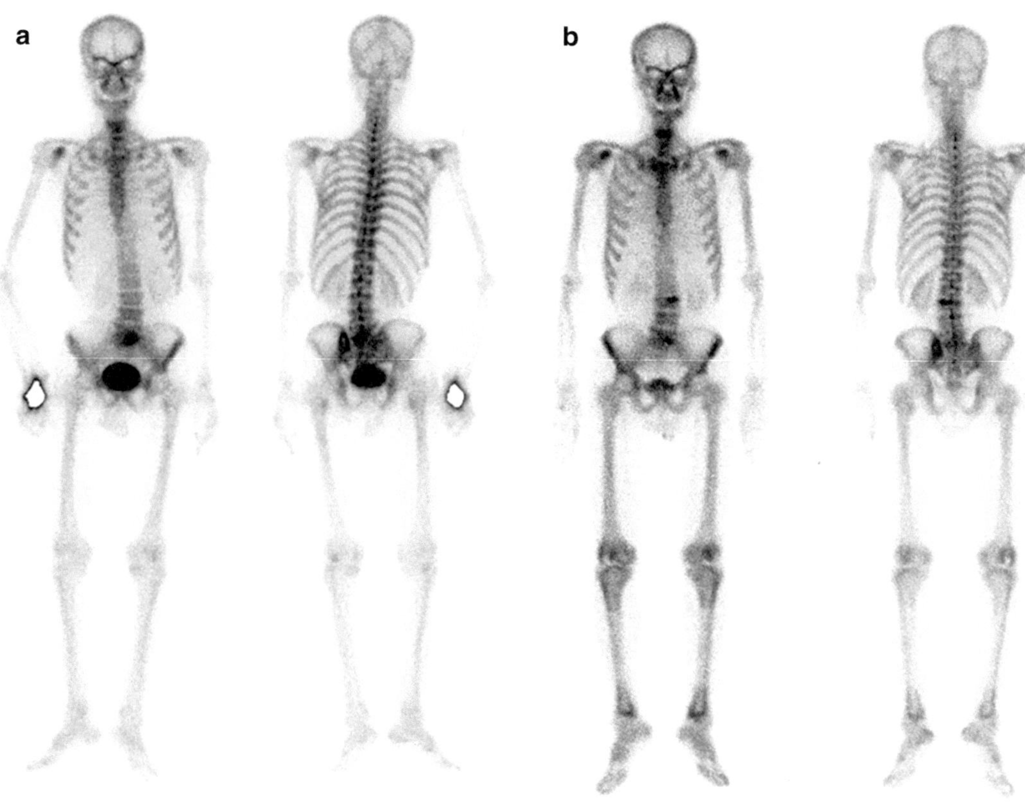

Fig. 5.5 The whole-body bone scan images for staging of initial diagnosis demonstrated the radiouptakes suggesting degenerative change in the L5-S1 spine and left sacroiliac joint and did not show any abnormal cortical radiouptake suggesting hypertrophic osteoarthropathy (**a**). On the whole-body bone scan taken 9 months later, the focal radiouptake in L3 spine suggesting bone metastasis and the diffuse cortical uptakes of both tibiae suggesting hypertrophic osteoarthropathy were shown (**b**). The size of metastatic subcarinal lymph node had increased significantly between the chest CT initial diagnosis (**c**) and the follow-up chest CT taken 9 months later (**d**)

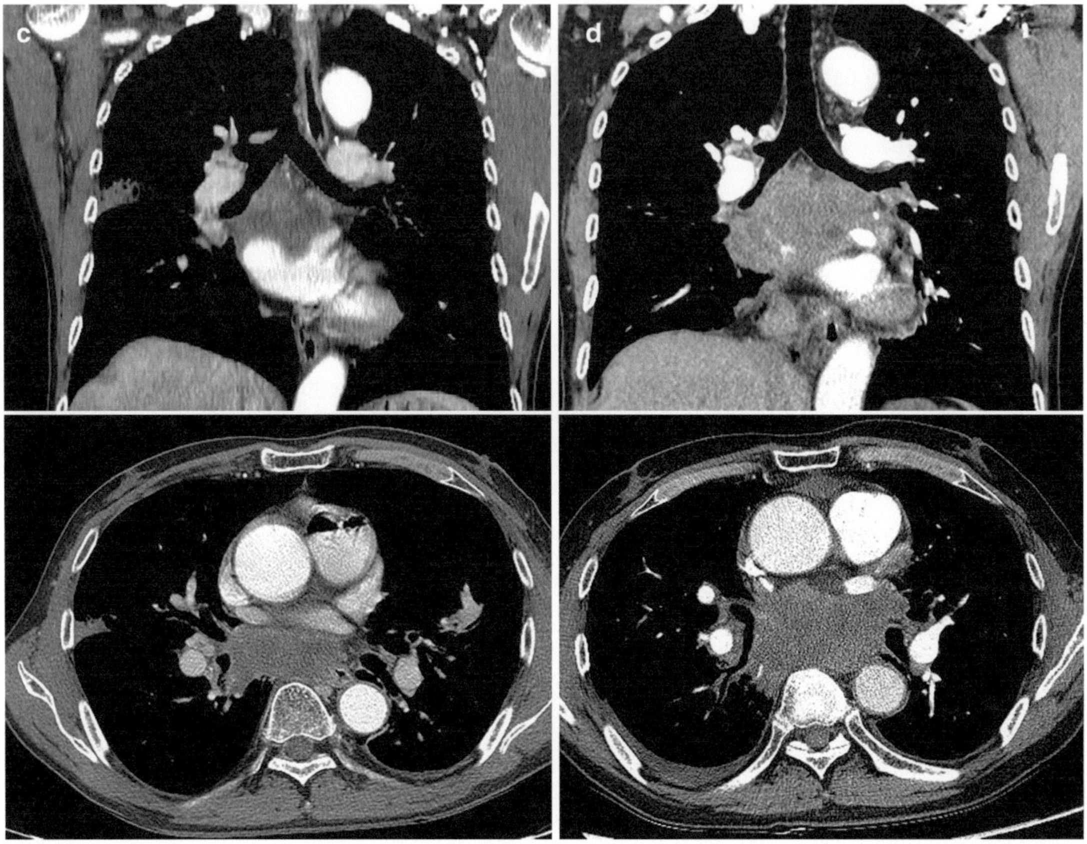

Fig. 5.5 (continued)

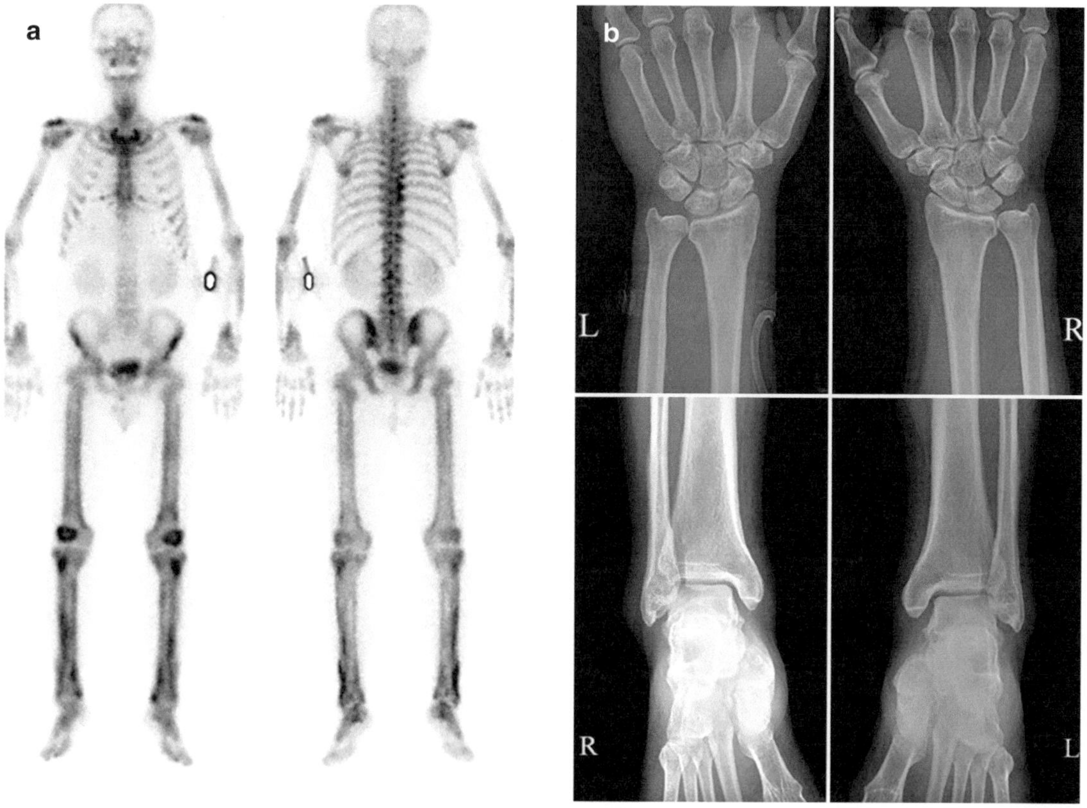

Fig. 5.6 Diffuse radiouptakes were seen on the cortices of long bones of bilateral upper and lower extremities. In particular, the uptakes of both tibiae were clearly increased (**a**). There was no demonstrable abnormal cortical thickening or cortical irregularity suggesting periosteal reaction on the X-ray images of both wrists and both ankles (**b**)

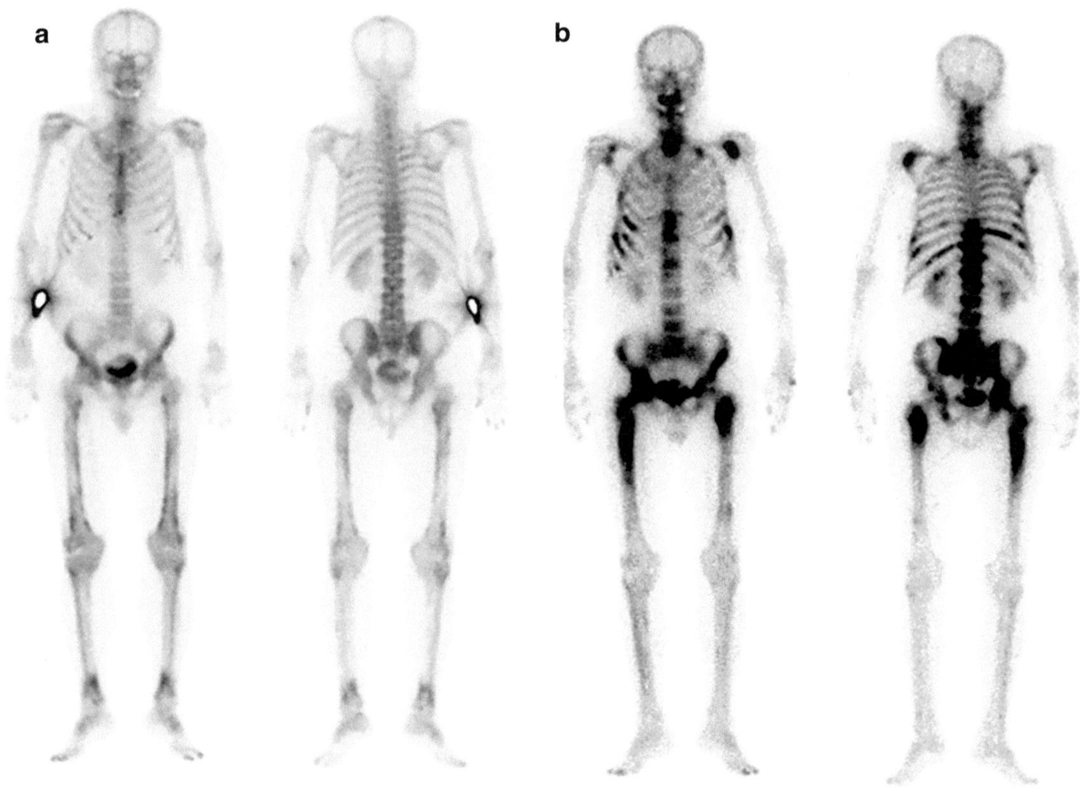

Fig. 5.7 Symmetric radiouptakes with uneven pattern were seen along the cortices of both femurs and both tibiae (**a**). Even considering the threshold difference due to intense radiouptake of metastatic lesions, the cortical radiouptakes of bilateral distal femurs and distal tibiae were decreased on the follow-up bone scan images (**b**)

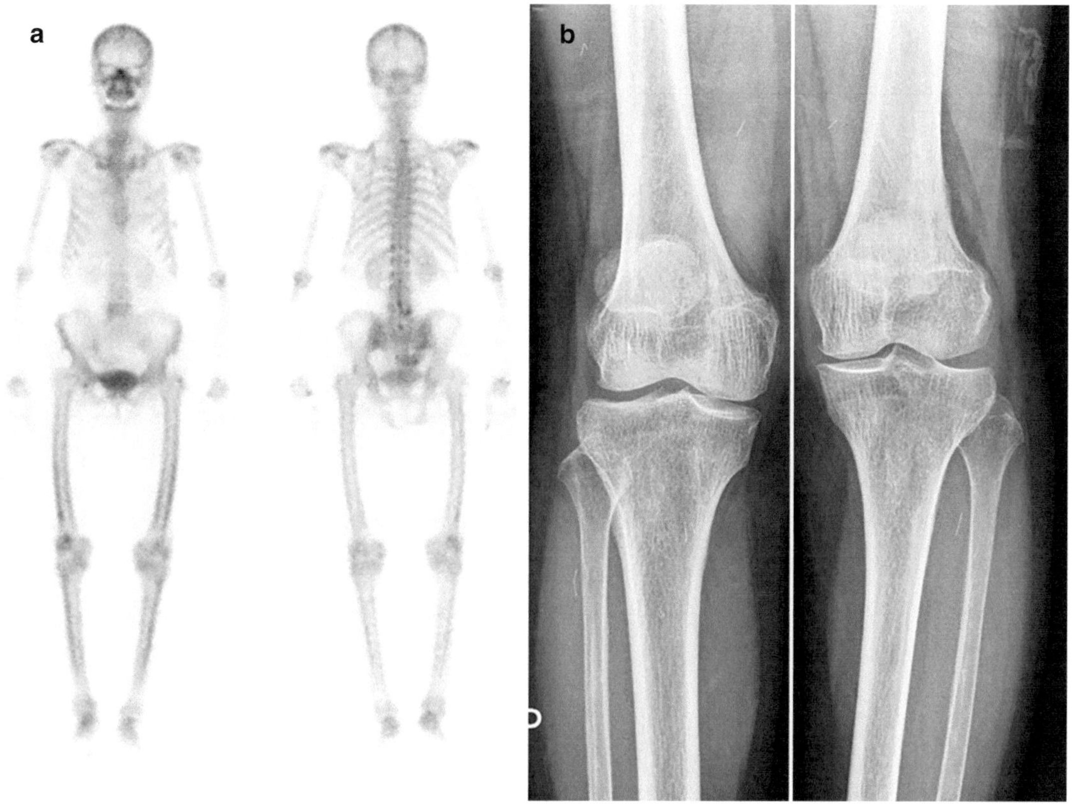

Fig. 5.8 Bone scan images showed the diffuse and symmetric radiouptakes described as "tram line" or "double stripe" along the cortices of bilateral femoral and tibial shafts (**a**). On the X-ray images of both knees, there was no significant sign of periosteal reaction in the cortices of both femurs and tibiae (**b**)

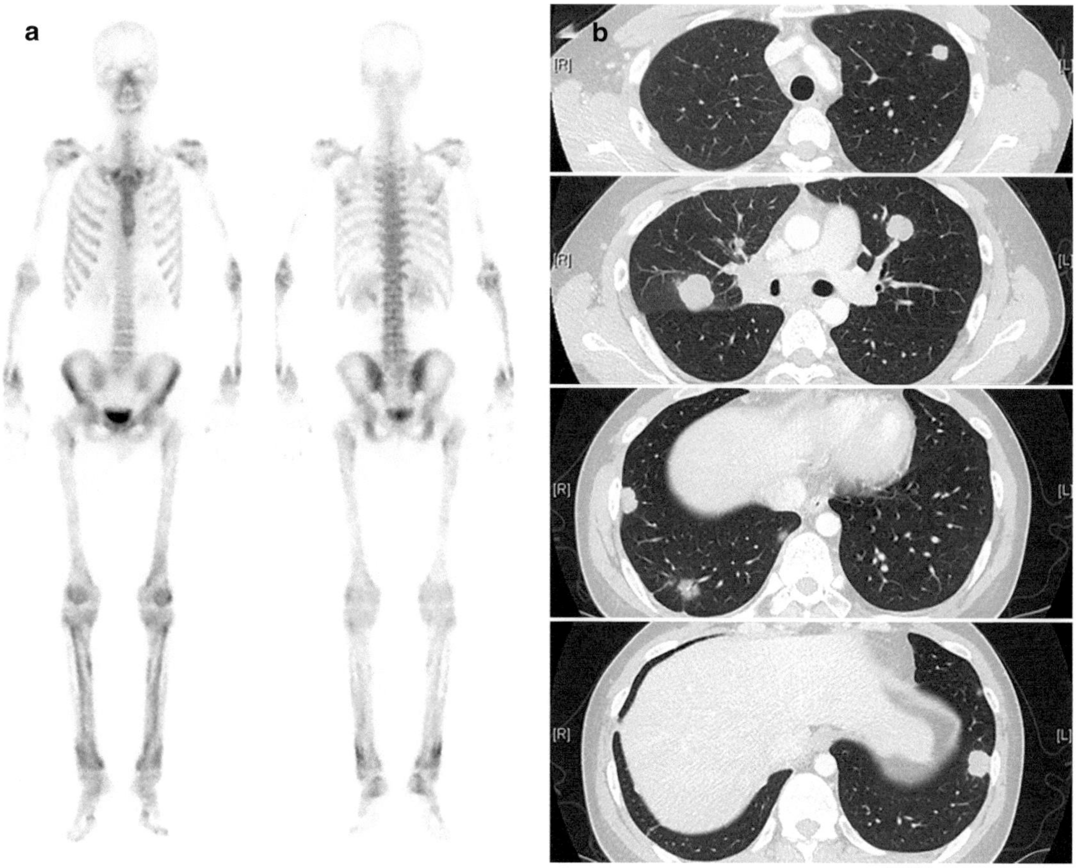

Fig. 5.9 Diffuse and symmetrical cortical uptakes in a heterogeneous pattern were shown in the long bones of bilateral upper and lower extremities (**a**). Multiple pulmonary nodules suggesting pulmonary metastasis of nasopharyngeal cancer were shown on chest CT (**b**)

References

1. Yap FY, Skalski MR, Patel DB, Schein AJ, White EA, Tomasian A, et al. Hypertrophic osteoarthropathy: clinical and imaging features. Radiographics. 2017;37:157–95.
2. Martinez-Lavin M. Hypertrophic osteoarthropathy. Best Pract Res Clin Rheumatol. 2020;34:101507.
3. Rana RS, Wu JS, Eisenberg RL. Periosteal reaction. AJR Am J Roentgenol. 2009;193:W259–72.
4. Greenfield GB, Warren DL, Clark RA. MR imaging of periosteal and cortical changes of bone. Radiographics. 1991;11:611–23. discussion 24
5. Rutherford GC, Dineen RA, O'Connor A. Imaging in the investigation of paraneoplastic syndromes. Clin Radiol. 2007;62:1021–35.
6. Russo RR, Lee A, Mansberg R, Emmett L. Hypertrophic pulmonary osteoarthropathy demonstrated on SPECT/CT. Clin Nucl Med. 2009;34:628–31.
7. Santhosh S, Bhattacharya A, Bhadada S, Kaur R, Singh M, Mittal BR. Three-phase skeletal scintigraphy in pachydermoperiostosis. Clin Nucl Med. 2011;36:e199–201.
8. Mohan HK, Groves AM, Clarke SE. Detection of finger clubbing and primary lung tumor on Tc-99 MDP bone scintigraphy in a patient with a scaphoid fracture. Clin Nucl Med. 2004;29:450–1.
9. Aparici CM, Bains S. Hypertrophic osteoarthropathy seen with NaF18 PET/CT bone imaging. Clin Nucl Med. 2011;36:928–9.
10. Makis W, Abikhzer G, Rush C. Hypertrophic pulmonary osteoarthropathy diagnosed by FDG PET-CT in a patient with lung adenocarcinoma. Clin Nucl Med. 2009;34:625–7.

Part II

Traumatic and Circulatory Disorders

6 Fracture, Non-union, and Bone Graft

Soon-Ah Park, Su Jin Lee, Hye Joo Son, and Jung Mi Park

Abstract

Bone fracture results from full or partial break in the continuity of bone in normal or pathologic conditions. In most of bone fractures, healing is a natural process. However, non-union of fracture sites can occur in the case with problems at the facture sites. The bone graft is commonly used for reconstruction of bony defect after oncology surgery. There are various nuclear medicine examinations such as planar or three-phase bone scan, bone SPECT, or SPECT/CT to evaluate detection of fracture site, reactive or atrophic non-union, and the viability of bone graft. Here, we introduce a variety of cases performed by nuclear medicine imaging to evaluate fracture sites, non-union, and bone graft. This chapter aims to inform you what points to keep in mind when evaluating trauma and bone graft with nuclear medicine imaging.

Keywords

Bone fracture · Non-union · Bone graft · Bone scan · Bone SPECT/CT

S.-A. Park (✉)
Department of Nuclear Medicine, Wonkwang University School of Medicine, Iksan, Republic of Korea
e-mail: nmbach@wku.ac.kr

S. J. Lee
Department of Nuclear Medicine, Ajou University School of Medicine, Suwon, Republic of Korea
e-mail: suesj202@ajou.ac.kr

H. J. Son
Department of Nuclear Medicine, Dankook University College of Medicine, Cheonan, Republic of Korea
e-mail: neuroscience@dankook.ac.kr

J. M. Park
Department of Nuclear Medicine, Soonchunhyang University Hospital, Bucheon, Republic of Korea
e-mail: jmipark@schmc.ac.kr

6.1 Bone Fracture

6.1.1 Etiology and Clinical Significance

A significant percentage of bone fractures occur in the normal bone due to prolonged minor stress or of a high force impact usually in the setting of trauma. However, a fracture may also be a result from a variety of settings: Firstly, some medical conditions weaken the bones such as osteoporosis and thus prone to be fractured from forces that would be insufficient to cause fractures in normal bones. These are known as insufficiency fractures. Secondly, the prolonged application of abnormal forces can result in the accumulation of the microfractures faster than healing, eventually resulting in macroscopic fracture. These are termed fatigue fractures. Thirdly, the bone may

S.-O. Yang et al. (eds.), *Atlas of Nuclear Medicine in Musculoskeletal System*,
https://doi.org/10.1007/978-981-19-2677-8_6

have some types of disease that focally weakens it (e.g., malignancy, bone cyst, etc.). These are known as pathological fractures.

In most of bone fractures, healing is a natural process that will generate proliferation of periosteal and endosteal connective tissue for the development of a cartilaginous matrix, formation of islands and bands of cartilage, and, in some cases, an osseous matrix [1]. The healing of fracture can take several weeks to several years, depending on which bone has become injured and whether there are any complications such as infection. The pathophysiological sequence of healing that occurs following a fracture can be divided into three main phases: Firstly, inflammatory phase shows local hyperemia beginning within a few hours after trauma onset. At the end of this phase, which usually takes approximately a week, soft tissue callus is present which is non-mineralized and not visible on radiography. Secondly, repair phase over the ensuing few weeks, this soft tissue callus is transformed into a bony callus by the activation of osteoprogenitor cells which stabilizes the fracture site. Thirdly, remodeling phase lasts many months and even years, and the union of the fracture fragment is formed by osteoblasts and osteoclasts. In most instances, remodeling can result in almost perfect healing. In some instances, however, particularly if the alignment is not perfect, a residual deformity will be remained.

6.1.2 Imaging

Bone scans visualize bone metabolic changes. Fractures are generally imaged using conventional radiographs for the identification fracture; however, in some cases that normal anatomy makes interpretation difficult (e.g., joints, wrist, feet, the base of skull, spine) and plain radiographs are insensitive to fracture, bone scans or bone SPECT can be useful to find missed or stress fractures that don't show up on the conventional radiography. Bone scans are commonly used for the examination of fracture sites to reveal all injuries due to its high sensitivity. And it can be especially useful in patients who cannot accurately describe symptoms clearly with brain injury or child abuse [2] and in orthopedic patients with plaster casts and metal splints which can interfere with examination of other radiographs [3].

Three-phase bone scanning has a narrower indication than single delayed phase imaging in patients with trauma. In cases of infection and/or inflammation, there will be asymmetric blood flow and blood pool activity showing preferentially to the affected region. In cases of fracture, however, immediately after a fracture, the area shows increased regional blood flow which is apparent in the first phase of three-phase bone scanning. This initial increase of blood flow to the affected regions subsides gradually over a few days following the trauma. In the second phase of three-phase bone scan, an increase in the tracer activity in the soft tissue of affected area can be seen. In the delayed phase of three-phase scanning, there is increased tracer uptake in the vicinity of the fracture. Whereas the initially increased blood flow gradually disappears after the fracture, callus continues to be formed at the fracture site. There are development of new vessels leading to increase in the local blood volume and formation of fibrous bone containing increased amounts of amorphous calcium phosphate with a high binding affinity for bone-seeking radiotracers. This increasing uptake on bone scanning in the initial weeks after trauma is a typical finding for a fracture.

Bone SPECT is useful, especially in injuries of the axial skeleton or base of the skull. The hybrid imaging with SPECT/CT has been particularly helpful in the evaluation of foot and ankle injuries and vertebral pathology. The physiological information and the anatomical detail allow a better understanding of injured sites and have proven to be useful in planning surgical intervention.

Case 6.1

A 58-year-old woman presented to the clinic due to chest pain after multiple contusions from

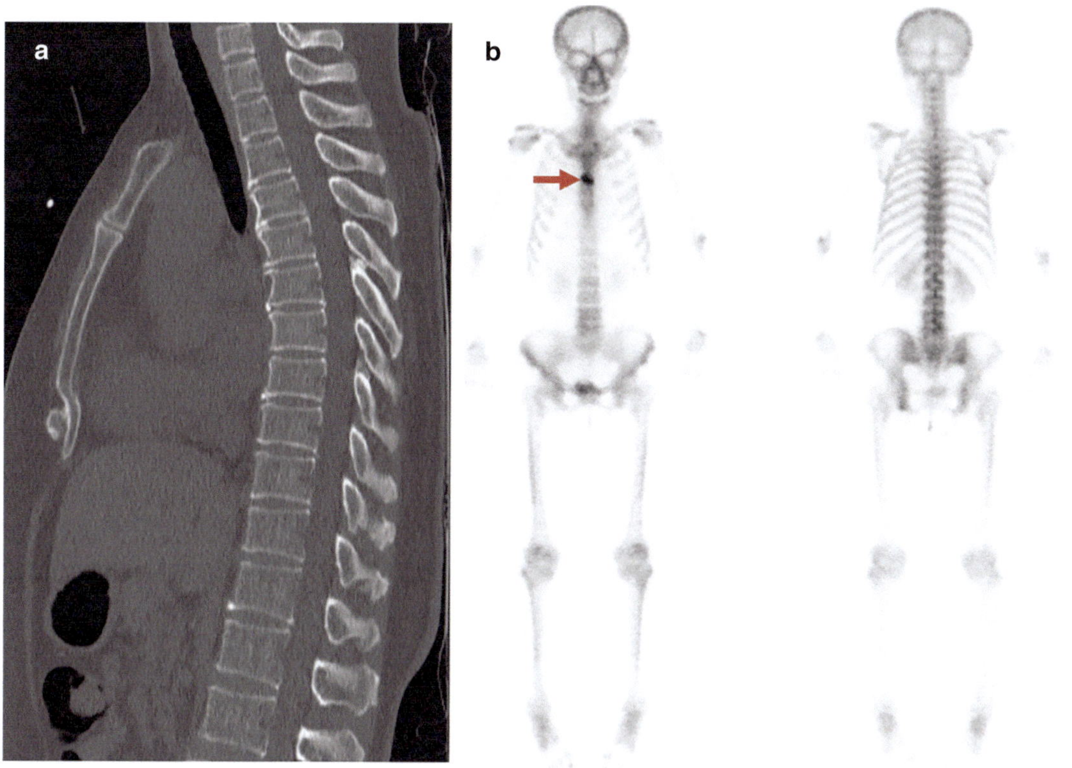

Fig. 6.1 A 58-year-old woman with the microfracture of sternum. The CT scan shows negative finding for fracture (**a**); however, a focal increased uptake indicating fracture (red arrow) is observed on bone scan (**b**). This case is micro- or missed fracture on the CT scan

car accident. Chest CT scan showed negative finding regarding fracture of sternum. Bone scan showed focal increased uptake in the sternum which is missed fracture on the CT scan (Fig. 6.1).

Case 6.2

A 49-year-old woman presented to the clinic due to persistent pelvic pain. Two months ago, she underwent pelvic radiograph to evaluate fracture of pelvic bone; however, it reveled negative finding. Bone SPECT/CT demonstrated active lesion in the left pubic bone and sclerotic change on the CT component (Fig. 6.2).

Case 6.3

A 53-year-old woman, who has been working in a bakery in a standing posture for a long time, underwent bone scan to rule out metastasis due to breast malignancy recently diagnosed. Bone scan revealed focal area of increased uptake in the lower portions of bilateral femoral neck and right proximal tibia. She had a history that she had bumped her hip joint area against the table while working at a crawl space. She underwent pelvic CT examination to further evaluate the lesions of pelvic bone on the same day. CT image revealed sclerotic change of subcortical bone of bilateral femoral necks, worse on the right. She was off the job after that time. Subsequent bone scan was performed 6 months later. Bone scan demonstrated almost normalized uptake uptake of both femora and right proximal tibia. This case was stress fractures in the neck of both femora and right proximal tibia shown positive findings on bone scan (Fig. 6.3).

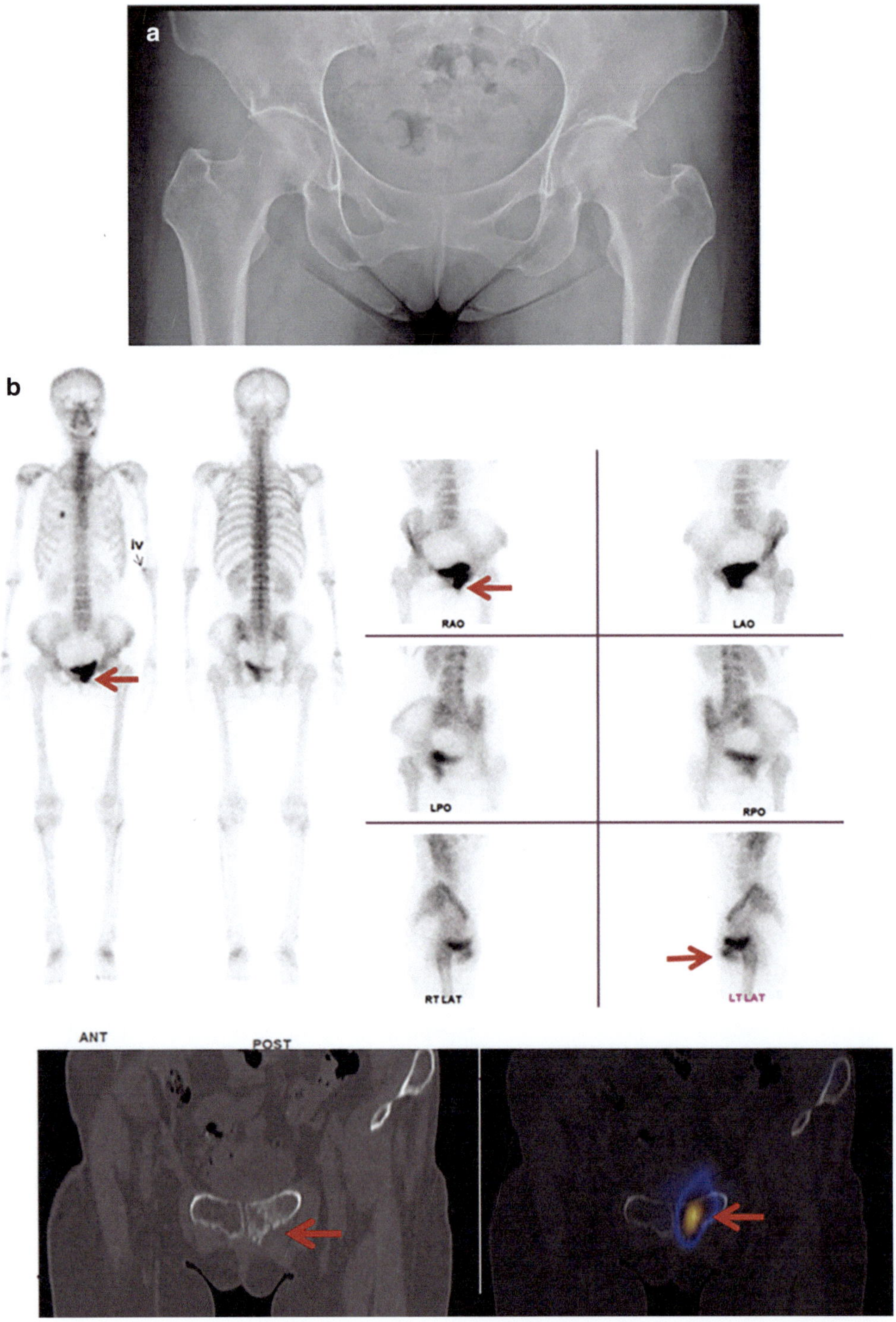

Fig. 6.2 A 49-year-old woman with missed left pubic bone fracture. Negative finding is observed on the pelvic conventional radiograph (**a**). A focal hot uptake lesion is shown in the left pubic bone (red arrow) on bone scan and SPECT/CT taken two months later, and sclerotic change suggesting posttraumatic change (red arrow) on the CT component of SPECT/CT (**b**). It is missed fracture on the conventional radiograph 2 months ago

Case 6.4
A 16-year-old boy was admitted for a head trauma caused by a traffic accident. Brain CT scan showed a depressed skull fracture with extension to the left parietal bone, left parieto-temporosphenoid bone, and left orbital wall and epidural hemorrhage and hemorrhagic contusion. At the time of arrival, he was not alert and could not communicate clearly. A neurologic examination revealed dysarthrosis, and he was not able to complain his dysfunction and/or pain clearly at that time. Bone scan was performed to rule out fracture sites throughout the whole skeletal system. Bone scan demonstrated more fracture or traumatic injury in the lower portion of manubrium, right proximal humerus, left scapula, and left upper ribs (Fig. 6.4).

6.2 Non-union

6.2.1 Etiology and Clinical Significance

Non-union is a serious complication of a fracture that persists for a minimum of 9 months without healing for 3 months [4]. Non-union results from multifactorial process when the bone lacks blood supply and adequate stability or both and gets infected. The major patent factor is the poor blood supply. This can occur with poor nutrition, smoking, and biologic causes of poor blood flow and poor bone healing. The other causes are inadequate stabilization of facture site and fracture types with fracture gap greater than 3 mm; lack of cortical continuity; highly comminuted, but-

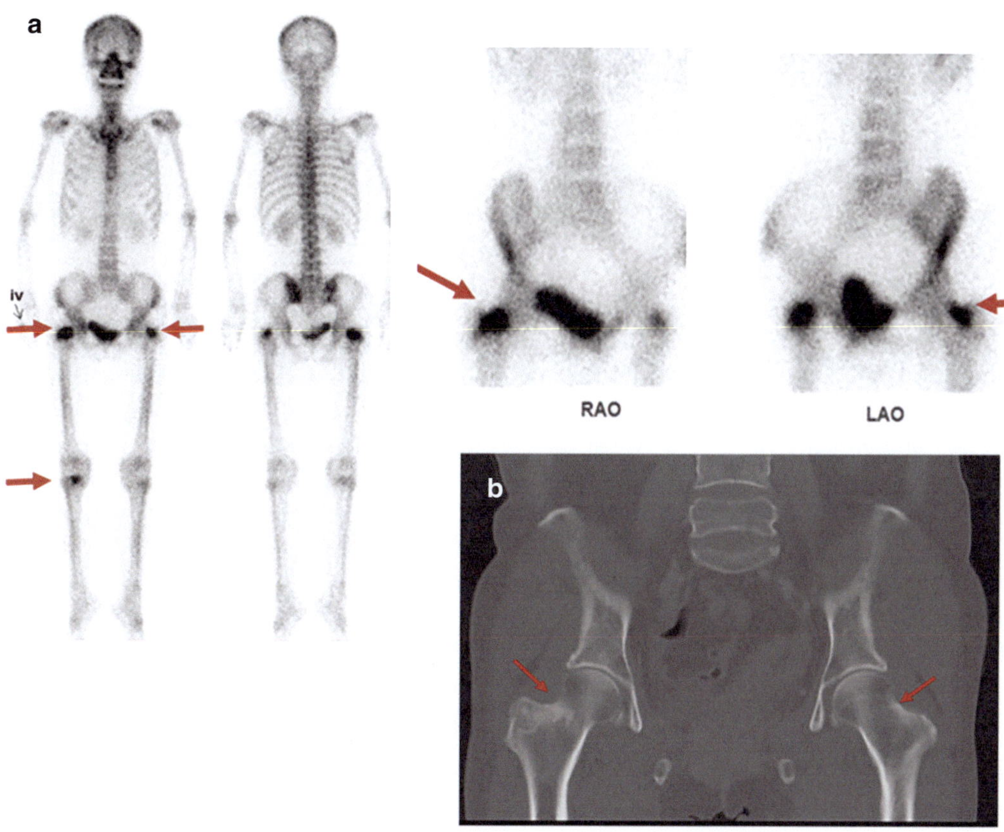

Fig. 6.3 A 53-year-old woman with stress fractures of the neck of both femora and right proximal tibia. Initial bone scan reveals focal area of increased uptake in the neck of both femora and right proximal tibia (red arrow) (**a**). Coronal CT image on the same day shows sclerotic change of subcortical bone of bilateral femoral necks, worse on the right (**b**). Bone scan taken 6 months later demonstrates almost normalized uptake of both femurs and right proximal tibia (**c**). Stress fractures appear to have occurred in normal bones due to persistent and repeated minor force in traumatic condition

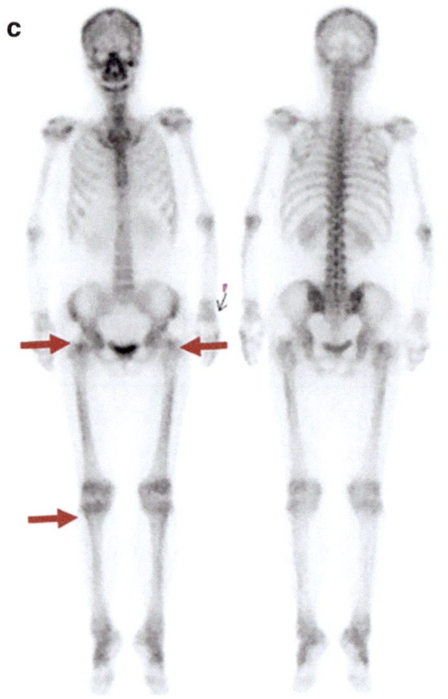

Fig. 6.3 (continued)

terfly fragments; and soft tissue compromised open fracture.

6.2.2 Imaging

Bone scan is useful in assessing atrophic non-unions. If a photon-deficient area between the fragments ends, it indicates a very low probability of union being achieved. The hypertrophic non-union shows persistent accumulation of tracer at the fragment ends. It reflects biological activity for blood flow and new bone formation.

Case 6.5
A 23-year-old woman was operatively treated with open reduction and internal fixation due to fractures after a skiing accident. The radiologist raised the possibility of non-union 10 months later. Then, she was diagnosed with a non-union at 13 months after trauma accident. The conventional radiograph showed fracture lines in the fibula and tibia, and bone scan revealed photon-deficient gap in the fracture site of tibia (Fig. 6.5).

6.3 Bone Graft

6.3.1 Etiology and Clinical Significance

The bone graft is commonly used for reconstruction of bony defect. The success of reconstruction depends on good blood supply to the bone graft. The vascular occlusion may result in necrosis and failure. It is important to assess vascularity and viability of the underlying bone.

6.3.2 Imaging

Bone scan can offer method for the assessment of the graft's physiologic status and viability [5]. Most allografts are not well microvascularized at the time of surgical insertion and depend on revascularization from surrounding blood vessel. In the early postsurgical phase, the graft demonstrates as a photon-deficient area. Subsequent bone scintigraphy is necessary for the ascertain sequential change of the increased perfusion, blood pool, and delayed uptake as revascularization progresses. Bone SPECT images can be useful to separate osseous activity from the adjacent normal bone and soft tissue activity.

Case 6.6
A 65-year-old man visited to the outpatient dental clinic for the evaluation of bone graft viability. He had a segmental mandibulectomy with fibular free flap for the osteosarcoma arising in the right mandible. Two weeks after operation, SPECT/CT fusion imaging showed diffusely increased radiotracer uptake at the vascularized fibular bone graft, which implies viable bone graft suggesting future good prognosis (Fig. 6.6).

Case 6.7
A 55-year-old man visited to the outpatient dental clinic for the evaluation of bone graft viability. He had a segmental mandibulectomy with fibular free flap for the squamous cell carcinoma arising in the right retromolar trigone. Two weeks after operation, SPECT/CT fusion imaging did not show the significant radiotracer uptake at the vascularized fibular bone graft, which implies non-viable bone graft suggesting future poor prognosis (Fig. 6.7).

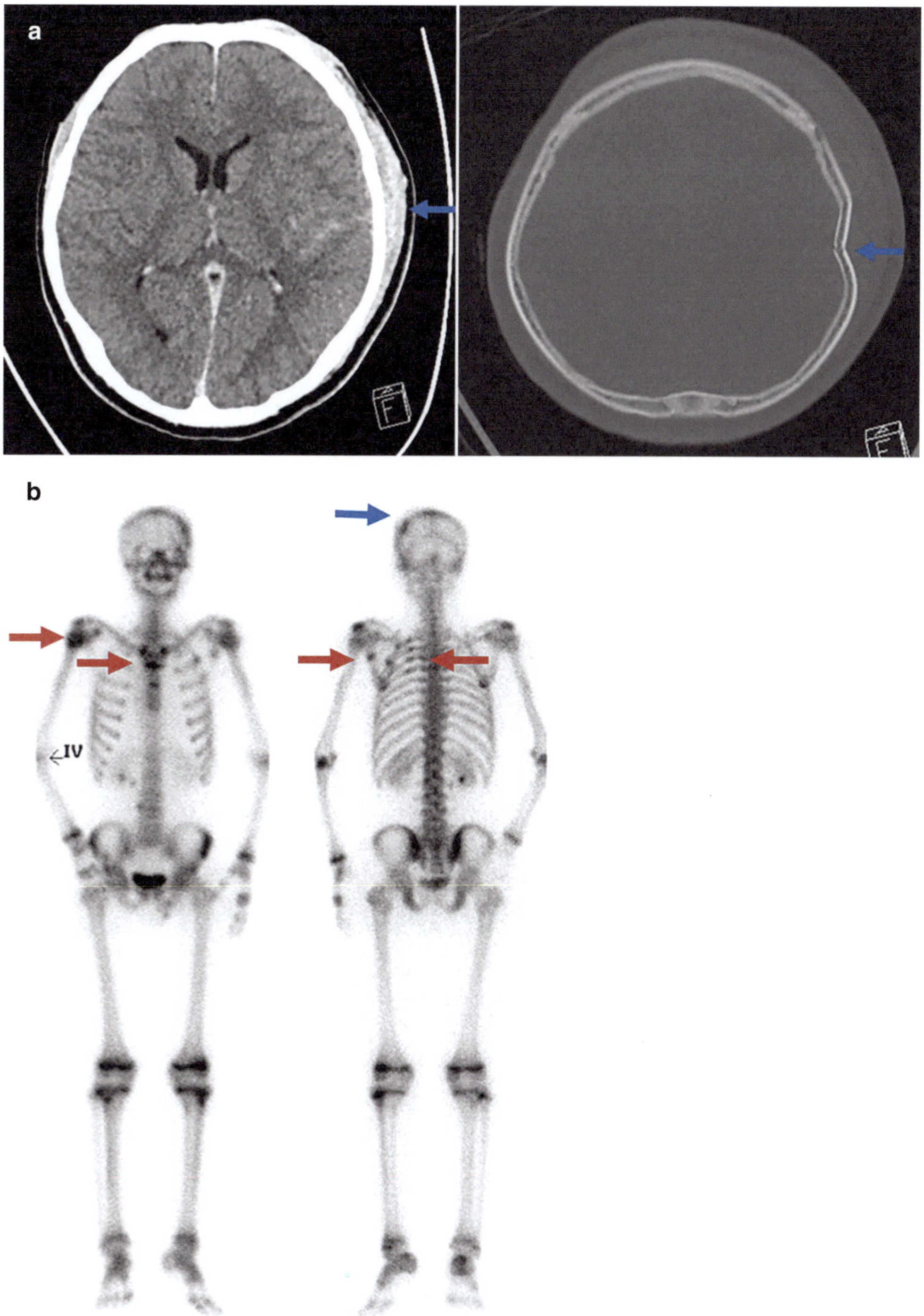

Fig. 6.4 A 16-year-old boy with head trauma who has additional fractures demonstrated by whole-body bone scan. Brain CT scan shows a depressed skull fracture (blue arrow) with extension to the left parietal bone, left parietotemporosphenoid bone, and left orbital wall and epidural hemorrhage and hemorrhagic contusion (**a**). Bone scan demonstrates more fractures or traumatic injury (red arrow) in the lower portion of manubrium, right proximal humerus, left scapula, and left upper ribs (**b**). In a patient with brain injury, bone scan can be useful imaging tool to evaluate further fracture sites

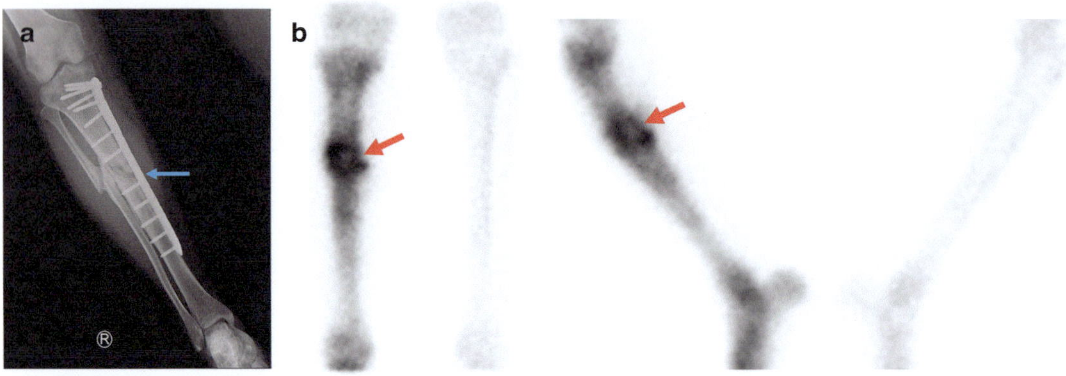

Fig. 6.5 A 23-year-old woman with atrophic non-union of right tibia fracture. The conventional radiograph demonstrates fracture line (blue arrow) following internal fixation of the right tibia (**a**). Bone scan reveals photon-deficient gap in the fracture site of tibia (red arrow) suggesting atrophic non-union (**b**)

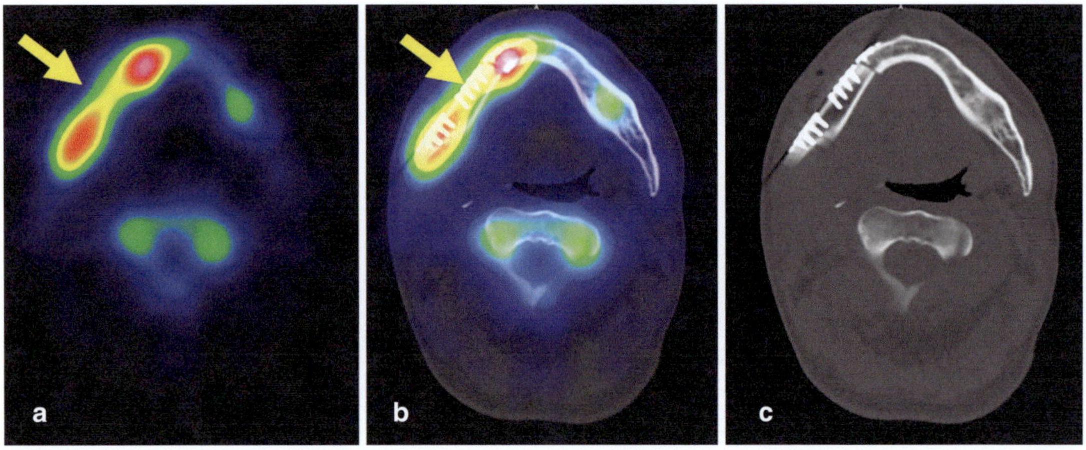

Fig. 6.6 A 65-year-old man with viable bone graft in the right side of mandible. SPECT (**a**), SPECT/CT (**b**), and CT (**c**) demonstrate increased tracer uptake (yellow arrow) suggesting viability of the bone graft of mandible

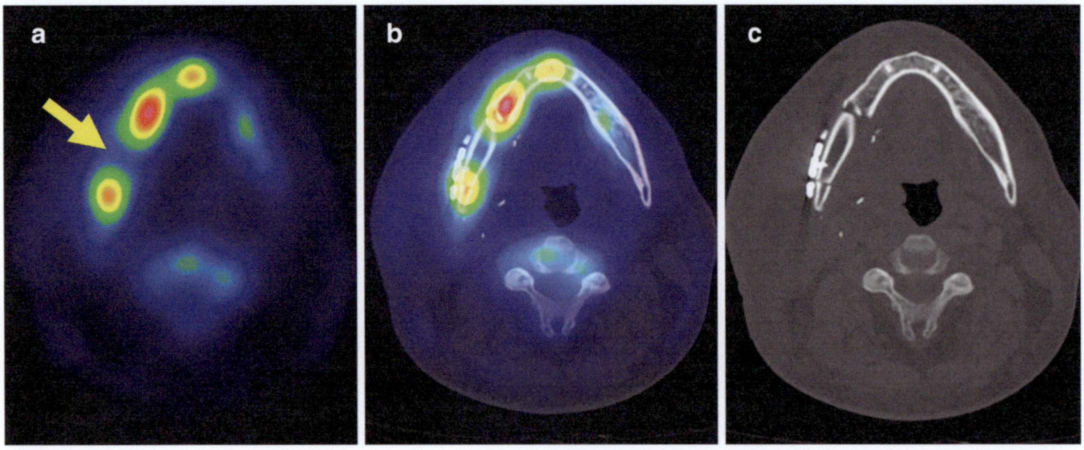

Fig. 6.7 A 55-year-old man with non-viable bone graft in the right side of mandible. SPECT (**a**), SPECT/CT (**b**), and CT (**c**) demonstrate cold defect (yellow arrow) suggesting non-viability of the bone graft of mandible

Teaching Points

- Bone scan is a highly sensitive tool for the diagnosis of fracture and can be helpful to demonstrate missed fracture which cannot be observed radiographically. Bone scan also can play an important role in the confirmation of suspected child abuse and in patients with brain injury.
- According to the fracture sites, the length of time of increased uptake is variable. Bone scan can provide information about the relative fracture age between old and acute fractures.
- There is a false-positive factor. It is immobilization and the resulting osteoporosis of disuse after fracture. False-negative finding in bone scans can result from a too-short time interval between the trauma and obtaining of a bone scan. Old and healed fractures also definitely show no increased tracer uptake.
- Bone scan has been used to provide information about the biological activity of the fracture site in treatment planning of fracture non-union.
- Bone scan can offer method for the assessment of the graft's physiologic status and viability. Superiority of SPECT or SPECT/CT providing three-dimensional information has been demonstrated to improve interpretation of the viability of bone grafts.

References

1. Cunningham BP, Brazina S, Morshed S, Miclau T. Fracture healing: a review of clinical, imaging and laboratory diagnostic options. Injury. 2017;48(Suppl 1):S69–75.
2. Seo Y, Whang K, Pyen J, Choi J, Kim J, et al. Missed skeletal trauma detected by whole body bone scan in patients with traumatic brain injury. J Korean Neurosurg Soc. 2020;63:649–56.
3. Krumme JW, Lauer MF, Stowell JT, Beteselassie NM, Kotwal SY. Bone scintigraphy: a review of technical aspects and applications in orthopedic surgery. Orthopedics. 2019;42:e14–24.
4. Brinker MR. Nonunions: evaluation and treatment. In: Trafton PG, editor. Skeletal trauma: basic science, management, and reconstruction. 3rd ed. Philadelphia: WB Saunders; 2003. p. 507–604.
5. Kim H, Lee K, Ha S, Shin E, Ahn K-M, Lee J-H, et al. Predicting vascularized bone graft viability using 1-week postoperative bone SPECT/CT after maxillofacial reconstructive surgery. Nucl Med Mol Imaging. 2020;54:292–8.

7 Stress Fractures and Sports Injury

Su Jin Lee

Abstract

Stress fractures, which appear as fatigue or insufficiency fractures, are common in athletes, military recruits, and the elderly population. Fatigue fractures usually occur in the lower extremities, while insufficiency fractures commonly involve the spine, pelvis, and ribs. If stress fractures are suspected, plain radiography should be the first test performed. However, a bone scan is much more sensitive than radiography for diagnosing stress fractures; therefore, if the plain radiograph shows no findings, or if an urgent diagnosis is needed, a bone scan can be useful. Application of single-photon emission computed tomography/computed tomography on bone scan is very useful in suspected fractures of the ankle, feet, and spine. This chapter briefly summarizes the pathophysiology of stress fractures and presents typical cases of stress fractures affecting various locations.

Keywords

Bone scan · Fatigue fracture · Insufficiency fracture · Stress fracture

S. J. Lee (✉)
Department of Nuclear Medicine, Ajou University School of Medicine, Suwon, Republic of Korea
e-mail: suesj202@ajou.ac.kr

7.1 Etiology and Pathophysiology

Stress fractures are caused by repetitive stress. When this occurs in a normal bone, the resulting fracture is called a fatigue fracture; however, when it occurs in an abnormal bone, such as a bone with osteoporosis, it is called an insufficiency fracture [1]. Fatigue fractures are common in athletes, military recruits, and dancers, with most cases affecting the lower extremities [2]. Insufficiency fractures are common in the elderly population and affect the spine, pelvis, and ribs, usually as a result of minor trauma or unnoticed trauma.

Stress fractures may occur as a result of repetitive or prolonged muscle action on a bone that has not adapted to the applied stress [3]. Repetitive stress may cause periosteal resorption that outperforms the rate of remodeling, weakening the cortex and leading to fractures. Histopathological studies have shown that stress fractures are linear regions of increased bone turnover. The initial change in the evolution of a stress fracture is the appearance of large resorption cavities. Next, a coupled osteoblastic response displaces some of the resorbed bone; however, the pace of bone formation cannot keep up with the resorption rate. A bone scan shows a very distinct line of this increased uptake attributable to the osteoblastic activity [4].

S.-O. Yang et al. (eds.), *Atlas of Nuclear Medicine in Musculoskeletal System*,
https://doi.org/10.1007/978-981-19-2677-8_7

7.2 Diagnosis

Patients with stress fractures will commonly complain of pain with ambulation [5]. Pain can manifest differently depending on the location of the fracture, such as groin pain with pelvic fracture, hip pain with femoral neck injury, and knee pain with proximal tibial injury [6].

Bone scans play an important role in the diagnosis of stress fractures because conventional radiographs require additional time to confirm fractures; bone scans may appear abnormal 6 weeks prior to the appearance of existing radiological changes [7]. Recently, the application of single-photon emission computed tomography/computed tomography (SPECT/CT) on bone scan has been very useful in the diagnosis of suspected fractures of the ankle, feet, and spine [8]. Magnetic resonance imaging (MRI) is also useful for diagnosing stress fractures because it has similar or slightly better sensitivity than bone scans, with a higher specificity [9, 10].

7.3 Bone Scan Findings of Specific Stress Fractures

7.3.1 Stress Fractures of the Tibia

The tibia is the most common site of stress fractures [11]. Most tibial stress fractures occur in the proximal or middle third of the bone and are either horizontal or oblique. Rarely, stress fractures at the distal third of the tibia have been reported in long-distance runners. Differentiating shin splints from stress fractures is important because the management of each is different. An untreated stress fracture can lead to a complete fracture, usually complicated by nonunion. A three-phase bone scan is a sensitive imaging modality for the diagnosis of tibial stress fractures and shin splints. Typical patterns of shin splints in three-phase bone scans are normal blood flow and blood pool and longitudinal increased uptake along the diaphysis commonly involving the posteromedial and anterolateral aspect of the tibial cortex. While a stress fracture in the acute stage showed focally increased blood flow, blood pool, and bone uptake, a stress fracture in the later stage may only show increased bone uptake on delayed phase.

Case 7.1

A 19-year-old male soldier complained of left lower leg pain for 6 weeks. The pain worsened with running. Whole-body bone scan (Fig. 7.1a) and regional medial view of both lower legs (Fig. 7.1b) showed focal increased uptake suggesting stress fractures in the proximal shaft of both tibiae. The pain was in the left lower leg; however, bone scan demonstrated stress fractures in both tibiae.

Case 7.2

A 20-year-old female soldier complained of right lower leg pain. Prolonged standing, running, and going uphill caused sharp pain. She underwent three-phase bone scan. There was no significant uptake at blood flow (not shown) and blood pool phase (Fig. 7.2a), but focal uptake was noted in the mid shaft of the right tibia at delayed phase image (Fig. 7.2b).

Case 7.3

A 26-year-old female soldier complained of chronic lower leg pain, especially in the mid tibia area. She regularly ran up to 6 miles at a time. A three-phase bone scan showed no significant increases in blood flow (not shown) and blood pool (Fig. 7.3a); however, it showed increased bone uptake suggesting stress fractures in both tibiae (Fig. 7.3b).

Case 7.4

A 37-year-old female patient complained of pain in both lower legs worsening with running. A three-phase bone scan demonstrated a linear pattern of increased uptake along the posteromedial part of both the tibiae on delayed phase only (Fig. 7.4b), with no alteration in blood pool (Fig. 7.4a). These findings are consistent with shin splints.

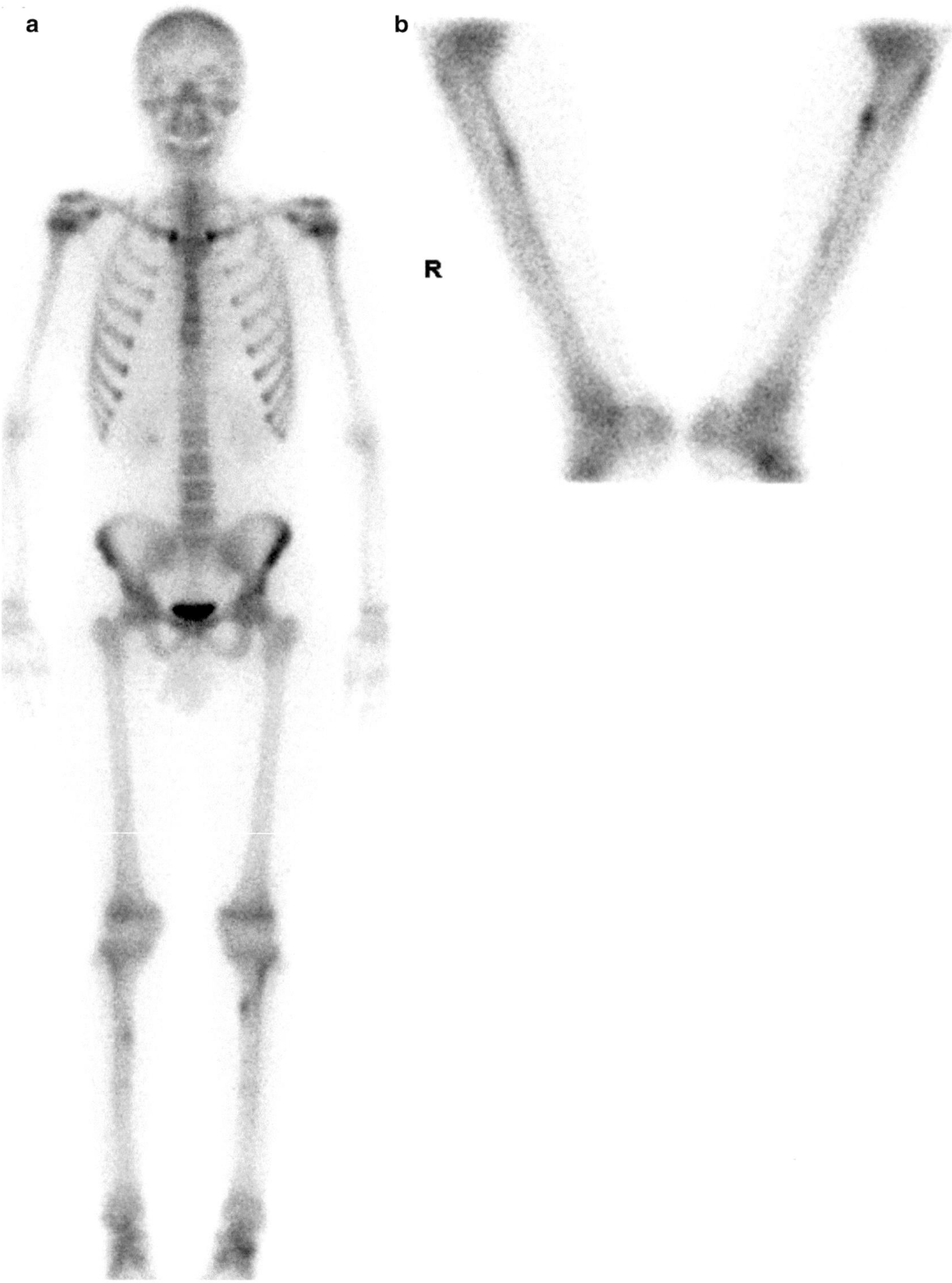

Fig. 7.1 Anterior view of whole-body bone scan (**a**) and regional medial view of both lower legs (**b**) in a 19-year-old male soldier show focal increased uptakes suggesting stress fractures in the proximal shaft of both tibiae

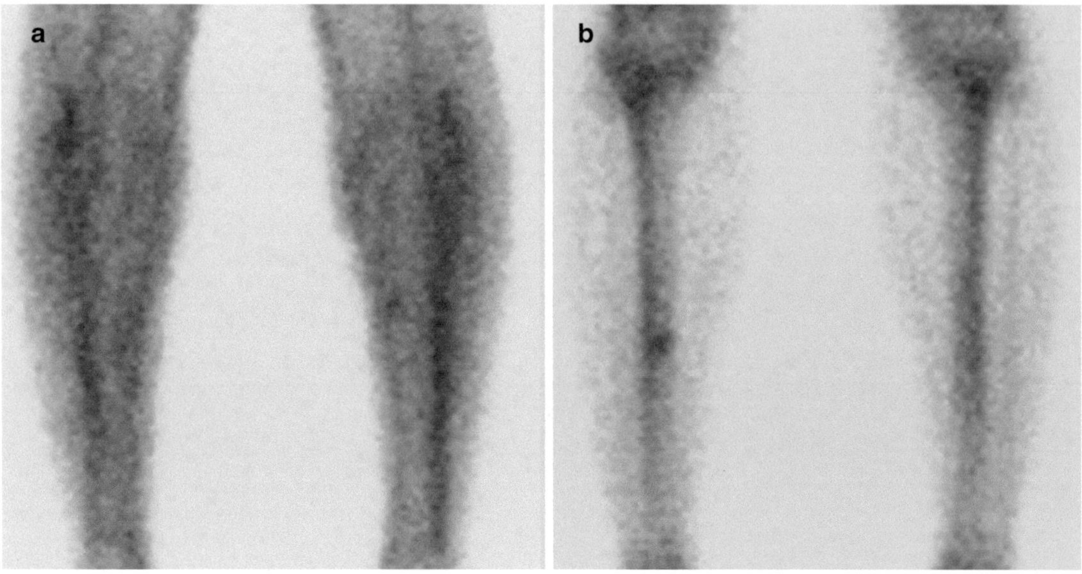

Fig. 7.2 Anterior regional blood pool and bone phase images of both lower legs in a 20-year-old female soldier. There is no significant uptake at blood pool phase (**a**), but focal uptake suggesting stress fractures is noted in the mid shaft of the right tibia at delayed phase (**b**)

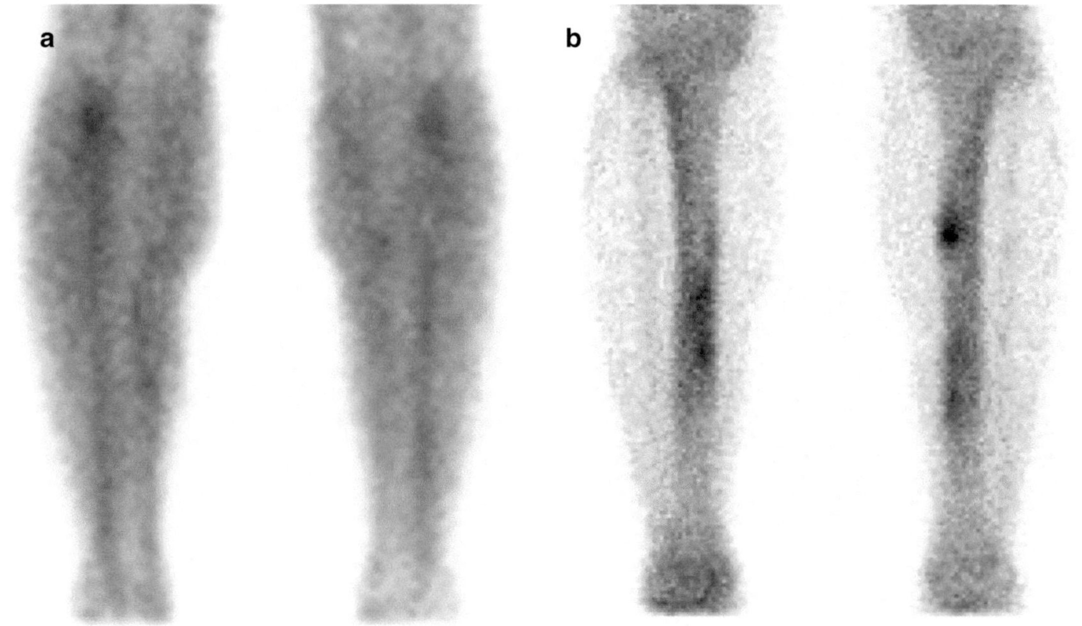

Fig. 7.3 Anterior regional blood pool and bone phase images of both lower legs in a 26-year-old female soldier. There is no significant uptake at blood pool phase (**a**), but focal uptakes are noted in the mid shaft of both tibiae at delayed bone phase (**b**)

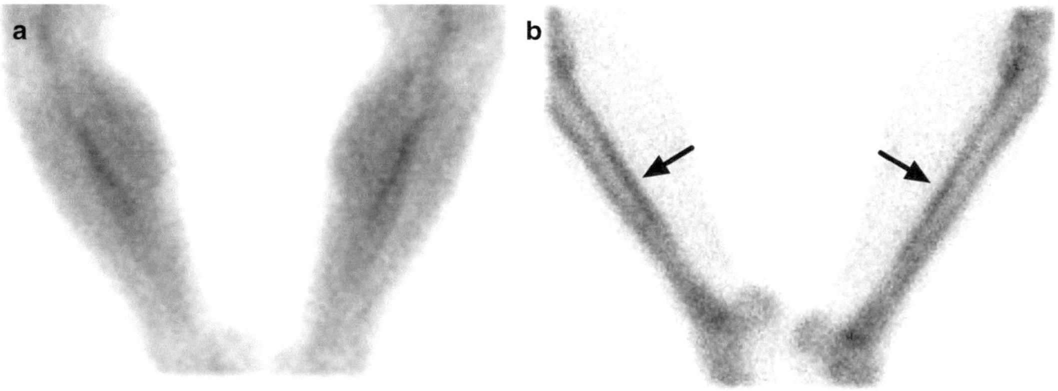

Fig. 7.4 Medial view regional blood pool (**a**) and bone phase (**b**) images of both lower legs showing shin splints. A three-phase bone scan demonstrates a linear pattern of increased uptake along the posteromedial part of both the tibiae on delayed phase only (**b**, arrow)

7.3.2 Stress Fractures of the Foot and Ankle

The majority of fibular stress fractures occur in the distal third portion of the bone; fractures in the proximal and middle thirds of the fibula are rare. The main sport involved in fibular stress fractures is running and jumping-related activities.

Metatarsal stress fractures may be the most common form of stress injury in the foot and ankle. These injuries mainly occur in athletes who participate in high-intensity sports, including running and jumping. These fractures primarily occur in the second and third metatarsal bones.

Case 7.5

A 21-year-old male soldier complained of left distal lower leg pain. The pain worsened with any impact activities including walking. A three-phase bone scan showed focally increased blood flow (not shown), blood pool (Fig. 7.5a), and bone uptake (Fig. 7.5b) in the left distal fibula.

Case 7.6

A 29-year-old female patient underwent right ankle reconstruction surgery about 1 year ago. She complained of acute worsening pain over the third metatarsal area. A bone scan revealed focal increased uptake suggesting fatigue fracture on the third metatarsal bone (Fig. 7.6a). A sagittal MRI scan (Fig. 7.6b) showed the fracture and bone marrow edema at the third metatarsal bone.

7.3.3 Stress Fractures of the Femur

The three femoral regions that are primarily prone to stress fractures are the neck, medial proximal shaft, and distal shaft [12]. Fractures may be fatigue fractures, which occur in athletes, or insufficiency fractures, which occur especially in the elderly population. Atypical femoral fractures (AFFs), also known as bisphosphonate-related proximal femoral fractures, are an example of insufficiency fractures [13].

Case 7.7

An 89-year-old female patient with osteoporosis visited the outpatient clinic with left thigh pain. She had a medication history of bisphosphonate for 5 years due to osteoporosis. An incomplete fracture line was suspected in the mid shaft of the left femur on X-ray (Fig. 7.7a), and focal increased uptake in the same area was seen on a whole-body bone scan (Fig. 7.7b). Based on her medical history and imaging findings, AFF was suspected.

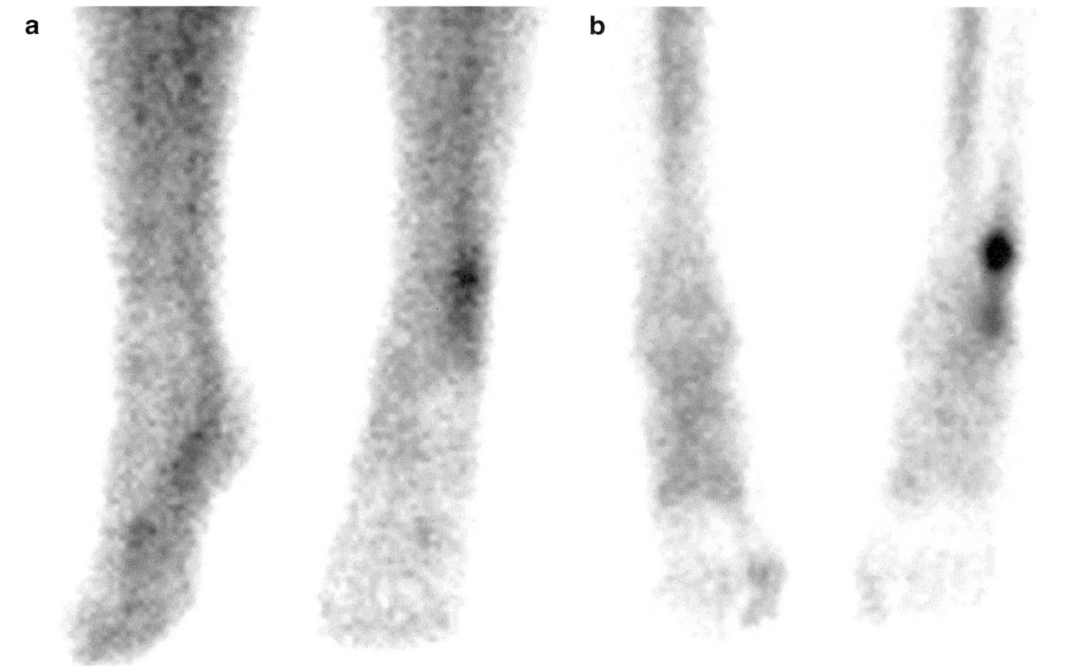

Fig. 7.5 Anterior view regional blood pool and bone phase images of both ankles in a 21-year-old male soldier with fibular stress fracture. Focally increased blood pool (**a**) and bone uptake (**b**) are noted in the left distal fibula

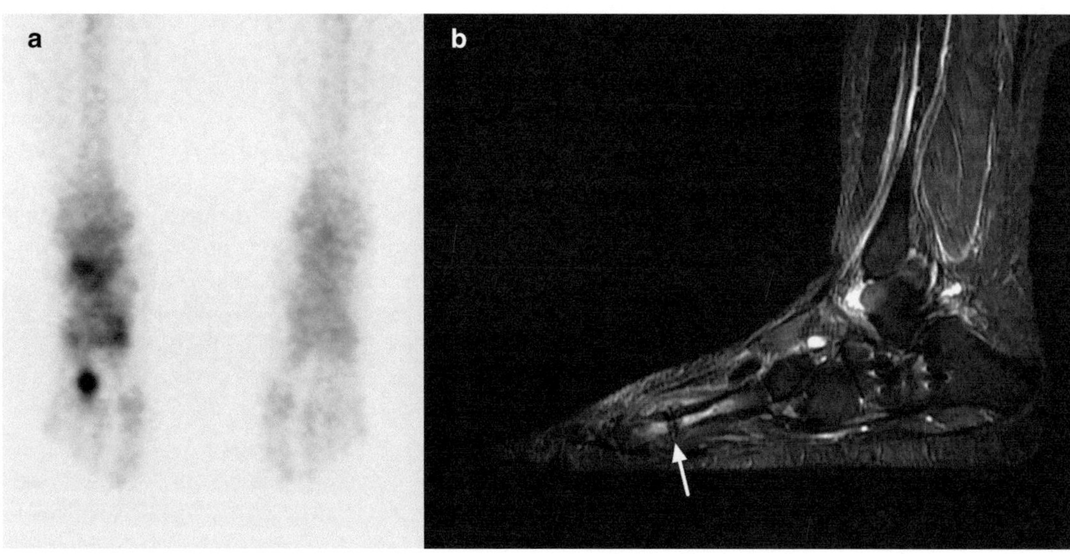

Fig. 7.6 A bone scan in a 29-year-old female patient shows focal increased uptake on the third metatarsal bone (**a**), and sagittal MRI scan (**b**) shows the fracture and bone marrow edema at the same bone

7.3.4 Stress Fractures of the Pelvis

Sacral stress fractures occur as fatigue fractures in young active persons and as insufficiency fractures among elderly osteoporotic patients. The typical patterns of bone scans are an H-shaped uptake (Honda sign) and its variants: unilateral vertical uptake, horizontal uptake, half H-shaped

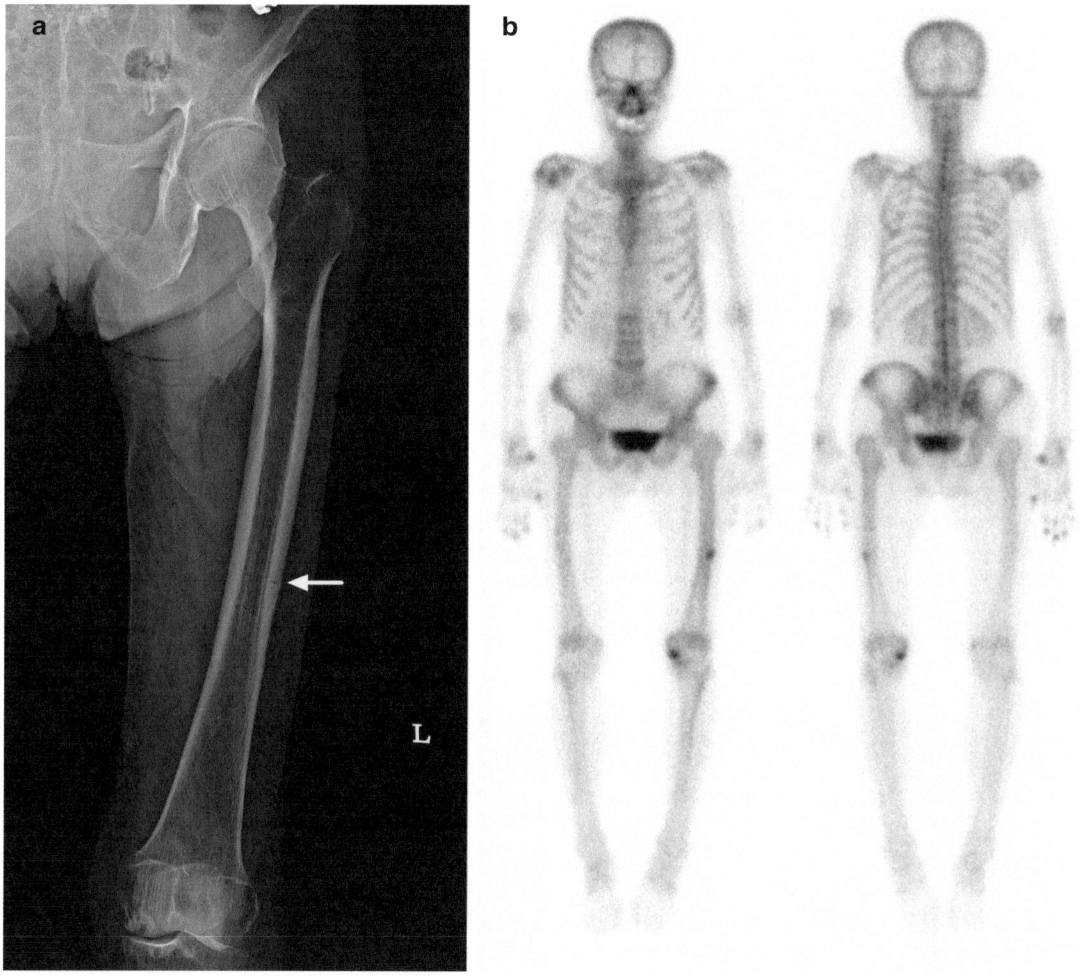

Fig. 7.7 An 89-year-old female patient with osteoporosis. An incomplete fracture line is suspected in the mid shaft of the left femur on X-ray (**a**, arrow), and focal increased uptake in the same area is seen on a whole-body bone scan (**b**)

uptake, and bilateral vertical uptake [1]. Pelvic insufficiency fractures usually occur in the sacroiliac joint and in the pubis.

Case 7.8

A 64-year-old female with osteoporosis complained of lower back pain. She had no trauma history. Increased uptake along the bilateral ala was noted on the posterior image of her bone scan (Fig. 7.8a). Another 80-year-old male complained of buttock pain and difficulty walking after hitting the buttock. Intense uptake was demonstrated in the right sacral ala, mid sacrum, left ilium, and left superior and inferior pubic rami on his bone scan (Fig. 7.8b).

Case 7.9

An 82-year-old female patient visited the outpatient clinic because she had difficulty walking after falling out of bed. No significant abnormalities were found on her pelvic X-ray. Whole-body bone scan and pelvis SPECT/CT revealed focal uptake in the left superior and inferior pubic rami (Fig. 7.9a–c). Whole-body bone scan additionally showed the insufficiency fracture at the right sixth rib (Fig. 7.9a). After a bone scan, a bone mineral density test was performed, and she was diagnosed with osteoporosis.

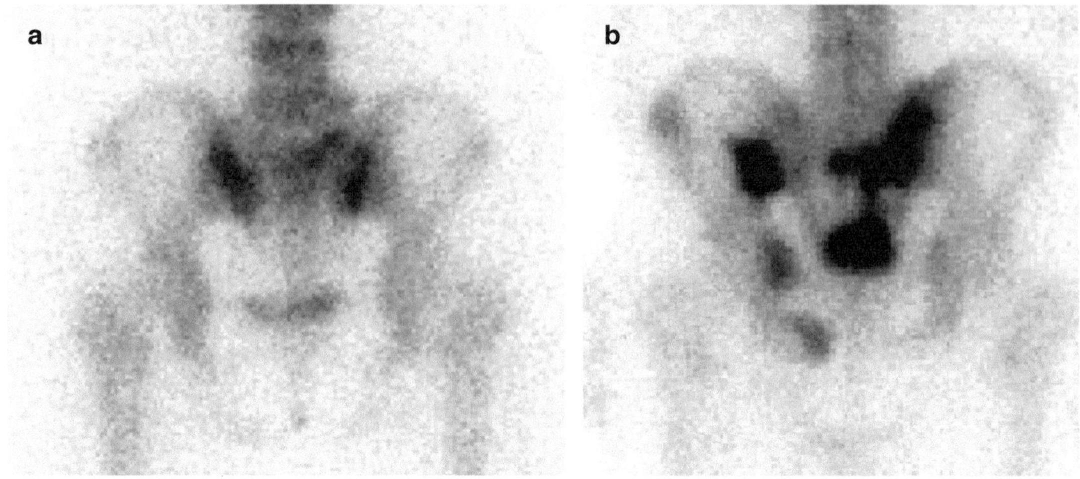

Fig. 7.8 Increased uptake along the bilateral sacral ala (bilateral vertical uptake variant of Honda sign) is noted on the posterior image of bone scan in a 64-year-old woman with osteoporosis (**a**). Intense uptake is demonstrated in the right sacral ala and mid sacrum (half H-shaped uptake variant) on the posterior image of bone scan in an 80-year-old man (**b**). Other uptakes suggesting insufficiency fractures are also noted in the left ilium and left superior and inferior pubic rami

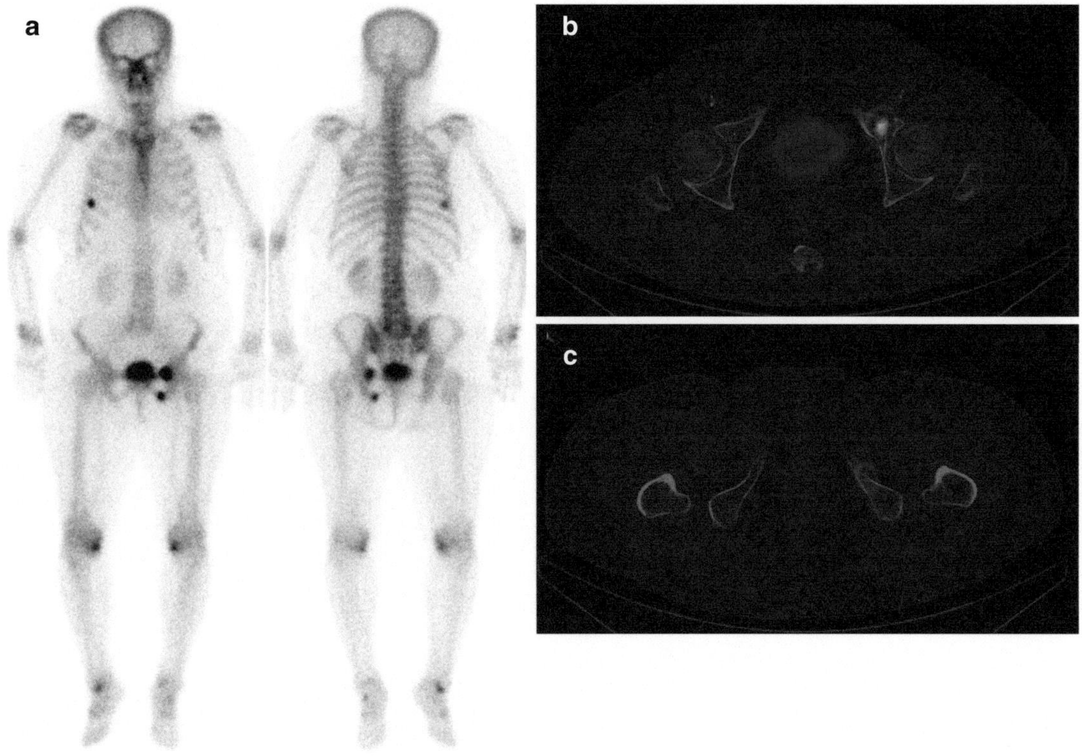

Fig. 7.9 Whole-body bone scan (**a**) and pelvis SPECT/CT (**b** and **c**) in an 82-year-old woman reveal focal uptakes in the left superior and inferior pubic rami. Whole-body bone scan additionally shows the insufficiency fracture at the right sixth rib

Teaching Points

- Stress fractures are common in athletes, military recruits, and the elderly population; fatigue fractures usually occur in the lower extremities, while insufficiency fractures commonly involve the spine, pelvis, and ribs.
- Bone scans play an important role in the diagnosis of stress fractures because conventional radiographs require additional time to confirm fractures.
- Recently, the application of SPECT/CT on bone scan has been very useful in the diagnosis of suspected fractures of the ankle, feet, and spine.

References

1. Elgazzar AH. Diagnosis of traumatic disorders. Orthopedic nuclear medicine. Springer; 2017. p. 147–89.
2. Liong SY, Whitehouse RW. Lower extremity and pelvic stress fractures in athletes. Br J Radiol. 2012;85:1148–56.
3. Daffner RH, Pavlov H. Stress fractures: current concepts. AJR Am J Roentgenol. 1992;159:245–52.
4. McCarthy EF. Histopathologic correlates of a positive bone scan. Semin Nucl Med. 1997;27:309–20.
5. Fredericson M, Bergman AG, Hoffman KL, Dillingham MS. Tibial stress reaction in runners. Correlation of clinical symptoms and scintigraphy with a new magnetic resonance imaging grading system. Am J Sports Med. 1995;23:472–81.
6. Niva MH, Mattila VM, Kiuru MJ, Pihlajamaki HK. Bone stress injuries are common in female military trainees: a preliminary study. Clin Orthop Relat Res. 2009;467:2962–9.
7. Norfray JF, Schlachter L, Kernahan WT Jr, Arenson DJ, Smith SD, Roth IE, et al. Early confirmation of stress fractures in joggers. JAMA. 1980;243:1647–9.
8. Scharf SC. Bone SPECT/CT in skeletal trauma. Semin Nucl Med. 2015;45:47–57.
9. Ishibashi Y, Okamura Y, Otsuka H, Nishizawa K, Sasaki T, Toh S. Comparison of scintigraphy and magnetic resonance imaging for stress injuries of bone. Clin J Sport Med. 2002;12:79–84.
10. Patel DS, Roth M, Kapil N. Stress fractures: diagnosis, treatment, and prevention. Am Fam Physician. 2011;83:39–46.
11. Gallo RA, Plakke M, Silvis ML. Common leg injuries of long-distance runners: anatomical and biomechanical approach. Sports Health. 2012;4:485–95.
12. Edwards WB, Gillette JC, Thomas JM, Derrick TR. Internal femoral forces and moments during running: implications for stress fracture development. Clin Biomech (Bristol, Avon). 2008;23:1269–78.
13. Toro G, Ojeda-Thies C, Calabro G, Toro G, Moretti A, Guerra GM, et al. Management of atypical femoral fracture: a scoping review and comprehensive algorithm. BMC Musculoskelet Disord. 2016;17:227.

Osteonecrosis

8

So Won Oh, Jee Won Chai, and Jung Mi Park

Abstract

Osteonecrosis is characterized by the death of cellular components of the bone that results from an interruption of the subchondral blood supply. Bone infarction and avascular necrosis are terms that may be used interchangeably. The risk factors of osteonecrosis are generally multifactorial, such as serious trauma, steroid medication, and alcohol consumption, but the etiology and pathogenesis remain unclear. The common sites for osteonecrosis are the femoral head, knee, talus, and humeral head. Osteonecrosis may lead to subchondral collapse, which threatens the viability of the involved joint. Therefore, early diagnosis is essential since it allows for the treatment of osteonecrosis and potentially improves the outcome.

Initial evaluation is conducted by plain radiographs demonstrating minimal osteopenia followed by variable changes, but it often appears normal in the early stages of the disease. In this regard, bone scintigraphy and MRI are preferred for the diagnosis of osteonecrosis at an earlier stage. MRI is the most sensitive diagnostic modality based on the high spatial resolution for the soft tissue as well as bone, and bone scintigraphy is quite sensitive and advantageous, allowing evaluation of multiple sites of the body. It is expected that bone SPECT/CT can improve the diagnostic accuracy of the evaluation of osteonecrosis, using the functional information of the SPECT images combined with the exact localization information of the CT images.

Keywords

Osteonecrosis · Bone scintigraphy · Bone SPECT/CT

8.1 Osteonecrosis of the Hip

8.1.1 Etiology and Clinical Significance

Avascular necrosis of femoral head (ANFH) is the bone death that results from the interruption of blood supply, mostly affecting the middle-aged male population. ANFH falls into two classes: traumatic or non-traumatic. Non-traumatic ANFH is associated with use of alco-

S. W. Oh (✉)
Department of Nuclear Medicine, Seoul National University Boramae Medical Center, Seoul, Republic of Korea

J. W. Chai
Department of Radiology, Seoul National University Boramae Medical Center, Seoul, Republic of Korea

J. M. Park
Department of Nuclear Medicine, Soonchunhyang University Hospital, Bucheon, Republic of Korea

S.-O. Yang et al. (eds.), *Atlas of Nuclear Medicine in Musculoskeletal System*,
https://doi.org/10.1007/978-981-19-2677-8_8

hol, glucocorticoids, and presence of hematologic disorders or metabolic disorders, but its etiology is unclear in about 30% of patients [1]. Idiopathic ANFH in the pediatric population is also known as Legg-Calve-Perthes (LCP) disease. The pathologic changes are equivalent to both ANFH in adults and pediatric LCP disease, except cortical maturity.

8.1.2 Imaging Findings

Diagnosis is normally made by images obtained through a non-invasive method, either with radiographs or MRI. When the disease begins, it may be undetectable on plain radiographs. However, early ANFH shows cystic and/or sclerotic changes in the femoral head followed by the crescent sign with disease progression. The crescent sign describes an area of subchondral radiolucency in the femoral head that indicates subchondral fracture due to bone necrosis and subsequent attempts at repair. ANFH at a later stage shows femoral head flattening, collapse, and degenerative changes. MRI is the modality of choice for patients with a suspicious history and physical examination with normal radiographs. Early ANFH usually presents as an area of low signal intensity (SI) on T1-weighted MR image and as a high SI on T2-weighted MR image.

Bone scintigraphy pattern depends on the pathophysiological stage of osteonecrosis, as osteonecrosis is an evolving process. Osteonecrosis initially appears as a photopenic area on the bone scintigraphy, and then increased radiotracer uptake is seen at the boundaries between the osteonecrotic site and the normal tissues due to osteoblastic activity. Increased radiotracer uptake starts to appear when bone collapse happens, and periarticular uptake is seen in both sides of the hip joints in advanced degenerative arthritic stage. However, diagnostic specificity of bone scintigraphy is low, and sensitivity of bone scintigraphy is variable according to the stage and etiology of osteonecrosis. Although MRI is the diagnosis of choice for osteonecrosis, bone scintigraphy has several roles in the management of ANFH. Bone scintigraphy may be helpful to provide information on viability, and it could be used in the evaluation of the fractured femoral neck with a metallic device. Recently, SPECT/CT is expected to enhance diagnostic performances by visualization of a central cold defect with/without surrounding increased uptake in the femoral head that is often masked by the adjacent normal bone in the early phase of osteonecrosis.

Case 8.1

A 52-year-old man was admitted to the orthopedic clinic for the treatment of right hip pain that had been recently aggravated. He used to stand all day because of his job, but he denied previous trauma history and substance abuse including alcohol. Except for antihypertensive medication, he had no history of treatment for chronic diseases such as diabetes or hepatitis. Imaging studies were performed, including plain radiography, hip MRI, and bone scintigraphy, and avascular necrosis (AVN) was demonstrated in the bilateral femoral heads (Fig. 8.1). Multiple drilling was undertaken for the treatment of the right ANFH, and close observation was chosen for the treatment of the left ANFH.

Case 8.2

A 41-year-old man visited the orthopedic clinic due to left inguinal area pain that had worsened 1 month previously. He denied a history of trauma and chronic diseases, including diabetes, hypertension, and chronic hepatitis. He was a chronic alcoholic who had drunk 1 or 2 bottles of Korean distilled spirits 4 or 5 days per week for 10 years. Imaging studies demonstrated AVN of the left hip (Fig. 8.2). He was admitted to the hospital for total hip replacement arthroplasty.

8.2 Osteonecrosis of Knee

8.2.1 Etiology and Clinical Significance

Osteonecrosis of the knee can occur in the epiphyseal or subarticular bone, often in the form of AVN. The literature on osteonecrosis of femoral condyles is often mixed with and sometimes dedicated entirely to spontaneous osteonecrosis of the knee (SONK). SONK was previously considered an idiopathic ischemic

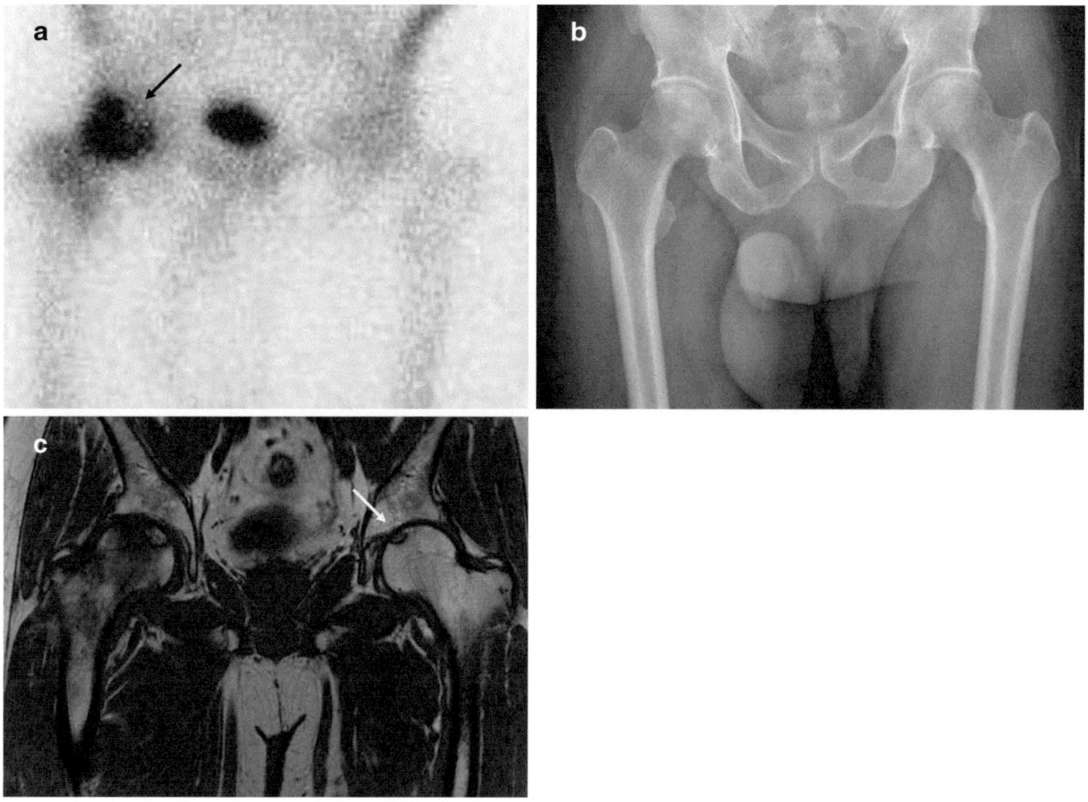

Fig. 8.1 Bone scintigraphy shows a small photopenic area (black arrow) that is surrounded by diffusely increased uptake in the right femoral head (**a**). Radiograph of the pelvis shows ill-defined sclerotic lesion in the right femoral head (**b**). MRI demonstrates a diffusely increased SI in the right femoral head, as well as a small lesion in the left femoral head (white arrow) (**c**). In contrast to the right femoral head lesion, the small left femoral lesion that is centrally located is easily missed by scintigraphy or plain radiograph

sequela that leads to the development of a crescent-shaped osteonecrosis lesion. At present, a more appropriate term for the condition is suggested since it represents a subchondral insufficiency fracture of the knee (SIFK) that progresses to subchondral collapse with secondary osteonecrosis [2]. By contrast, primary AVN results from a reduction of the blood supply, and its clinical significance is different from SONK. Moreover, MRI features of these two lesions have been shown to be profoundly different from each other. Primary AVN of the knee is known to share the established features of AVN of other sites, but SONK is associated with marked bone marrow edema emanating from the subchondral region and extending over large areas [2].

SIFK is seen more frequently in women, and up to 94% of cases affect the medial femoral condyle (MFC) [3]. Patients with SIFK complain of knee pain that typically gets worse at night and on weight bearing, and the onset is usually acute without prior trauma, mostly unilateral. Due to its similarity with clinical symptoms, SIFK is often mistakenly identified as a medial meniscus tear. The natural course of SIFK varies from complete recovery to total joint collapse, in cases where the biomechanics of the knee joint is altered due to structural changes, and joint destruction may eventually occur.

8.2.2 Imaging

Typical radiographic findings, including flattening of the MFC, subchondral bony radiolucency, and complicating subchondral fracture, become overt in advanced stages, although

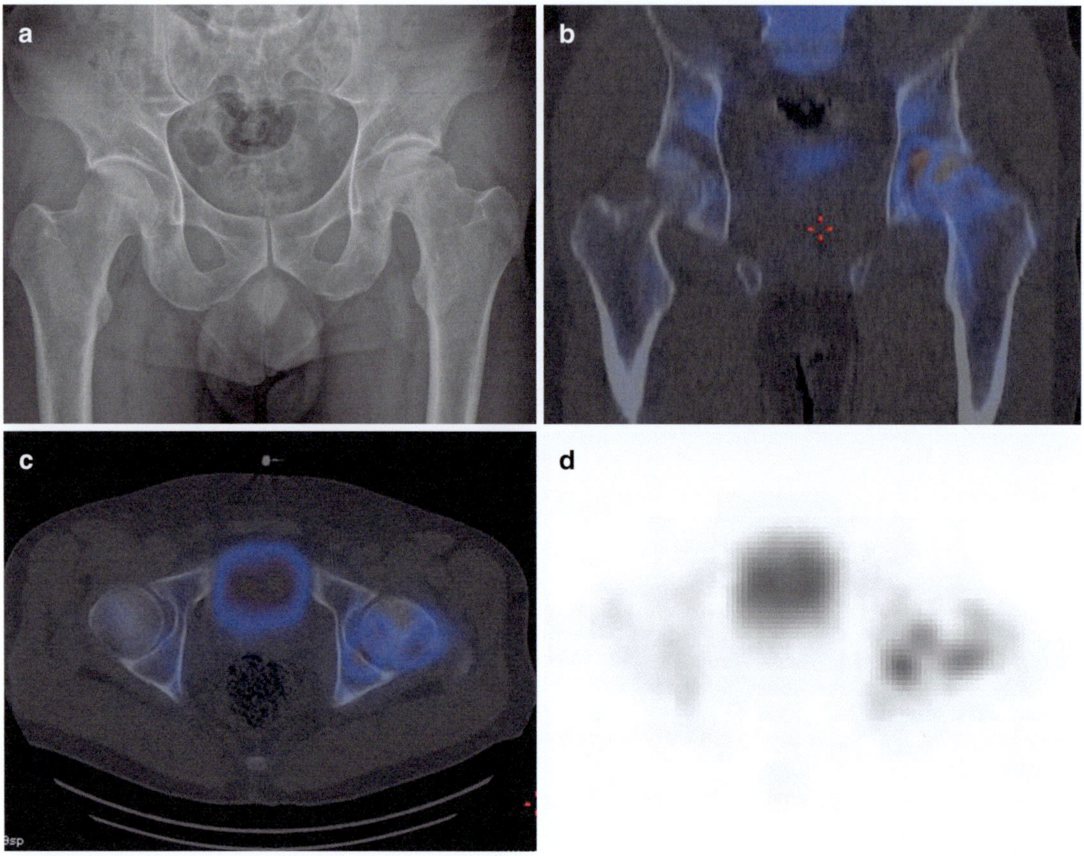

Fig. 8.2 Radiograph of the pelvis shows a sclerotic lesion in the left femoral head with articular surface collapse (**a**). Bone SPECT/CT demonstrates a photopenic area in the left femoral head superolateral aspect that is surrounded by irregularly increased uptake (**b**–**d**)

they are often negative in the early stages. MRI findings can vary according to stage, and it is important to determine the extent of the disease for advanced stages. SIFK is associated with marked bone marrow edema emanating from the subchondral region and extending over large areas, often involving the entire femoral condyle. This differs from the more localized bone marrow edema lesion subjacent to cartilage loss in osteoarthritis. In general, osteonecrosis is seen as a sharply demarcated photon defect that is surrounded by intense uptake in the reparative and reactive zone in bone scintigraphy. SIFK usually shows a focally increased uptake, which the likely pathogenesis of microfracture that is related with vascular disruption might be reflected by bone scintigraphy. In this regard, bone scintigraphy is a more sensitive modality and helpful in early detection of SIFK.

Case 8.3

A 63-year-old man was managed for sudden onset of left knee pain that developed 2 months ago. Knee MRI was taken because his knee pain persisted for 9 months. MRI showed middle and posterior one-third large bone marrow edema in the left MFC with focal subcortical fracture. Bone scintigraphy showed focal intense increased uptake in the left MFC. Knee MRI and bone scintigraphy suggest subchondral insufficiency fracture of the knee (Fig. 8.3).

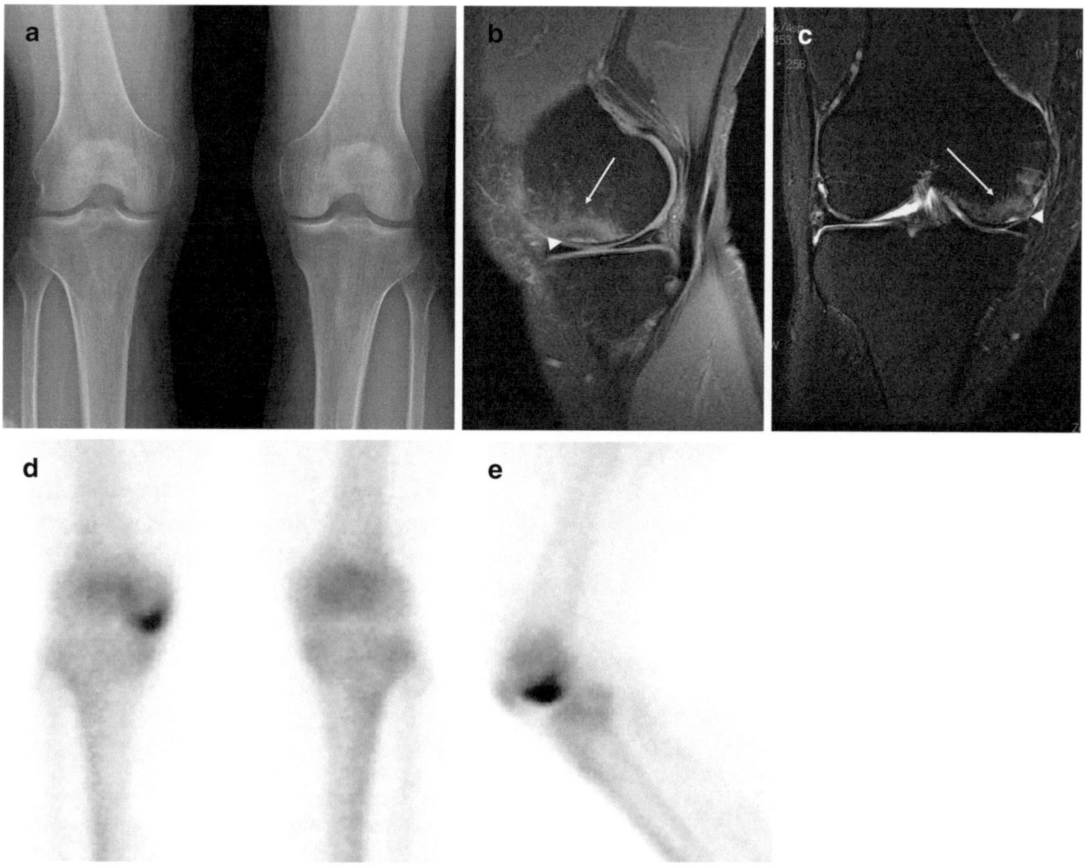

Fig. 8.3 The knee AP view shows no significant abnormality in both knees (**a**). Knee MRI demonstrates diffuse bone marrow edema: coronal and sagittal spin-echo fat-suppressed proton density images (**b**, **c**) show high SI suggesting bone marrow edema in the subchondral bone of the right MFC (arrows) and low SI linear fracture line in the trabecular cancellous bone beneath the subchondral bone plate without disruption of the articular surface (arrowheads). Bone scintigraphy shows focal increased uptake in the subchondral bone area of the right MFC (**d** anterior image of both knees, **e** medial image of the right knee)

Case 8.4

A 69-year-old woman visited to the outpatient clinic due to right knee pain that developed 6 months ago, and she denied trauma history to the knees. Physical examination revealed swelling and tenderness over the medial side of the right knee. Imaging workups including radiographs and bone SPECT/CT were performed, and it demonstrated SIFK of the right MFC associated with mild osteoarthritis of the medial tibiofibular compartment (Fig. 8.4). Based on the clinical diagnosis, medication with NSAID was chosen for the patient, instead of surgical treatment.

8.3 Osteonecrosis of the Hand and Foot

8.3.1 Etiology and Clinical Significance

Kienböck disease is known as osteonecrosis of the lunate or lunatomalacia, which can lead to progressive wrist pain and abnormal carpal motion, particularly in the dominant wrist of young male patients. The exact pathophysiology has not been fully elucidated, but it is thought to be an interplay between altered vascular perfu-

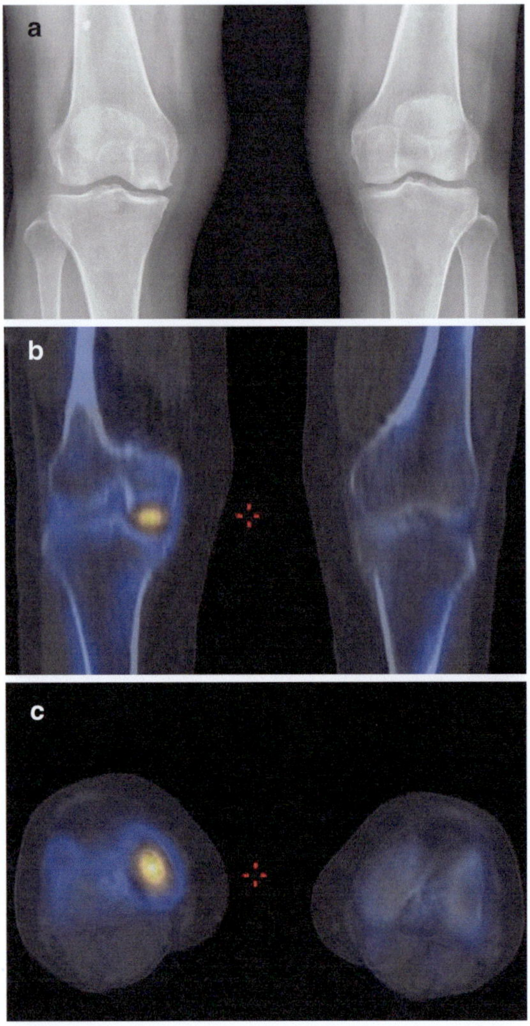

Fig. 8.4 The knee AP view demonstrates articular surface depression with a focal subchondral bony radiolucency in the right MFC accompanied by mild osteoarthritic changes in the medial tibiofemoral compartment, but there is no evidence of typical osteoarthritic changes in the contralateral knee (**a**). Bone SPECT/CT shows focally increased uptake that matched with a subchondral bony lesion in the right MFC; otherwise no significant abnormalities are observed (**b**, **c**)

sion, repetitive microtrauma, variable lunate anatomy, altered loading and kinematics, and potential systemic disease. The lunate typically has both palmar and dorsal blood supplies; 20%–26% of lunates may have a singular palmar blood supply, increasing their risk for osteonecrosis [4]. In addition, the negative ulnar variance is present as a predisposing factor in around 75% of cases of Kienböck disease.

8.3.2 Imaging

Radiographs show that osteonecrotic changes start with sclerosis of the lunate and leads to lunate collapse, fracture, scaphoid flexion, loss of carpal height, and carpal arthritis [5]. Advanced imaging, such as CT or MRI, is helpful, often resulting in upgrading to Kienböck disease, especially in patients with lunate collapse not seen on plain radiographs. Since MRI is the most sensitive tool, it may facilitate the diagnosis of osteonecrosis in patients without other radiographic changes. In the MRI, the pattern of lunate bone signal change allows the condition to be differentiated from ulnar impaction syndrome, the major differential diagnosis.

Case 8.5

An 81-year-old woman visited the outpatient clinic due to worsening left wrist pain. She had complained of left wrist pain since she had injured the left wrist a few decades before. Imaging studies, including plain radiography, MRI, and SPECT/CT, suggested osteonecrotic changes in the lunate. Kienböck disease was diagnosed based on the imaging studies (Fig. 8.5).

Case 8.6

An 83-year-old woman was taken to the emergency room after she was found collapsed in a nursing home. She presented with right wrist pain accompanied by swelling, tenderness, and bruising. Radiographs showed a right distal radius fracture, and bone scintigraphy was performed to diagnose hidden fractures of the whole body. Bone scintigraphy incidentally detected a suspicious lesion in the left distal tibia, and further imaging studies including radiography and MRI followed (Fig. 8.6). Osteonecrosis of the distal tibia was diagnosed based on the imaging studies.

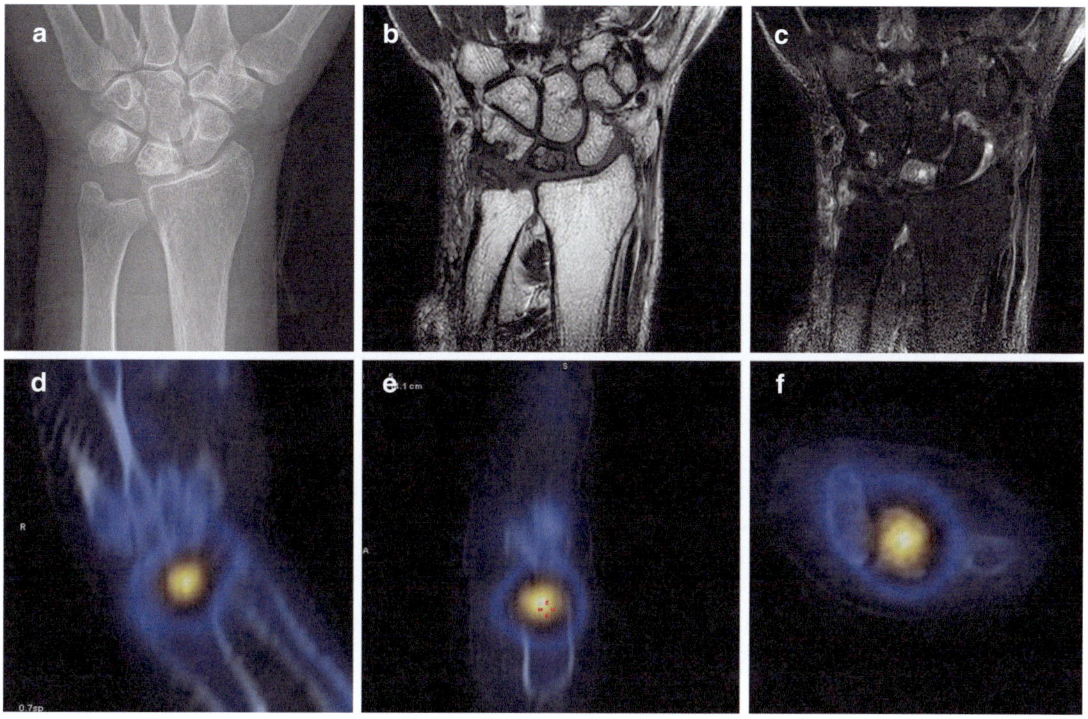

Fig. 8.5 The wrist PA view shows sclerotic changes of the lunate (**a**). MRI T1 and T2 fat-saturated images demonstrate T1 low and T2 high SI in the lunate (**b**, **c**). SPECT/CT shows focally increased uptake in the lunate (**d** coronal, **e** sagittal, **f** transverse)

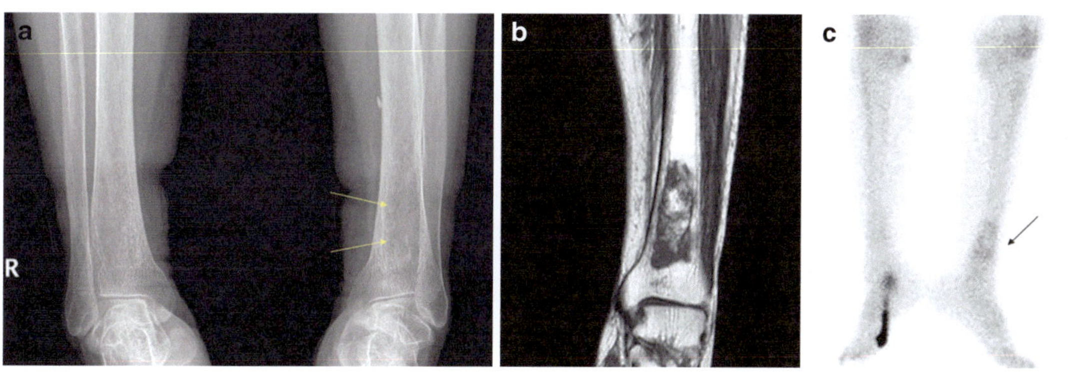

Fig. 8.6 The lower leg AP view radiograph shows an ill-defined osteolytic lesion (yellow arrows) in the left distal tibia without periosteal reaction nor cortical thickening around the lesion (**a**). MR T1 coronal image demonstrates a geographic intramedullary lesion in the left distal tibia with remaining hyperintense fat signal in the center of the lesion (**b**). Bone scintigraphy shows the oval shape of increased uptake in the left distal tibia (black arrow) and linear shape of increased uptake on the right foot indicating the radiopharmaceutical injection site (**c**)

8.4 Osteonecrosis of the Jaw

8.4.1 Etiology and Clinical Significance

Bisphosphonate-induced osteonecrosis of the jaw is a potential complication associated with long-term use of bisphosphonates, especially pamidronate and zoledronate. Medication-related osteonecrosis of the jaw (MRONJ) has become the preferred term since other medications, such as anti-resorptive and anti-angiogenic agents, have been implicated as etiologic agents. Although the etiology and pathogenesis of MRONJ remain obscure, it has been proposed that the jaw bones are highly susceptible to osteonecrosis due to certain anatomical and physiological factors [6]. Drugs are highly concentrated in the jaw because of high vascularity, and the forces of mastication and periodontal ligament around numerous teeth ensure rapid bone turnover around the periodontium, potentially inducing microfractures in MRONJ.

8.4.2 Imaging

Conventional orthopantomography provides an excellent general assessment of the entire jaw, but mineral loss must be as high as 30–50% to be visible [7]. Thus, radiographs may not visualize subtle changes in the early disease, but mottled bone similar to diffuse osteomyelitis and widening of periodontal ligament space become overt in extensive bone involvement. However, radiographic findings and clinical symptoms are often non-specific even in the full-blown stages; thus, meticulous clinical examination, including medication history, should be considered for an accurate diagnosis.

Case 8.7

A 75-year-old woman visited the dental clinic due to gingival inflammation developed 2 weeks before. She had a history of bisphosphonate medication for 5 years for the treatment of osteoporosis. Her medical history and imaging study findings strongly suggested osteonecrosis of the jaw (Fig. 8.7).

Teaching Points

- Osteonecrosis is an evolving process, and thus bone scintigraphy findings may differ by stage. Initially, osteonecrosis appears as a photopenic area and progresses to increased bony uptake at the boundaries between the osteonecrotic site and the normal tissues. As osteonecrosis leads to subchondral bone collapse, bone scintigraphy demonstrates irregularly increased uptake in the whole femoral head. Further, periarticular uptake is seen in both sides of the hip joints in advanced degenerative arthritic stage.
- Since bone SPECT/CT provides cross-sectional images combined with anatomical CT information, it is advantageous to evaluate the centrally located structure, such as the femoral head. Thus, SPECT/CT improves both sensitivity and specificity, compared to bone scintigraphy.

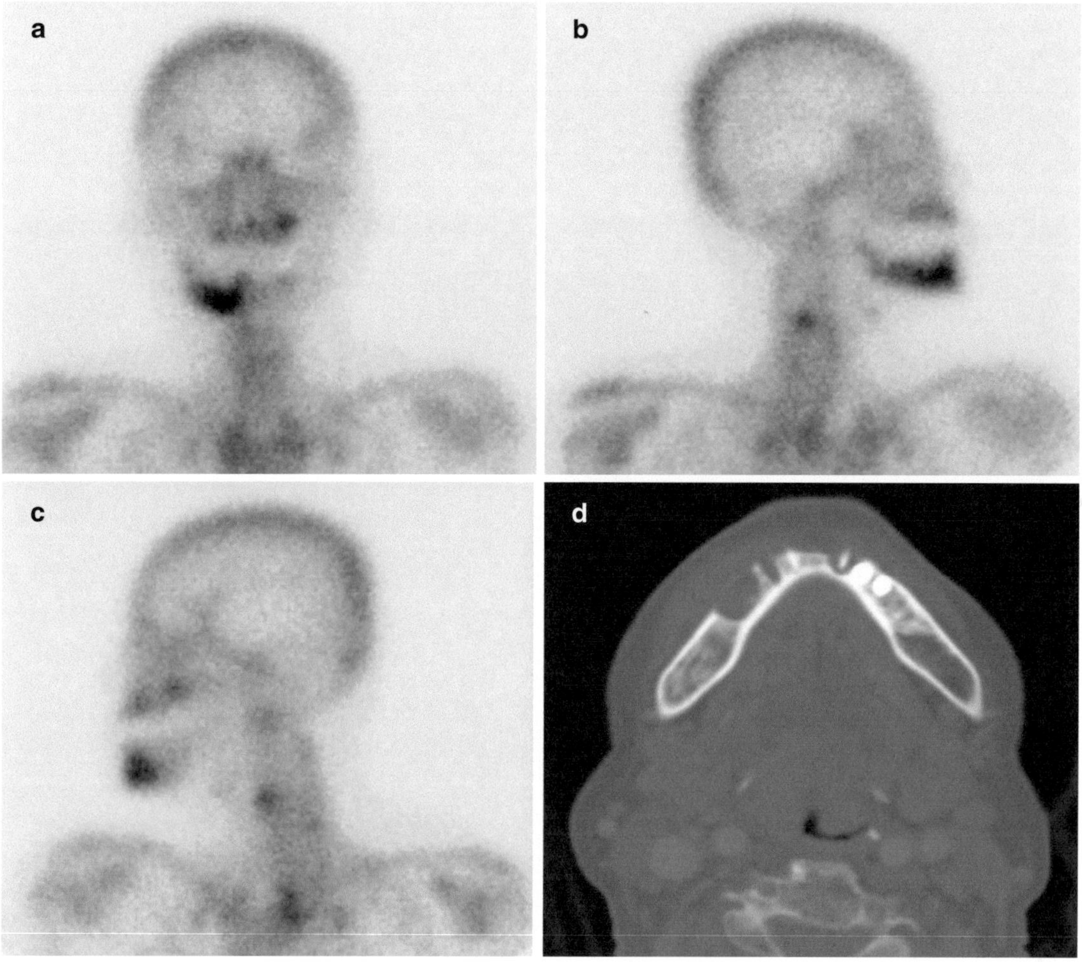

Fig. 8.7 Bone scintigraphy shows diffusely increased uptake in the right mandibular body (**a–c**). Mandible CT demonstrates irregular bony destruction in the right mandibular body with soft tissue abscess formation (**d**)

References

1. Sen RK. Management of avascular necrosis of femoral head at pre-collapse stage. Indian J Orthop. 2009;43:6–16.
2. Gorbachova T, Melenevsky Y, Cohen M, Cerniglia BW. Osteochondral lesions of the knee: differentiating the most common entities at MRI. Radiographics. 2018;38:1478–95.
3. Zaremski JL, Vincent KR. Spontaneous osteonecrosis of the knee. Curr Sports Med Rep. 2016;15:228–9.
4. Lamas C, Carrera A, Proubasta I, Llusa M, Majo J, Mir X. The anatomy and vascularity of the lunate: considerations applied to Kienbock's disease. Chir Main. 2007;26:13–20.
5. Rioux-Forker D, Shin AY. Osteonecrosis of the lunate: Kienbock disease. J Am Acad Orthop Surg. 2020;28:570–84.
6. Varun B, Sivakumar T, Nair BJ, Joseph AP. Bisphosphonate induced osteonecrosis of jaw in breast cancer patients: a systematic review. J Oral Maxillofac Pathol. 2012;16:210–4.
7. Koth VS, Figueiredo MA, Salum FG, Cherubini K. Bisphosphonate-related osteonecrosis of the jaw: from the sine qua non condition of bone exposure to a non-exposed BRONJ entity. Dentomaxillofac Radiol. 2016;45:20160049.

9 Complex Regional Pain Syndrome

Joon-Kee Yoon, Soon-Ah Park, Young Seok Cho,
Jung Mi Park, and Jang Gyu Cha

Abstract

Complex regional pain syndrome (CRPS) is a chronic pain condition caused by a variety of diseases. The pathophysiology of CRPS is uncertain, and the diagnosis depends on clinical criteria. Three-phase bone scintigraphy (TPBS) using ^{99m}Tc-diphosphonates is helpful in documenting the symptoms and signs of CRPS and in the differential diagnosis of extremity pain. The typical pattern of TPBS in patients with CRPS is diffusely increased blood flow, blood pool, and delayed periarticular bone uptake in the affected extremity. In this chapter, we introduce several cases to help understand the findings and clinical usefulness of TPBS in patients with CRPS.

Keywords

Three-phase bone scintigraphy · Complex regional pain syndrome · Reflex sympathetic dystrophy · Extremity pain

J.-K. Yoon (✉)
Department of Nuclear Medicine, Ajou University Medical Center, Suwon, Republic of Korea
e-mail: jkyoon3@ajou.ac.kr

S.-A. Park
Department of Nuclear Medicine, Wonkwang University School of Medicine, Iksan, Republic of Korea
e-mail: nmbach@wku.ac.kr

Y. S. Cho
Department of Nuclear Medicine, Samsung Medical Center, Seoul, Republic of Korea
e-mail: ysnm.cho@samsung.com

J. M. Park
Department of Nuclear Medicine, Soonchunhyang University Hospital, Bucheon, Republic of Korea
e-mail: jmipark@schmc.ac.kr

J. G. Cha
Department of Radiology, Soonchunhyang University Hospital, Bucheon, Republic of Korea
e-mail: mj4907@schmc.ac.kr

9.1 Etiology and Pathophysiology

Complex regional pain syndrome (CRPS) refers to a chronic pain condition in injured limbs that is characterized by allodynia (pain in response to a non-painful stimulus), hyperalgesia (exaggerated pain in response to a painful stimulus), color and temperature changes in the skin, swelling, autonomic dysfunction, sensory motor changes, and trophic changes. Patients may complain of movement disorders. A variety of diseases may cause CRPS: trauma, or surgery to the extremities, stroke, and myocardial infarction [1, 2].

CRPS is more common in women than in men and is more likely to occur in middle-aged people. It affects the upper extremities more frequently than the lower extremities. Manifestations of this condition in other body parts are uncommon [2, 3].

S.-O. Yang et al. (eds.), *Atlas of Nuclear Medicine in Musculoskeletal System*,
https://doi.org/10.1007/978-981-19-2677-8_9

In 1864, Silas Weir Mitchell first described the specific nature of "severe burning pain" caused by a gunshot injury. In 1946, James A. Evans termed this pain syndrome "*reflex sympathetic dystrophy (RSD)*" to elucidate the symptoms associated with the sympathetic dysfunction. Subsequently, this has also been called by various names such as "causalgia," "Sudeck's atrophy," and "shoulder-hand syndrome." The term "CRPS" was designated to describe RSD and similar disorders in a consensus meeting by the International Association for the Study of Pain (IASP) in 1994 [3–5].

CRPS is further classified into CRPS-1 and CRPS-2; CRPS-1, previously known as "RSD," is not associated with major nerve injury (nociceptive pain), whereas CRPS-2, previously known as "causalgia," is associated with peripheral nerve damage (neuropathic pain). CRPS-1 occurs more frequently than CRPS-2.

No single definite mechanism for the development of CRPS has been suggested. Proinflammatory neuropeptides released from peripheral nerve endings induce inflammatory responses at the site of tissue injury (*neuroinflammation*), which reduces the pain threshold (*nociceptive sensitization*), leading to allodynia and hyperalgesia [6]. For autonomic dysfunction in CRPS, a decrease in the circulating norepinephrine increases the peripheral catecholamine sensitivity in the affected area, which results in vasoconstriction (cool skin) and hyperhidrosis [1]. Symptoms such as motor dysfunction, neglect, and impaired recognition suggest the involvement of the central nervous system in the development of CRPS [6]. There have also been reports that autoimmune and psychological factors contribute to the development and progression of CRPS.

Table 9.1 Symptoms and signs categories in Budapest Criteria for CRPS

Symptoms categories	
Sensory	Hyperesthesia, allodynia
Vasomotor	Temperature asymmetry, skin color changes, skin color asymmetry
Sudomotor/edema	Edema, sweating changes, sweating asymmetry
Motor/trophic	Decreased range of motion, motor dysfunction (weakness, tremor, dystonia), trophic changes (hair, nail, skin)
Signs categories	
Sensory	Hyperalgesia (to pinprick), allodynia (to light touch, temperature sensation, deep somatic pressure, joint movement)
Vasomotor	Temperature asymmetry (>1 °C), skin color changes, skin color asymmetry
Sudomotor/edema	Edema, sweating changes, sweating asymmetry
Motor/trophic	Decreased range of motion, motor dysfunction (weakness, tremor, dystonia), trophic changes (hair, nail, skin)

9.2 Diagnosis

The clinical course of CRPS varies from a self-limiting, mild disease to chronic, and debilitating status. The diagnosis of CRPS depends on the clinical criteria. The IASP first developed the diagnostic criteria for CRPS in 1994, which had high sensitivity, but limited specificity. In 2003, the diagnostic criteria were redefined to improve specificity, and these are the current diagnostic standard for CRPS ("Budapest Criteria"). In the Budapest Criteria, CRPS is defined as continuing pain, which is disproportionate to any inciting event, which must report at least one symptom in three of four categories, and must display at least one sign in two of four categories (Table 9.1). CRPS is diagnosed when there is no other diagnosis that better explains the signs and symptoms [3].

In 2010, a quantitative parameter, the CRPS severity score (CSS), was also designed to assess severity and monitor the therapeutic response of CRPS. CSS is composed of 17 self-reported or observed CRPS symptoms.

9.3 Three-Phase Bone Scintigraphy in the Diagnosis of CRPS

Although there is no validated diagnostic test for CRPS, imaging tests (radiographs, bone scintigraphy, magnetic resonance imaging [MRI]), skin temperature measurement (infrared thermography, laser Doppler flowmetry), sudomotor function test, and neurophysiologic tests (electromyography, nerve conduction velocity) can help outline the symptoms and signs of CRPS [4]. Among these imaging tests, three-phase bone scintigraphy (TPBS) is the most helpful diagnostic test for CRPS. TPBS using ^{99m}Tc-labeled diphosphonates consists of blood flow, blood pool, and delayed bone phases and is widely accepted for the evaluation of soft tissue and bone infection/inflammation. Blood flow images can be acquired in a dynamic mode over the first 60 s, whereas blood pool images are obtained in a static mode immediately after the acquisition of flow images. Both images provide information regarding soft tissue hyperemia. Delayed bone images are acquired 2–4 h after the injection of a radiotracer, which reflects osteoblastic activity and bone turnover. TPBS is also useful in the differential diagnosis between CRPS and other etiologies in patients with extremity pain. However, TPBS is not recommended for monitoring the treatment response.

The typical pattern of TPBS in CRPS is '*diffusely increased uptake at the blood flow and pool phases and increased periarticular uptake at the delayed bone phase*' in the affected extremities. However, the uptake is dependent on the clinical course of CRPS [1, 4, 7–9]. In the acute stage of CRPS, increased radiotracer uptake in all three phases of TPBS is observed in the affected extremities. In contrast, in the chronic stage, the uptake pattern is more variable [10]. In the blood flow and pool phases, the uptake is decreased or normal due to vasoconstriction, whereas delayed bone uptake is either increased or normal. In the early acute stage (<6 weeks), the uptake is normal or minimally increased in all three phases [8]. An atypical pattern of TPBS, which is the decreased uptake in all three phases in the affected extremity, is frequently observed in children with CRPS and can also be seen in adults with chronic CRPS [11, 12]. The diagnostic performance of TPBS varies according to the clinical stage, diagnostic criteria, location, and age at onset of CRPS [1, 2]. Scan interpretation criteria may also affect the diagnostic performance. The accuracy of TPBS is higher in the acute stage than in the chronic stage. The scan findings are less consistent in the lower extremities than in the upper extremities. Among the three phases, the delayed bone phase is more reliable for the diagnosis of CRPS than the blood flow and pool phases.

Case 9.1

A 21-year-old man complained of painful swelling of the left lower leg. He underwent surgery on the left knee for meniscal injury. ^{99m}Tc-MDP TPBS revealed diffusely increased blood flow in the left foot and ankle, increased blood pool, and delayed bone uptake in the left foot, ankle joint, and metatarsophalangeal joints (Fig. 9.1). TPBS findings were suggestive of acute stage CRPS. He underwent physical therapy and lumbar sympathetic plexus block.

Case 9.2

A 48-year-old man underwent external ventricular drainage and gross total tumor resection due to hemorrhagic glioblastoma in the right basal ganglia. Two months after surgery, he complained of tenderness and swelling in his left hand. Presuming CRPS, ^{99m}Tc-DPD TPBS was performed. TPBS revealed diffusely increased blood flow and blood pool in the left hand, and prominent periarticular bone uptake in the small joints of the hand, left wrist joint, left elbow joint, and left shoulder joint (Fig. 9.2). He received steroid pulse therapy and complex exercise therapy due to CRPS and left hemiplegia. Tenderness and swelling improved on the third day of therapy.

Case 9.3

A 51-year-old woman presented with a throbbing pain and burning sensation in her right forearm after housework. As MRI findings were suggestive of reactive tenosynovitis, she took medication to control her pain. Four months later, swelling, tenderness, and trophic skin changes developed. Functional changes (weakness and limited range of motion) in the right hand and right shoulder joints were also detected. The patient underwent ^{99m}Tc-DPD TPBS, which revealed increased periarticular bone uptake in the small joints of the right hand, right wrist joint, right elbow joint, and right shoulder joints

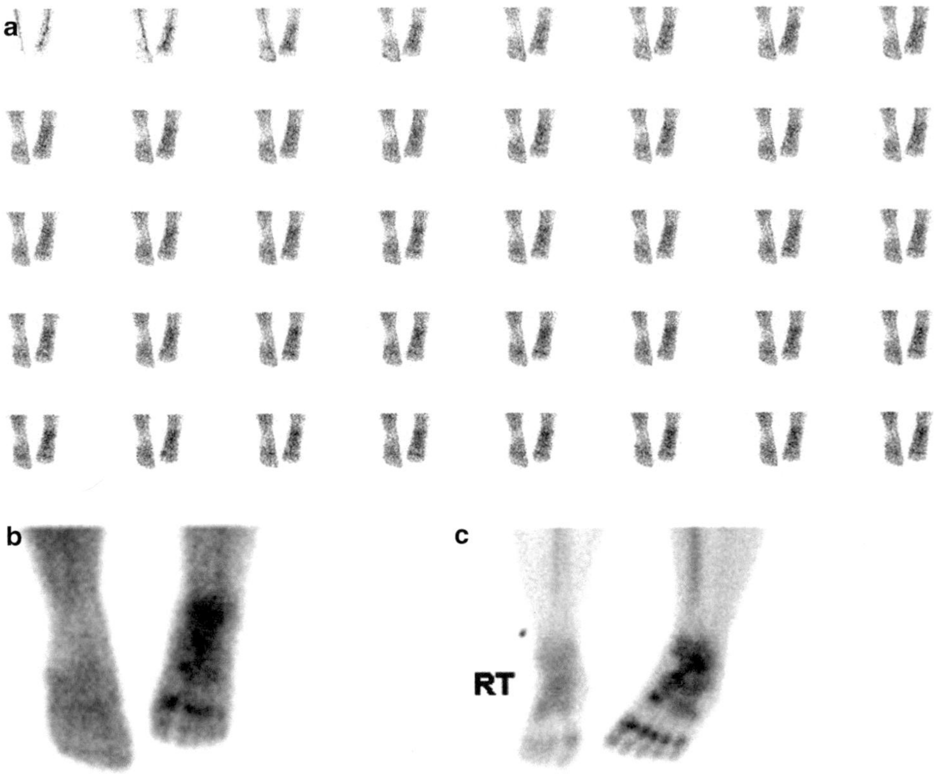

Fig. 9.1 A case of acute stage CRPS in the lower extremity. A 21-year-old male patient with left leg swelling after knee surgery. ^{99m}Tc-MDP TPBS reveals diffusely increased blood flow in the left foot and ankle (**a**), increased blood pool (**b**), and delayed bone uptake (**c**) in the left foot, ankle joint, and metatarsophalangeal joints. *MDP* methylene diphosphonate

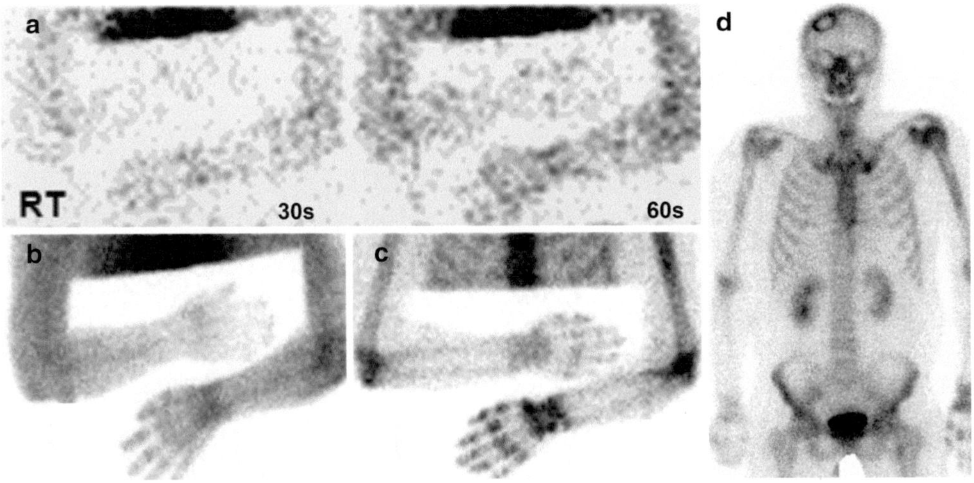

Fig. 9.2 A case of acute stage CRPS in the upper extremity. ^{99m}Tc-DPD TPBS was performed in a 48-year-old patient with tenderness and swelling of the left hand which developed after the resection of hemorrhagic glioblastoma. ^{99m}Tc-DPD TPBS reveals diffusely increased blood flow (**a**) and blood pool (**b**) in the left hand. Prominent periarticular bone uptake is also seen in the small joints of the hand, left wrist joint, left elbow joint, and left shoulder joint (**c**, **d**), suggesting acute stage CRPS. Round-shaped bone uptake due to postoperative change is seen on the right side of the skull. *DPD* 3,3-diphosphono-1,2-propanodicarboxylic acid

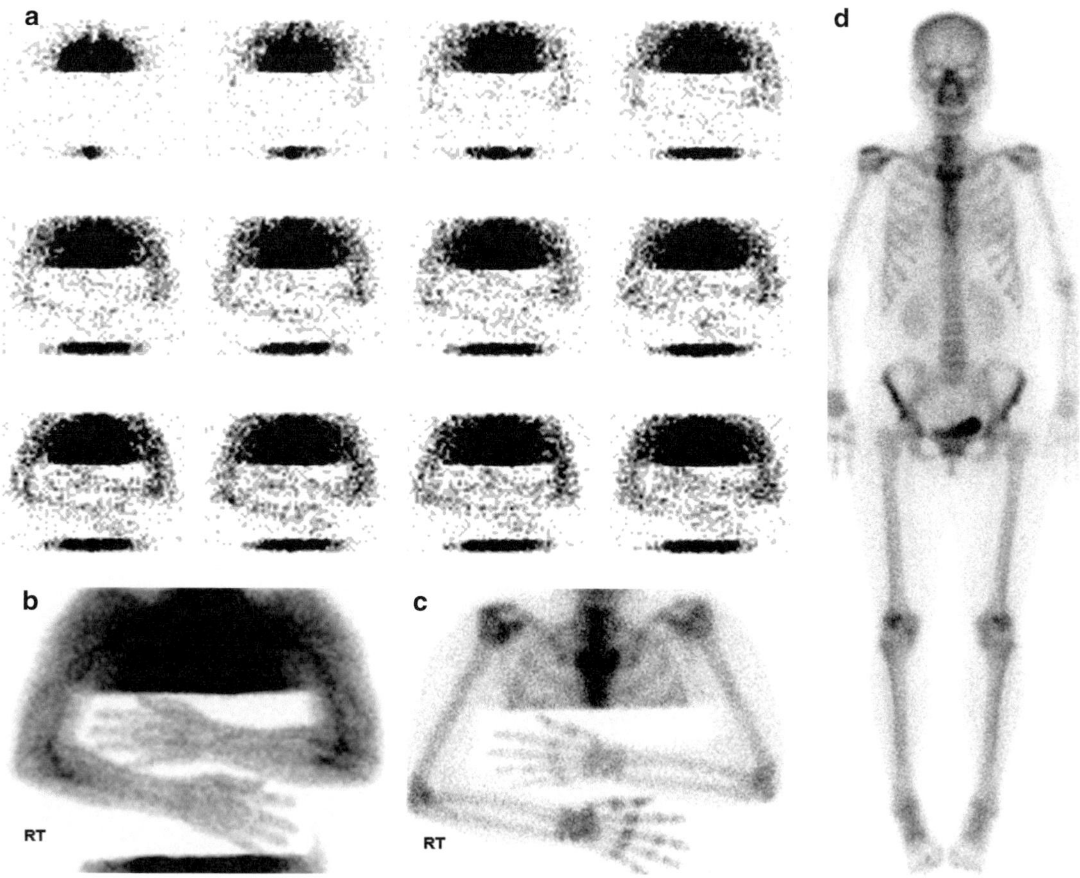

Fig. 9.3 A case of chronic stage CRPS in the upper extremity. ^{99m}Tc-DPD TPBS was performed in a 51-year-old woman with swelling, tenderness, trophic skin changes, and limited function in the right hand. ^{99m}Tc-DPD TPBS reveals symmetric blood flow (**a**) and blood pool (**b**) in both hands. However, periarticular uptake in the delayed bone phase (**c**, **d**) is observed in the small joints of the right hand and right wrist-elbow-shoulder joints (**c**, **d**). *DPD* 3,3-diphosphono-1,2-propanodicarboxylic acid

(Fig. 9.3). However, the blood flow and blood pool in both hands were symmetric. Clinical and scintigraphy findings favored chronic stage CRPS. The patient's symptoms improved after medication for a few months.

Case 9.4

A 40-year-old man visited the hospital with a complaint of burning pain, allodynia, and hypoesthesia in the left lower leg, which occurred after a car ran over his foot. He underwent a lumbar sympathetic ganglion block and received an intravenous injection of ketamine. However, as the pain did not subside, ^{99m}Tc-DPD TPBS was used for the evaluation of the pain. On TPBS, the blood flow, blood pool, and delayed bone uptake decreased diffusely in the left lower leg (Fig. 9.4a–d), which was inconsistent with typical CRPS. The intravenous injection of ketamine was continued, and the symptoms improved partially. Three months later, the patient revisited the hospital because of persistent pain, tenderness, allodynia, and trophic changes. Follow-up TPBS revealed improved bone uptake in the left lower leg, whereas hypoperfusion had not changed (Fig. 9.4e–h). He was diagnosed with CRPS and underwent lumbar epidural blocks.

Case 9.5

A 46-year-old male patient with right hemiplegia due to acute left thalamic infarction was referred for ^{99m}Tc-DPD TPBS for the evaluation of possible CRPS. ^{99m}Tc-DPD TPBS was performed at 2 weeks (early acute phase, Fig. 9.5a–c) and 4 months (acute phase, Fig. 9.5d–f) after disease onset. On TPBS in the early acute phase, the blood flow and blood pool were asymmetrically decreased in the right hand (Fig. 9.5a, b), whereas delayed periarticular bone uptake was increased (Fig. 9.5c). Conversely, in the acute phase, the uptake was increased in the right hand in all three phases (Fig. 9.5d–f) which was compatible with CRPS. This is a representative case indicating that an atypical uptake pattern can be observed in the early acute phase of CRPS. The delayed bone phase is more reliable in the diagnosis of CRPS, and serial TPBS imaging may be helpful in such cases.

Case 9.6

A 41-year-old man complaining of pain in the left hand after a road traffic accident was referred to undergo ^{99m}Tc-DPD TPBS. A tendon injury in the second finger was detected on the radiographic images. CRPS was presumed becuase of swelling and allodynia of the left hand, and a limited range of motion in the left shoulder. ^{99m}Tc-DPD TPBS was performed 3 months after the traffic accident, and the findings were consistent with CRPS (Fig. 9.6a–c). The patient underwent a sympathetic ganglion block and an intravenous injection of lidocaine. The symptoms partially improved. Fourteen months after onset, pain and skin changes in the left hand were not evident, and the motor function recovered to grade 3–4. Compared with the bone uptake on pretreatment TPBS, the asymmetry in the periarticular bone uptake was reduced on the follow-up TPBS (Fig. 9.6d). Scintigraphic findings were consis-

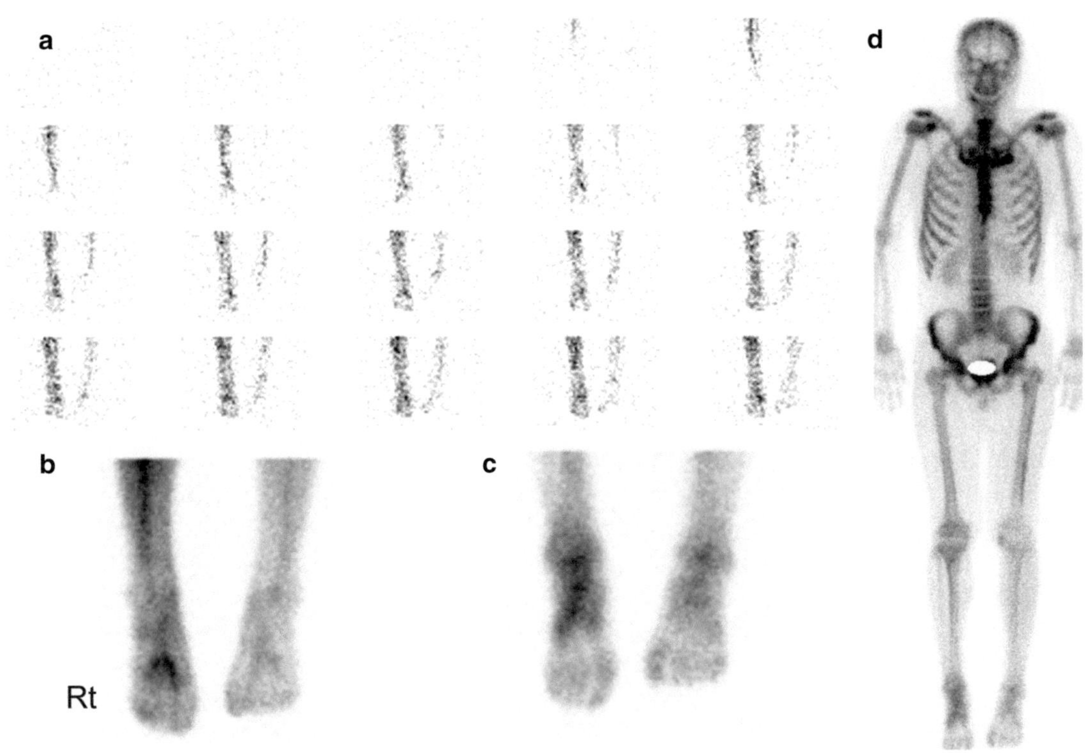

Fig. 9.4 A case of atypical CRPS in the lower extremity. ^{99m}Tc-DPD TPBS was performed in a 40-year-old male patient with burning pain, allodynia, and hypoesthesia in the left lower leg. On the baseline TPBS, the blood flow (**a**), blood pool (**b**), and delayed bone uptake (**c**, **d**) were decreased in the left lower leg. Three months later, follow-up TPBS reveals that bone uptake of the left lower leg (**g**, **h**) is improved. However, the blood flow (**e**) and blood pool (f) did not change. *DPD* 3,3-diphosphono-1,2-propanodicarboxylic acid

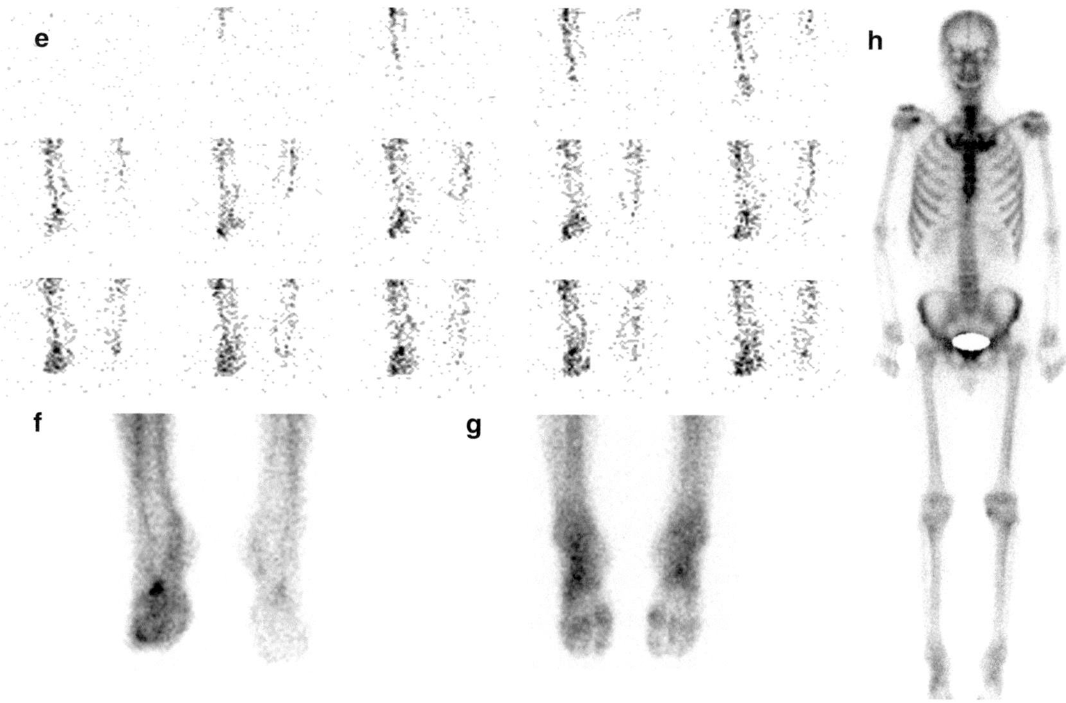

Fig. 9.4 (continued)

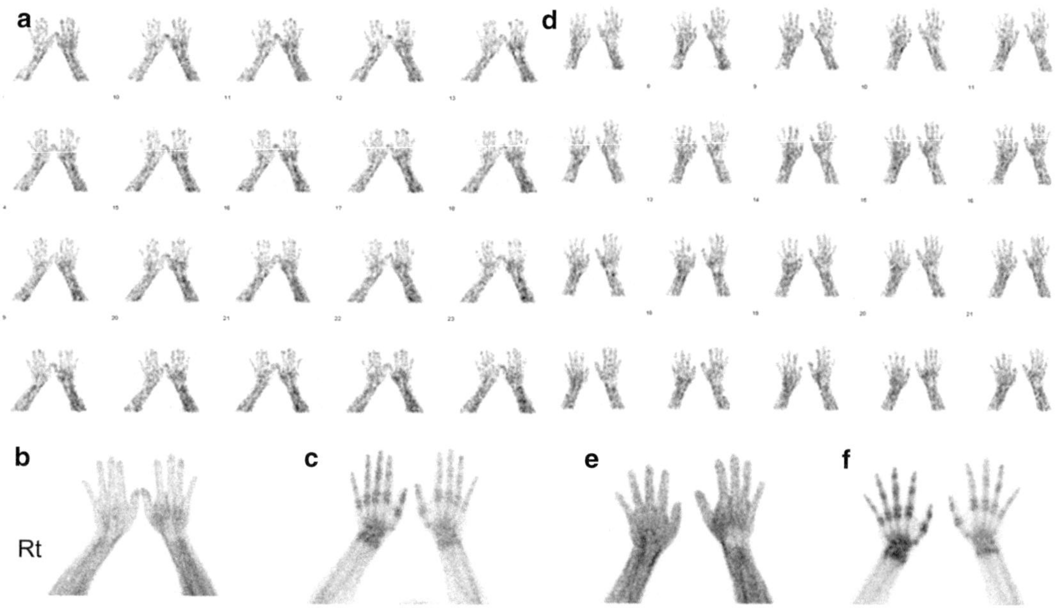

Fig. 9.5 A case for the serial scintigraphic changes of CRPS in the upper extremity. ^{99m}Tc-DPD TPBS was performed in a 46-year-old male patient with acute left thalamic infarction. In the early acute phase, the blood flow (**a**) and blood pool (**b**) were asymmetrically decreased in the right hand, whereas delayed bone uptake was increased in the periarticular area of small joints and the wrist (**c**). In the acute phase, the blood flow (**d**) and blood pool (**e**) were asymmetrically increased in the right hand (wrist), and delayed bone uptake became more prominent (**f**). *DPD* 3,3-diphosphono-1,2-propanodicarboxylic acid

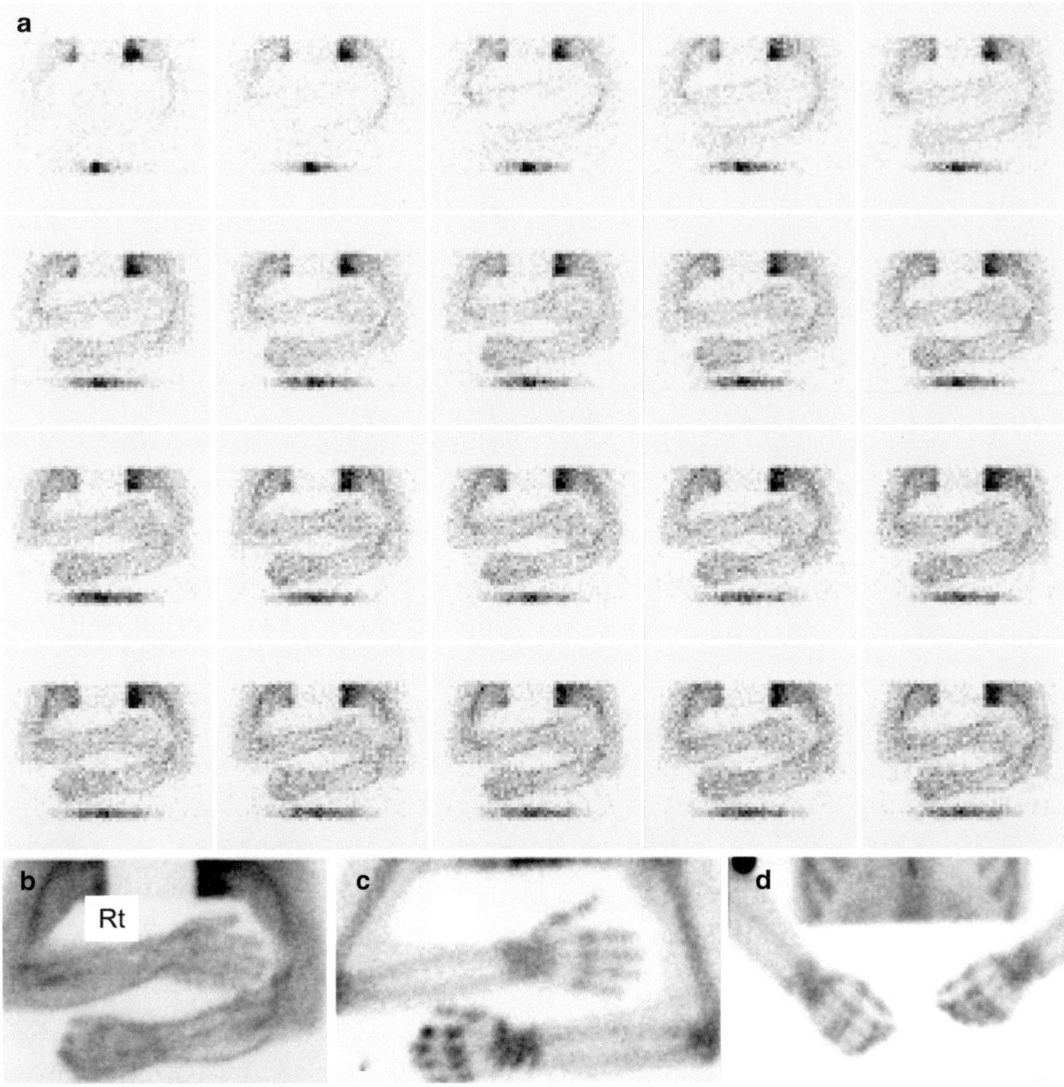

Fig. 9.6 A case of monitoring therapeutic response using TPBS in CRPS. A 41-year-old male patient with lefth and pain underwent ^{99m}Tc-DPD TPBS. On pretreatment TPBS, the blood flow (**a**), blood pool (**b**), and delayed bone uptake (**c**) were asymmetrically increased in the left hand. After treatment for CRPS, the periarticular bone uptake in the left hand and wrist joint was less prominent (**d**). *DPD* 3,3-diphosphono-1,2-propanodicarboxylic acid

tent with symptomatic and functional improvement. Although monitoring the treatment response of CRPS using TPBS is not generally accepted, it may be helpful in some patients.

Case 9.7

A 63-year-old man present with left shoulder and hand swelling and pain due to left hemiplegia after a spontaneous intracranial hemorrhage in the right basal ganglia 3 months earlier. The patient was diagnosed with CRPS. His TPBS revealed diffusely decreased bone uptake in his left hand and decreased perfusion in his left fourth and fifth fingers (Fig. 9.7a–c). This finding suggested that CRPS was associated with combined ulnar nerve palsy. His clinical symptoms,

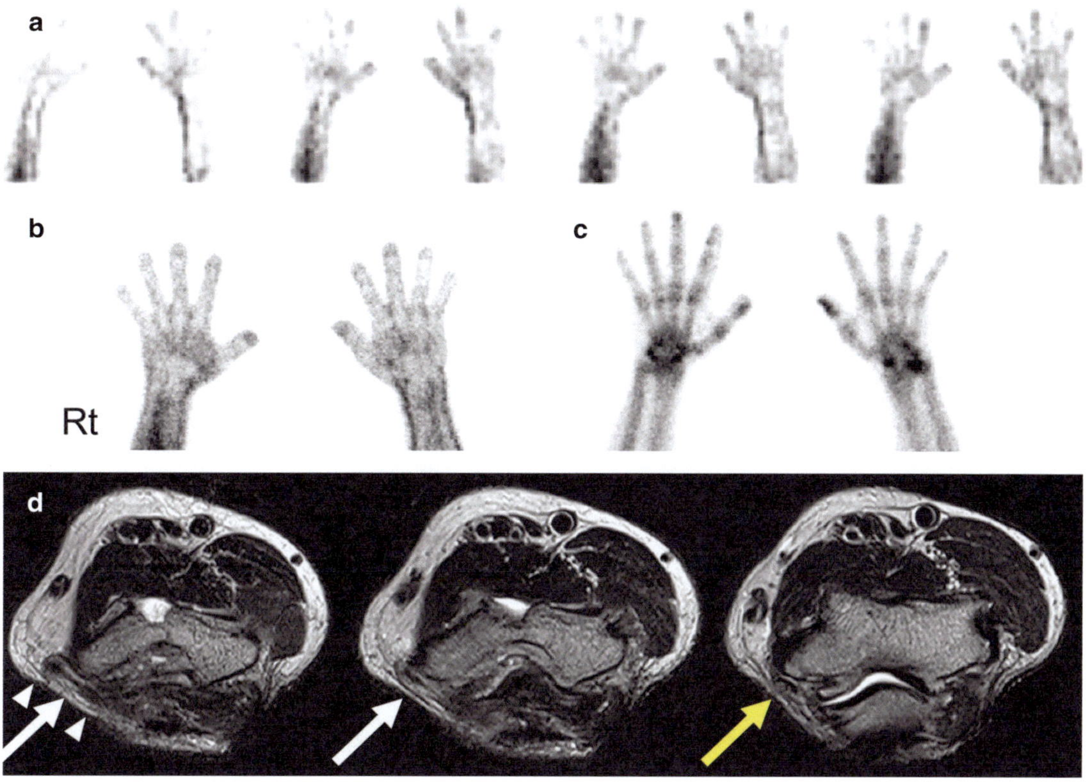

Fig. 9.7 A case of a patient with mixed CRPS-1 and CRPS-2. ^{99m}Tc-DPD TPBS reveals a diffusely decreased blood flow (**a**), blood pool (**b**), and delayed bone uptake (**c**) in the left hand, especially in the fourth and fifth fingers. T2 axial MRI images (**d**) reveal hypertrophy (arrowheads) and high SI (white arrow) of the left ulnar nerve. The yellow arrow points to the normal ulnar nerve

such as tingling sensations and stiffness of the left fourth and fifth fingers, were newly developed when he was followed up 3 months later. Electromyography revealed left ulnar nerve lesion at the elbow level. This resulted in cubital tunnel syndrome with axonal degeneration. The patient underwent anterior subcutaneous ulnar nerve transposition surgery. Preoperative MRI of the left elbow revealed hypertrophic changes and high SI of the ulnar nerve at the cubital tunnel on the T2 axial images (Fig. 9.7d), which was considered as an ulnar nerve impingement. He was diagnosed with mixed CRPS-1 and CRPS-2, which resulted from peripheral nerve injury (Fig. 9.7).

Teaching Points

- The diagnosis of CRPS is based on clinical criteria.
- TPBS is helpful in outlining the symptoms and signs of CRPS and the differential diagnosis of extremity pain.
- The typical pattern of TPBS of CRPS is diffusely increased uptake in the blood flow, blood pool, and delayed bone phases in the affected extremity.
- The uptake pattern of TPBS varies according to the clinical stage, diagnostic criteria, location, and age.

References

1. Fournier RS, Holder LE. Reflex sympathetic dystrophy: diagnostic controversies. Semin Nucl Med. 1998;28:116–23.
2. Howard BA, Roy L, Kaye AD, Pyati S. Utility of radionuclide bone scintigraphy in complex regional pain syndrome. Curr Pain Headache Rep. 2018;22:7.
3. Shim H, Rose J, Halle S, Shekane P. Complex regional pain syndrome: a narrative review for the practising clinician. Br J Anaesth. 2019;123:e424–e33.
4. Intenzo CM, Kim SM, Capuzzi DM. The role of nuclear medicine in the evaluation of complex regional pain syndrome type I. Clin Nucl Med. 2005;30:400–7.
5. Lee GW, Weeks PM. The role of bone scintigraphy in diagnosing reflex sympathetic dystrophy. J Hand Surg Am. 1995;20:458–63.
6. Urits I, Shen AH, Jones MR, Viswanath O, Kaye AD. Complex regional pain syndrome, current concepts and treatment options. Curr Pain Headache Rep. 2018;22:10.
7. Demangeat JL, Constantinesco A, Brunot B, Foucher G, Farcot JM. Three-phase bone scanning in reflex sympathetic dystrophy of the hand. J Nucl Med. 1988;29:26–32.
8. Park SA, Yang CY, Kim CG, Shin YI, Oh GJ, Lee M. Patterns of three-phase bone scintigraphy according to the time course of complex regional pain syndrome type I after a stroke or traumatic brain injury. Clin Nucl Med. 2009;34:773–6.
9. Shin SH, Kim SJ. Bone scintigraphy in patients with pain. Korean J Pain. 2017;30:165–75.
10. Cheon M, Kang HJ, Do KH, Yang HS, Han EJ, Yoo J. Diagnostic performance of three-phase bone scintigraphy and digital infrared thermography imaging for chronic post-traumatic complex regional pain syndrome. Diagnostics (Basel). 2021;11:1459.
11. Goldsmith DP, Vivino FB, Eichenfield AH, Athreya BH, Heyman S. Nuclear imaging and clinical features of childhood reflex neurovascular dystrophy: comparison with adults. Arthritis Rheum. 1989;32:480–5.
12. Laxer RM, Allen RC, Malleson PN, Morrison RT, Petty RE. Technetium ^{99}m-methylene diphosphonate bone scans in children with reflex neurovascular dystrophy. J Pediatr. 1985;106:437–40.

Part III

Spine and Joint Disorders

Spine

10

Tae Joo Jeon

Abstract

Spine is one of the most important structures supporting our body and which is continuously stressed by various postures as well as gravity. These various stresses can affect the stability of spine and can cause many problems. Lower back pain is the most common disease, and its overall prevalence has been known to be over 10% of population. Although many of patients with this symptom can be successfully cared by conservative management, not small portion of the patients require surgical intervention such as internal fixation or spinal fusion. At this time, imaging modalities such as CT, MRI, and SPECT/CT have important roles to assess the exact conditions of spine before and after the surgery, predict the prognosis, and made decision for follow-up management plan. All these modalities have their own benefits and limitations as is well known, and SPECT/CT can play special role due to highly sensitive detection rate of early bone change and less metal artifacts despite the relative low special resolution. In this chapter we will review the role of SPECT/CT mainly in the evaluation of the spine after surgical intervention and add some brief discussion about other conditions such as spondylolysis and fractures.

Keywords

SPECT/CT · Spine · lumbar fusion · Fracture
Trauma · Hybrid imaging · Spondylolysis
Failed back surgery syndrome

10.1 Evolution of Bone SPECT

Before the 1990s, plain radiography and planar bone scintigraphy were the imaging procedures of choice for the evaluation of patients with orthopedic problems of spine, and this trend has not been changed much for a long time, even after the development of SPECT technique, because this new technique was not widely applied to the clinical field of bone disease, despite its high detectability of bone change by tomographic data, due to relatively low spatial resolution and long scan time. Meanwhile, magnetic resonance imaging (MRI) emerged as a choice of modality for spine evaluation.

However, introduction of hybrid bone imaging using SPECT and CT made robust change in many aspects [1]. For example, advanced reconstruction algorithm has significantly improved image quality compared to conventional filtered back projection (FBP) technique. Introduction of

T. J. Jeon (✉)
Department of Nuclear Medicine, Gangnam Severance Hospital, Yonsei University College of Medicine, Seoul, Republic of Korea
e-mail: tjeonnm@yuhs.ac

S.-O. Yang et al. (eds.), *Atlas of Nuclear Medicine in Musculoskeletal System*,
https://doi.org/10.1007/978-981-19-2677-8_10

attenuation correction and scatter correction also contributed to achieving better image quality, and image fusion with CT data resulted in improving localization power [2]. Under the all these progressions, some investigators suggest that SPECT/CT is clinical routine in spine and pelvis imaging [3].

Furthermore, quantitative analysis technology in SPECT/CT made it possible to measure SUV in Tc-99m diphosphonates bone images as F-18 FDG PET/CT does, and this new technology can be applied to traumatic bone disease as well as oncologic cases. This new technology can make it possible to monitor the serial bone changes after spine surgery by objectively measured data, not by only visual evaluation [4, 5].

10.2 Diagnosis of Spine Disease After Various Operations

Although we will focus on the spine after surgery such as interbody fusion, screw fixation, etc., SPECT/CT has been also reported to be useful in the evaluation of low back pain in young people with stress fracture, spondylolysis, and benign bone lesion [6, 7].

In patients with spinal fusion surgery, degenerative changes commonly affect the segment above or below the fusion site which is an important type of failed back surgery syndrome. Usually this is known to be developed with time-related process. Most common affecting sites are facet joint and end plate of vertebra which will be demonstrated by many cases later. Progression of degenerative changes in these areas with the passage of time can lead to spondylolisthesis which may be above and/or below the fused segment [8]. The incidence of this change in lumbar spine has been reported to be about 70% at 10 years after the surgery, and SPECT/CT can play an important role in early detection of this change and providing the information for appropriate management [9].

According to the American College of Radiology (ACR) Appropriateness Criteria, bone SPECT/CT is useful to detect and localize the pseudarthrosis lesion with pain [10].

10.3 Abnormalities in Fused Segments

Spinal fusion is a complicated procedure using diverse metallic devices, and various problems can occur after this surgery.

One of important problems is non-union, failure of osseous bridging to inserted metal even 1 year after the surgery and which commonly produces pain and its incidence varies according to patient's factors and the properties of used materials. Secondly, fracture of metallic devices also can be a possible side effect, and SEPCT/CT is useful to detect the secondary bone change as well as the problem of metallic device per se. The loosening of prosthesis is also an important condition which should be carefully checked when interpreting the bone SPECT/CT. The evaluation of the exact phase of these problems can make it possible to choose the best treatment option at each time point [11–13].

10.4 Evaluation of Spondylolysis and Other Traumatic and Degenerative Changes

Spondylolysis is also an important cause of back pain which is defined as break in the pars interarticularis of neural arch. The importance of this disease entity is that this can commonly occur in children to young adults as well as elderlies because this area is weak during developmental phase before the achievement of full maturation of skeletal system. The etiologies of spondylolysis are varied, such as continuous stress, trauma, and developmental problem. The role of SPECT/CT in spondylolysis is to identify the stress of pars interarticularis before apparent spondylolysis and differentiate acute spondylolysis from chronic non-union.

SPECT/CT also plays an important role in early detection of degenerative changes in end-plate of vertebral bodies as well as osteophyte formation, and both sclerotic change information from CT part and radiotracer uptake representing bone metabolic activity from SPECT data will provide us better option for interpretation of various spinal diseases.

Teaching Points

- Hybrid bone SPECT/CT image is a useful modality in evaluation of spine after surgery.
- Degenerative change affecting the segment above or below the fusion is important type of failed back surgery syndrome.
- Failed back syndrome is a time-related process.
- Common affecting sites of failed back syndrome after spinal fusion are facet joint and endplate.
- Bone SPECT/CT has high sensitivity and specificity in detecting the screw loosening of spine.
- SPECT/CT is also useful in evaluating the spectrum of spondylolysis, only stress reaction without spondylolysis, spondylolysis, and non-union.

Case 10.1

An 81-year-old man presented to the hospital due to upper back pain developed 2 days ago. He underwent multilevel lumbar pedicle fixation surgery 1 year ago and got a slip down injury recently. Planar bone scintigraphy showed increased uptake in T12 to L1 vertebrae (a). MIP image obtained from SPECT data reveals stronger uptake in that lesion with additional hot lesions in the remaining lumbar spine (b). Sagittal reconstruction CT image revealed anterior wedging deformity of T12 vertebral body and multiple mild compression fractures of L1, 3, 5 vertebral bodies (c). Fusion SPECT/CT images show intense uptake in T12 body and relatively strong uptake in L1 body, while only mild uptakes are noted in L3 and L5 bodies (d). These SPECT/CT findings were not clearly defined by planar scintigraphy only. Considering all these results, only T12 and L1 vertebral bodies got recent traumatic insults, while the other lesions in compressed L3, 5 vertebral bodies with minimal uptake are supposed to be old compression fractures. Otherwise, all these compression fractures have different severity of insults if all these injuries occurred in the same time. This case is one of good example representing that SPECT/CT provides us important information about exact phase of bone disease by collaboration of anatomical and functional data (Fig. 10.1).

Case 10.2

An 87-year-old woman visited to the outpatient clinic due to chronic back pain. She underwent posterior screw fixation at the L4, 5 level of spine.

SPECT/CT images reveal no significant bone uptake in the operation site, but strong uptake can be seen in Lt. facet joint of L1/2 level, and fused SPECT/CT images show asymmetric sclerotic change of the Lt. facet joint as well. Facet joint is a common site of secondary degenerative change after spine fusion surgery as previously mentioned. Like this case, SPECT/CT can accurately localize the sclerotic bone changes on CT images (a), and fusion images provide the exact localization of affected site on axial (b) and sagittal (c) plane, while planar images failed to depict the facet joint problem (d).

According to SPECT/CT finding, Lt. facet joint lesion appears to be active phase of disease in spite of sclerotic change, and this cannot be validated by CT and planar scintigraphic data only (Fig. 10.2).

Case 10.3

A 55-year-old woman with history of total hip replacement on Lt. side presented to the outpatient clinic due to low back pain. Planar bone scintigraphy shows focal hot uptake in L3 vertebra (a), and coronal fusion SPECT/CT images represent more clearly defined hot uptake in the same area (b). Sagittal reconstruction CT image reveals only mild compression of upper margin of L3 vertebral body (c); however SPECT/CT image shows intense radiotracer uptake in posterior portion of L3 vertebral body as well as upper margin of the vertebral body (d). Although upper margin of sacrum has sclerotic bone changes on

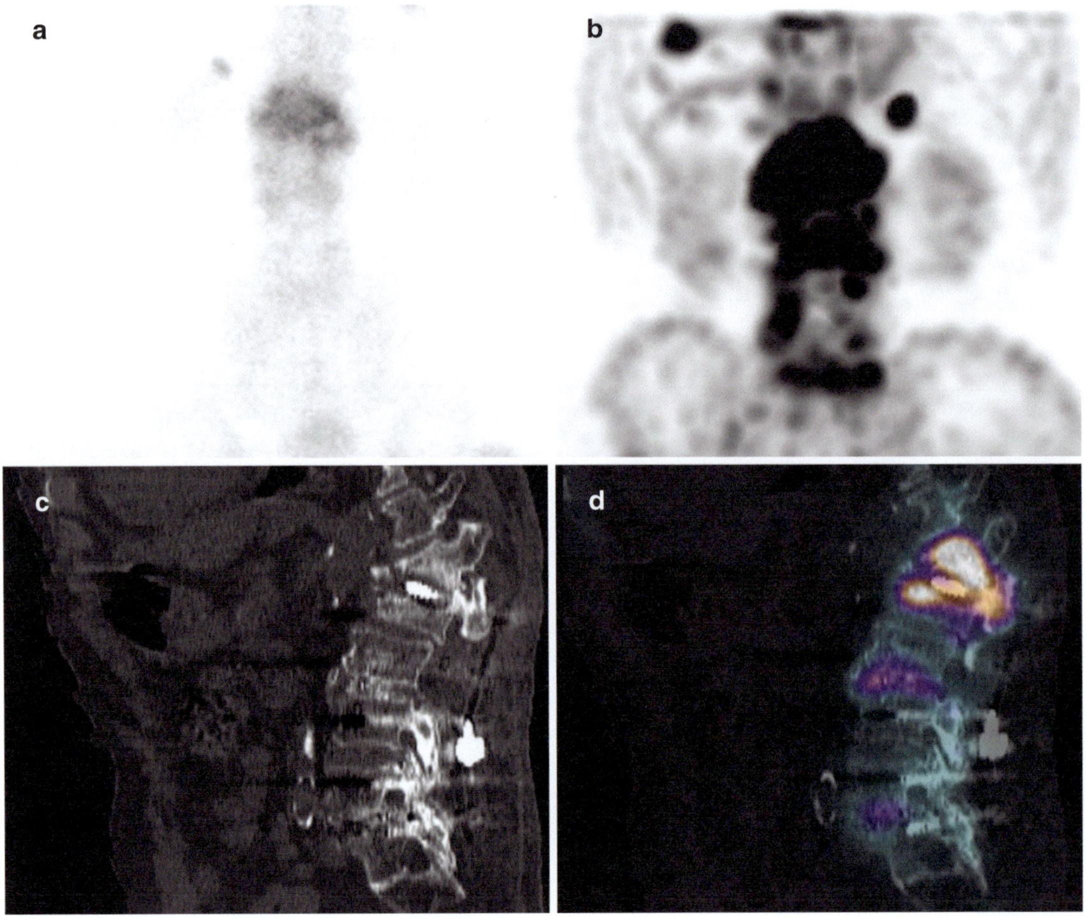

Fig. 10.1 Planar scintigraphy (**a**) shows only mild uptake in T12, L1 level compared to MIP SPECT image (**b**), and CT scan can only provide the information of anatomic changes of spine (**c**), while SPECT reveals different activity in multiple compression fracture of vertebrae, very strong uptake in T12, strong uptakes in L1, and mild uptakes in L3, 5 vertebral bodies (**d**)

CT scan (c), SPECT image reveals no visible hot uptake in this area (d). All these findings mean that SPECT/CT is a very useful modality that can validate the exact extent of bone disease as well as the exact phase of bone injury. SPECT images are known to have higher resolution as well as higher sensitivity compared to those of planar scintigraphy in the evaluation of deep structure according to using tomographic data set. Rapid progression of hardware and software technology of SPECT/CT will definitely exaggerate these results in the near future (Fig. 10.3).

Case 10.4

An 83-year-old woman with history of total hip replacement on Rt. side and posterior screw fixation of L2–L4 came to the clinic due to back pain. Planar bone scintigraphy reveals increased uptake only in part of L2, 3 vertebrae (a); however MIP image of SPECT shows more intense uptakes in this area and additional hot uptake in L4, 5, and Rt. acetabulum (b). Sagittal reconstruction CT image shows sclerotic changes in upper and lower portion of L2 and upper margin of L3 vertebral bodies (c). Fusion SPECT/CT images

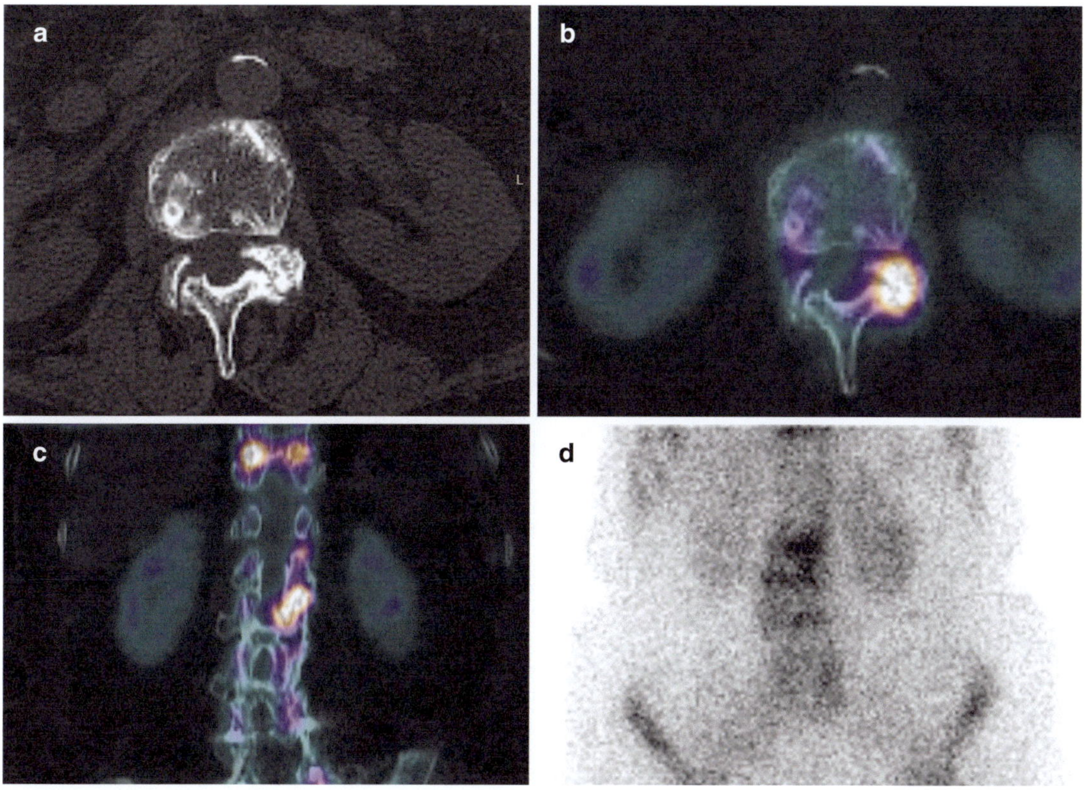

Fig. 10.2 Asymmetric sclerotic changes of Lt. facet joint are noted on axial CT image (**a**), and axial fusion SPECT/CT image shows strong uptake in the Lt. facet joint, but only minimal radiotracer uptakes are noted in another small round sclerotic lesions of vertebral body (**b**). More exact extent of hot uptake can be estimated by coronal reconstruction image (**c**), while planar scintigraphy failed to localize the facet lesion, and only degenerative change of vertebral body can be suspected by this image (**d**)

reveal localized hot uptakes in the endplate of L2/3 vertebral body with sclerotic changes and additional hot uptakes in facet joints of L3/4 and L4/5 (d). This is another case demonstrating typical findings of failed back syndrome with hot uptakes above and below level of fusion and adjacent facet joints. In the interpretation of cases with failed back syndrome, knowledge about commonly affected site will be very helpful and essential (Fig. 10.4).

Case 10.5

A 70-year-old woman with history of posterior screw and rod fixation of L2 to L4 presented to the clinic due to back pain. Axial CT image (a) shows periscrew lucency in Rt. side (arrow), and fusion SPECT/CT images reveal strong focal uptakes in both screws, especially in Rt. side (b).

These findings can be due to screw loosening, and the incidence of this event is reported to be 0.6% to 11%, and bone SPECT/CT has known to have excellent sensitivity (100%) and specificity (89.7%) in detecting loosening of screw in spine [14]. In the interpretation of loosening, CT images must be very important like in other diseases. Although only planar scintigraphy and plain radiography were available in the past, now SPECT/CT images provide much more useful information for this problem.

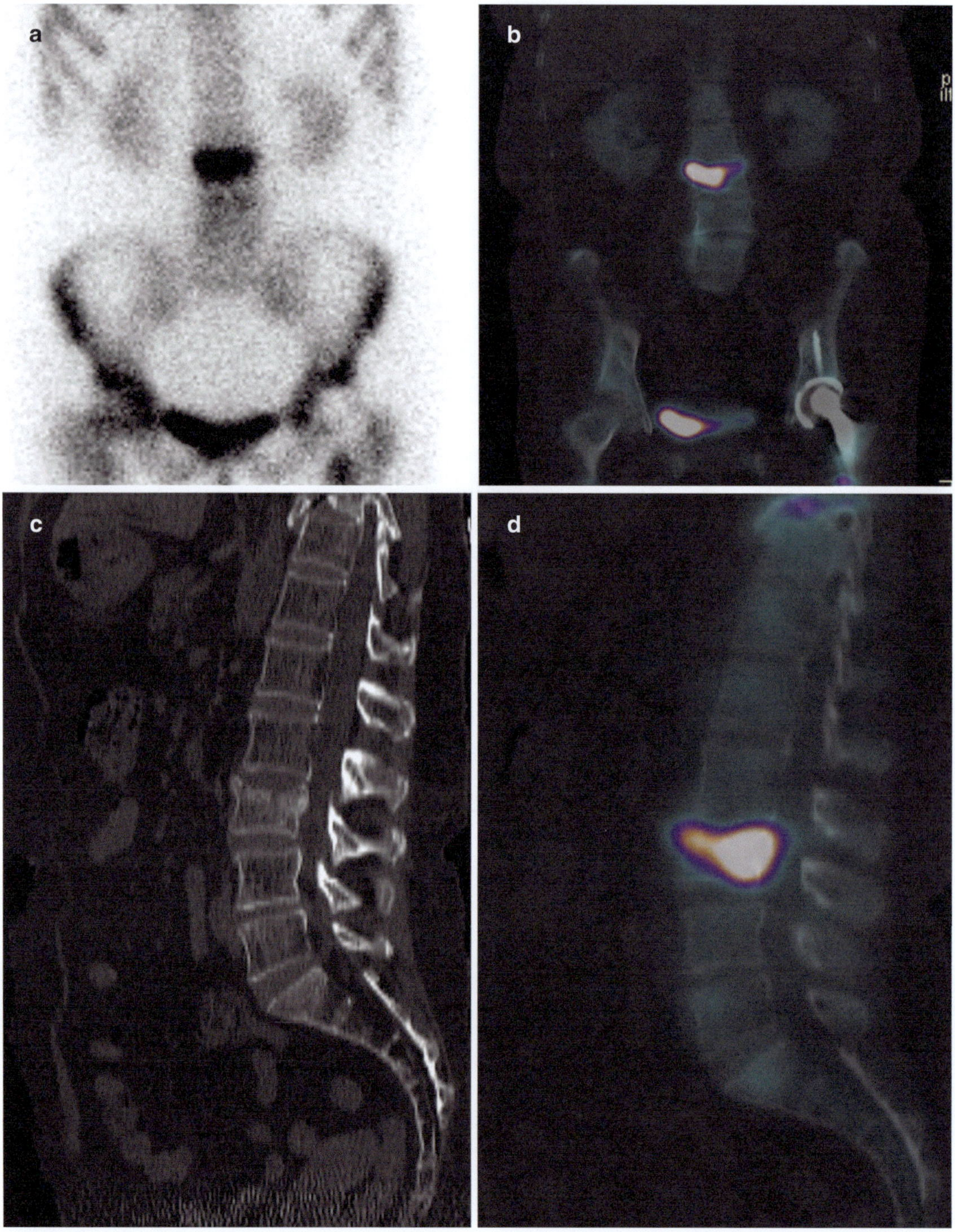

Fig. 10.3 Nearly all part of L3 body seems to be involved by hot uptake on planar scintigraphy due to blurring of image (**a**); however only part of L3 body was involved by hot uptake on SPECT image fused to CT (**b**). Sagittal reconstruction CT represents mildly increased bone density in upper margin of L3 body (**c**), while SPECT/CT image reveals some discrepancy, strong uptake in the posterior portion of vertebral body (**d**)

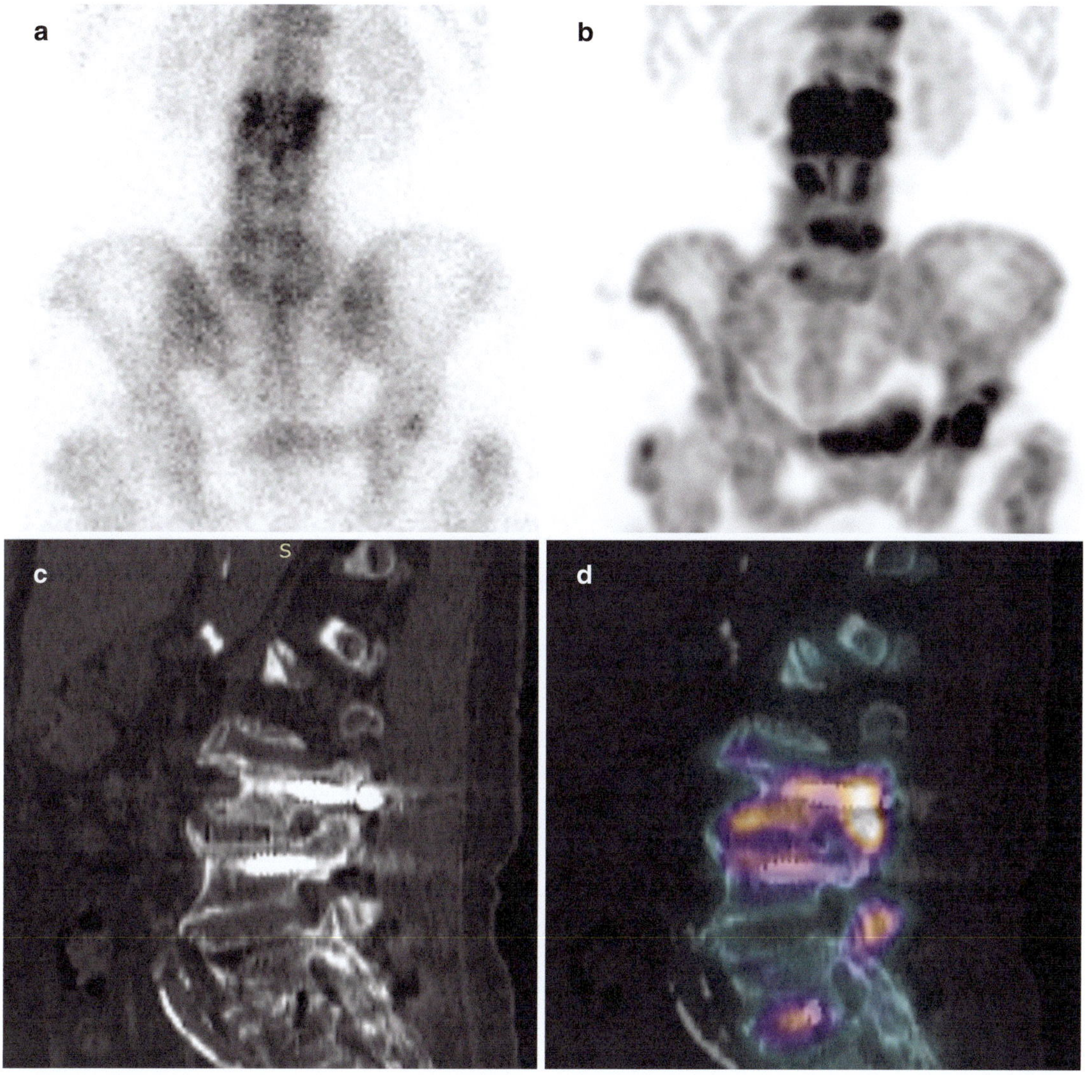

Fig. 10.4 Planar scintigraphy shows focal hot uptakes only in the lateral margins of L2, 3 vertebrae with mild focal uptakes in L4, 5 vertebrae, and only minimal focal uptake is noted in Lt. acetabulum (**a**). However, MIP SPECT images show stronger and larger hot lesions in all these areas (**b**). Mild sclerotic bone changes of L2, 3 vertebral bodies are well defined by sagittal reconstruction CT images (**c**), and increased uptakes are noted in the lower margin of L2 and upper margin of L3 vertebral bodies (**d**)

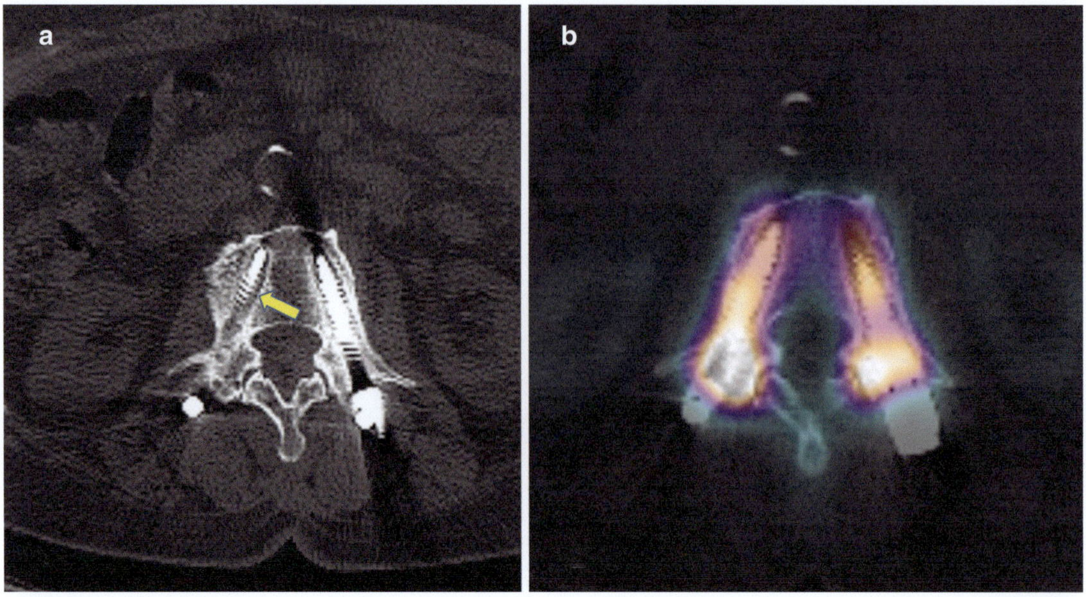

Fig. 10.5 Axial CT image (**a**) reveals periscrew lucency of Rt. side (arrow), and strong radiotracer uptakes are noted in both sides of screws, especially in Rt. side (**b**). According to both anatomic and functional imaging findings, more exact evaluation of loosening and disease activity can be achieved

Especially loosening of posterior fixation of vertebral body by screw like in this case is commonly missed by planar scintigraphy, although longitudinal pattern of loosening case such as total hip replacement can be more easily detected by planar technology only. Hybrid tomographic imaging SPECT/CT provides tomographic images of three axial plane, and any plane of loosening of device is readily detectable (Fig. 10.5).

Case 10.6

A 50-year-old man with history of bilateral total hip replacement surgery was admitted to the clinic due to low back pain. Axial CT image shows bony defects in bilateral pars interarticularis of L5 vertebra with mild sclerotic changes (a). However, fusion SPECT/CT image reveals asymmetric focal tracer uptake only in the Lt. part interarticularis (b). Sagittal CT (c) and fusion SPECT/CT (d) image of Rt. pars interarticularis at the same level represents focal bone defect without significant radiotracer uptake. These findings suggest the possibility of different time of event in these two spondylolysis lesions although anatomic image reveals similar findings in both pars interarticularis lesions of L5 vertebra.

SPECT/CT is also useful in the evaluation of exact phase of various spinal fractures such as spondylolysis, vertebral pedicle fracture, and avulsion fracture of spinal spinous process. Even small uptakes in fracture lesions can be easily detected and exactly localized by this hybrid imaging technique, and the accumulation of knowledge about this condition will make SPECT/CT provide proper treatment guideline in the future (Fig. 10.6).

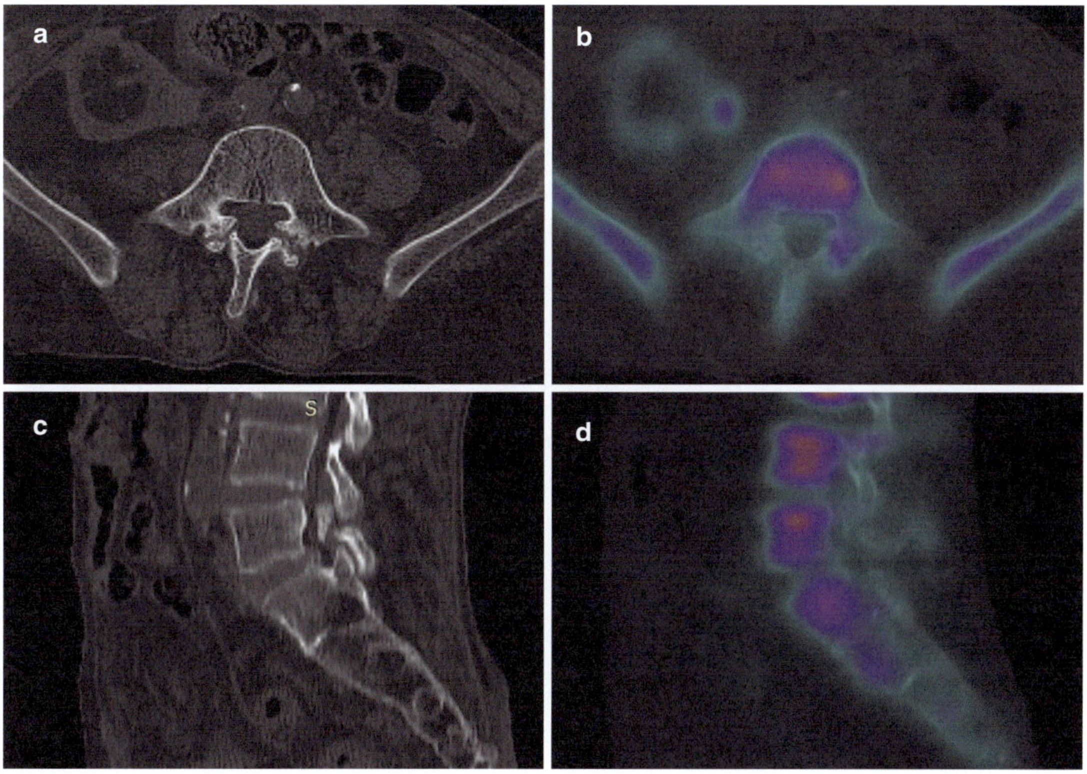

Fig. 10.6 Axial CT image (**a**) shows breaks in the pars interarticularis of both sides (L5 level) with mild sclerotic changes, and asymmetrically increased uptake is noted in defect of Lt. side on axial fusion image (**b**). These findings suggest the possibility of chronic non-union of Rt. pars interarticularis, and fusion images demonstrate different status of bilateral pars interarticularis defects although CT scan reveals similar findings. Sagittal reconstruction CT and fusion SPECT/CT at the level of Rt. pars interarticularis reveal well-defined bony defect (**c**) and no significant uptake in this area (**d**)

References

1. Utsumomya D, Shiraishi S, Imuta M, Tomiguch S, Kawanak K, Morishita S, et al. Added value of SPECT/CT fusion in assessing suspected bone metastasis: comparison with scintigraphy alone and non fused scintigraphy and CT. Radiology. 2006;238:264–71.
2. Miyaji N, Miwa K, Tokiwa A, Ichikawa H, Terauchi T, Koizumi M, et al. Phantom and clinical evaluation of bone SPECT/CT image reconstruction with Xspect algorithm. Eur J Nucl Med Mol Imaging Res. 2020;10:71.
3. Scheyerer MJ, Pietsch C, Zimmermann SM, Osterhoff G, Simmen HP, Werner CM. SPECT/CT for imaging of the spine and pelvis in clinical routine: a physician's perspective of the adoption of SPECT/CT in a clinical setting with a focus on trauma surgery. Eur J Nucl Med Mol Imaging. 2014;41(Suppl 1):S59–66.
4. Tbotta F, Jreige M, Schaefer N, Becce F, Prior J, Laonde M. Quantitative bone SPECT/CT: high specificity for identification of prostate cancer bone metastases. BMC Musculoskelet Disord. 2019;20:619.
5. Huang K, Feng Y, Liu D, Liang W, Li L. Quantification evaluation of Tc-99m MDP concentration in the lumbar spine with SPECT/CT: compare with bone mineral density. Ann Nucl Med. 2020;34:136–43.
6. Matesan M, Behnia F, Bermo M, Vesselle H. SPECT/CT bone scintigraphy to evaluate low back pain in young athletes: common and uncommon etiologies. J Orthop Surg Res. 2016;11:76.

7. Trout AT, Sharp SE, Anton CG, Gelfand MJ, Mehlman CT. Spondylolysis and beyond: value of SPECT/CT in evaluation of low back pain in children and young adults. Radiographics. 2015;35(3):819–34.
8. Levin DA, Hale JJ, Bendo JA. Adjacent segment degeneration following spinal fusion for degenerative disc disease. Bull NYU Hosp Jt Dis. 2007;65(1):29–36.
9. Lee I, Budiawan H, Moon JY, Cheon GJ, Kim YC, Paeng JC, et al. The value of SPECT/CT in localizing pain site and prediction of treatment response in patients with chronic low back pain. J Korean Med Sci. 2014;29(12):1711–6.
10. Patel ND, Broderick DF, Burns J, Deshmukh TK, Fries IB, Harvery HB, et al. ACR appropriateness criteria low back pain. J Am Coll Radiol. 2016;13(9):1069–78.
11. Al-Riyami K, Van den Wyngaert GG, T, Bomanji J. Bone SPECT/CT in the postoperative spine: a focus on spinal fusion. Eur J Nucl Med Mol Imaging. 2017;44(12):2094–104.
12. Sumer J, Schmidt D, Ritt P, Lell M, Forst R, Kuwert T, et al. SPECT/CT in patients with lower back pain after lumbar fusion surgery. Nucl Med Commun. 2013;34(10):964–70.
13. Waldman LE, Scharf SC. Bone SPECT/CT of the spine, foot, and ankle: evaluation of surgical patients. Semin Nucl Med. 2017;47(6):639–46.
14. Hydyana H, Maes A, Vandenberghe T, Fidlers L, Sathekge M, Nicolai D, et al. Accuracy of bone SPECT/CT for identifying hardware loosening in patients who underwent lumbar fusion with pedicle screws. Eur J Nucle Med Mol Imaging. 2016;43(2):349–54.

11 Hip

Sun Jung Kim and So Won Oh

Abstract

Hip replacement and internal fixation are major surgeries commonly performed in the hip region. Total hip arthroplasty (THA) is one of the most successful and cost-effective surgical procedures. The main indications are osteoarthritis, avascular necrosis, femur neck fracture, and inflammatory arthritis. The incidence of THA has increased dramatically over the past 20 years, despite a variety of early and late complications. Accordingly, the increase of revision arthroplasty has followed. It is still challenging to identify the cause of pain and failure in THA despite the advances in radiologic and nuclear imaging techniques. Internal fixation is widely used in treatment of hip fractures. Hip fractures are a common injury, and femur neck fractures are associated with high levels of patient morbidity and mortality after surgery. In this chapter, we present a brief review of cases to assess the cause of pain and complications after hip surgery rather than dealing with primary hip diseases.

Keywords

Total hip arthroplasty · Internal fixation · Complications · Nuclear imaging · SPECT/CT · Fracture

11.1 Loosening in THA

Loosening of the prostheses is one of the major complications of THA and accounts for about 70% cases of revision arthroplasty [1]. Aseptic loosening is loss of fixation of the implant, which can be caused by inadequate initial fixation, mechanical loss of fixation overtime, or biologic loss of fixation due to particle-induced osteolysis around the implant. The Hip Society has defined it as confirmed intraoperatively or identified radiographically as a change in implant position or a progressive radiolucent line at the bone-cement or bone-implant interface [2]. Thus, it is important to check serial radiographs with clinical follow-up.

Reproducible assessment of periprosthetic lucency uses the standardized zones proposed by Gruen (zones 1–7) for the femur and DeLee and Charnley (zones I–III) for the acetabulum (Fig. 11.1a) [3, 4]. A lucent zone greater than

S. J. Kim (✉)
Department of Nuclear Medicine, National Health Insurance Service Ilsan Hospital, Goyang, Republic of Korea
e-mail: sunjk32@nhimc.or.kr

S. W. Oh
Department of Nuclear Medicine, Seoul National University Boramae Medical Center, Seoul, Republic of Korea

S.-O. Yang et al. (eds.), *Atlas of Nuclear Medicine in Musculoskeletal System*,
https://doi.org/10.1007/978-981-19-2677-8_11

2 mm in diameter around the prosthesis is a common sign of loosening on radiography.

In bone scan, loosening is suspected when there is an increased uptake in around the entire or near entire periprosthetic area. Bone scan (including triple phase) has slightly lower diagnostic performance than radiography to detect loosening of prosthesis: a sensitivity of 67% and specificity of 75% for acetabular cup and 85% and 72% for femoral stem, respectively [5, 6]. Increased uptake around prosthesis on vascular and blood pool image of triple-phase bone scan (TPBS) is likely not aseptic loosening. It is challenging to distinguish between aseptic and septic loosening. In nuclear imaging, white blood cell (WBC) scan can be useful, and ^{18}F-FDG PET/CT seems to be needed by further research.

Case 11.1

A 55-year-old man who underwent bilateral hip arthroplasty visited the outpatient clinic complaining of worsening right hip pain for 1 month. The right one was operated 3 years ago and the left one 13 years ago.

Radiograph showed periprosthetic radiolucency in entire zones around the right femoral stem and periosteal reaction in zones 2, 3, 5, and 6 of the right femur. Osteolysis was observed in zones I and II of the left acetabulum (Fig. 11.1b). Bone scan showed increased uptake in most of zone around the right femur stem (Fig. 11.1c). CT showed well radiolucent zone around prosthesis of the right femur (Fig. 11.1e) and periosteal reaction around lower prosthesis (Fig. 11.1d). An osteolytic lesion was seen in zones I and II of the left acetabulum (Fig. 11.1f, g).

These findings are reasonable for loosening of the right femoral stem and asymptomatic osteolysis in the left acetabulum. He underwent revision surgery for the painful right femur component. There were quite a few inflammatory debris in the femur where the femur stem was located. Frozen biopsy of several periprosthetic soft tissues during operation showed polymorphonuclear leukocytes/high-power field microscopic examination in some materials, but the criteria for infection were not reached.

11.2 Chronic Expanding Hematoma in THA

Chronic expanding hematoma (CEH) is a rare entity that often results from trauma, surgery, anticoagulation therapy, or bleeding disorders [7]. In addition, periprosthetic chronic expanding hematoma after THA is very rare. To the best of our knowledge, only a few cases of CEH after THA were reported to date, which was accompanied by progressive osteolysis [8, 9]. In reported cases, there was no clear trigger for hematoma formation, and the cause was unknown. In contrast to pseudotumor that occurs around replaced hip joint, there was no histiocytic infiltration and very little evidence of particulate or metal debris on histological findings.

Clear preoperative diagnosis could be difficult to determine. The differential diagnosis to be considered is as follows: acute local tissue reaction (ALTR) known as pseudotumor, benign and malignant soft tissue tumor, and deep infection.

Case 11.2

Eight years after the patient of Case 11.1 undergoing revision arthroplasty on the right femur, he revisited the outpatient clinic due to worsening left hip pain that developed 2 weeks prior. He occasionally felt discomfort in the left groin after 2 years since the revision surgery. On radiograph, the preexisting osteolytic lesion in the left acetabulum appeared slightly larger than 8 years ago (Fig. 11.2a). Bone scan showed no abnormal uptake in the left acetabulum (Fig. 11.2b). CT obtained 8 months later revealed a large cystic mass in the left iliac fossa extending from the left iliac bone to the anterior aspect of the ipsilateral hip joint coursing below the heads of the iliopsoas muscle (Fig. 11.2d–f, h–j). The cystic mass was abutting to the osteolytic lesion

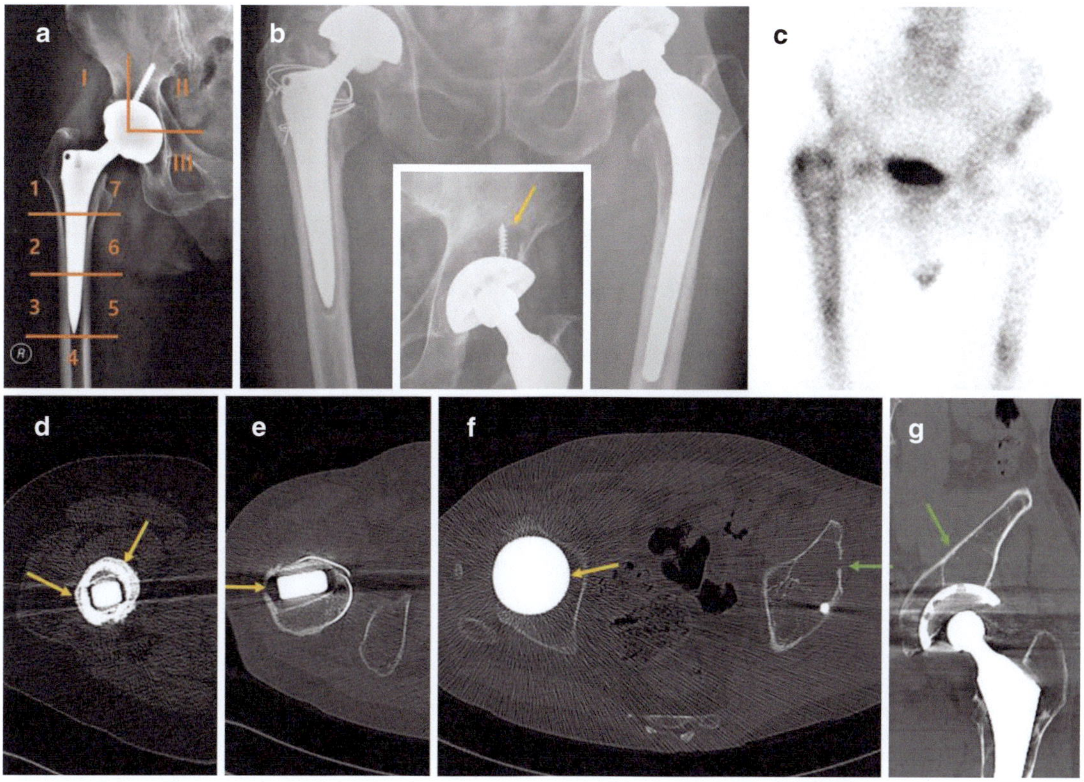

Fig. 11.1 (**a**) The Charnley-DeLee numbering system for acetabular cups and the Gruen zone numbering for femoral stems in the anterior-posterior plane. (**b**) Radiograph shows periprosthetic radiolucency in entire zones around the right femoral stem and periosteal reaction in zones 2, 3, 5, and 6. Osteolysis (arrow) in zones I and II of the left acetabulum (inset). (**c**) Bone scan shows increased uptake in most of zone of the right femur stem, suggesting loosening. Focally increased uptake in zone 4 of the left femoral stem is still seen even 13 years after surgery. (**d**) Axial CT image of lower level of prosthesis shows periosteal bone formation (arrow), which is often seen in periprosthetic infection. (**e**) Axial CT of upper level of prosthesis shows well radiolucent zone (yellow arrow) greater than 2 mm around prosthesis. (**f**), (**g**) The right acetabular cup is well fixed (yellow arrow) and an osteolysis with thin sclerotic rim and cortical breakdown (green arrows) in zones I and II of the left acetabulum on axial and sagittal CT images

grown in the left superior acetabulum and iliac bone (Fig. 11.2e, f, i, j). MRI showed a mixture of fresh and old blood indicating repeated bleeding (Fig. 11.2g, k). He underwent surgery to remove the cystic mass, which had separated into two lumens, filled with old blood and clots. Histopathologic report revealed hematoma with thick capsule. He replaced the left acetabular cup and the femur head due to prolonged osteolysis and loosening confirmed during surgery.

He had no previous history of trauma and anticoagulation therapy. Laboratory data showed normal coagulation profiles. Unlike previous reports, osteolysis did not progress significantly.

11.3 Periprosthetic Joint Infection in THA

Periprosthetic joint infection (PJI) is one of the most dreaded complications. This is because several stages of surgery may be necessary instead of once and the subsequent increase in morbidity and the outcome of the prosthesis may be poor. The diagnosis of PJI is difficult and not standardized. At least six different definitions of PJI were released by independent societies, but most of them do not include imaging techniques, except for the recently released World Association against Infection in Orthopaedics and Trauma

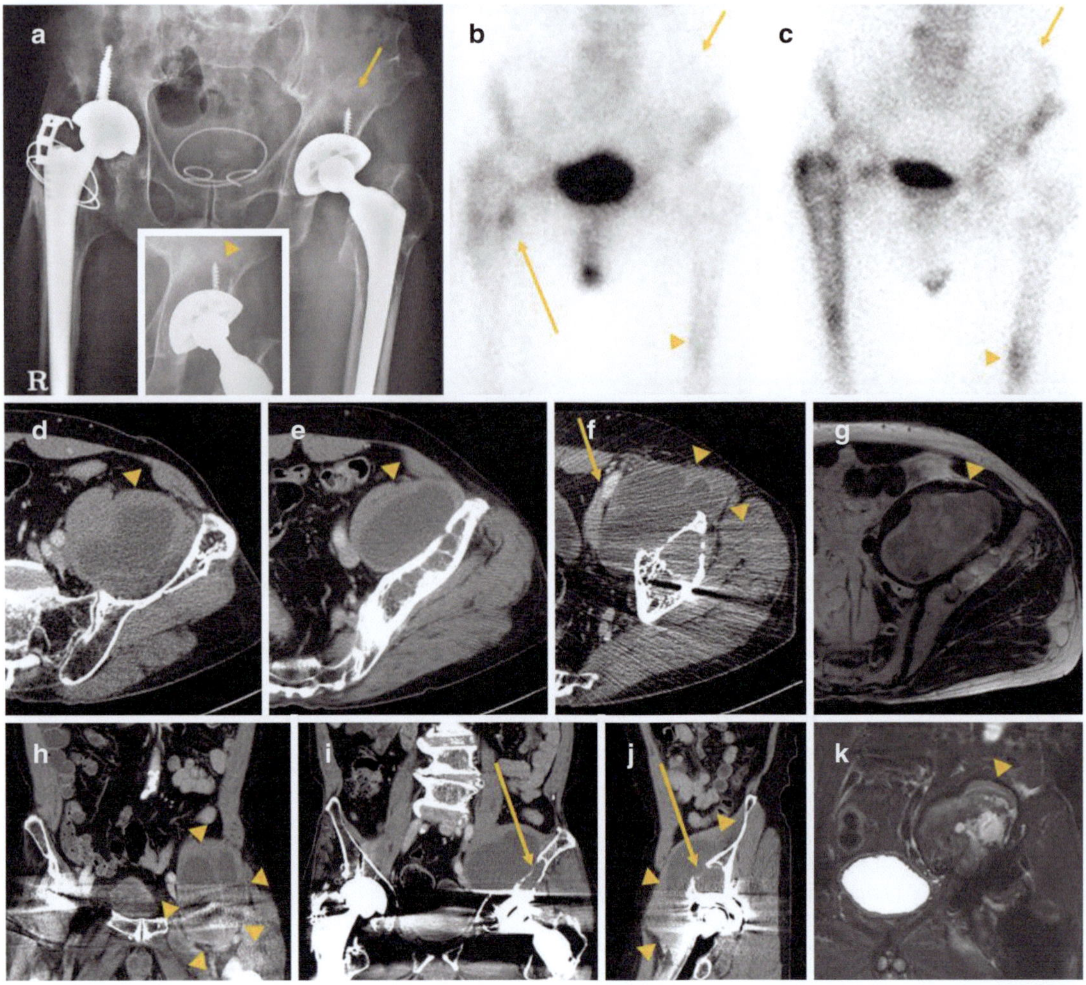

Fig. 11.2 (**a**) Radiograph shows an osteolytic lesion (arrow) larger than 8 years ago (inset, arrow head) in zones I and II the left acetabulum. (**b**) Bone scan shows no abnormal uptake in the left hip area. Cortical margin of the left iliac crest is not clearly visible (arrow). Slightly increased uptake in zones 1 and 7 of the right femur (long arrow) even after 8 years of revision. Uptake in zone 4 (arrow head) of the left femur stem reduced, compared to previous bone scan that acquired 8 years ago before the revision (**c, same image of Fig. 11.1** (**c**)). (**d**)–(**f**) Axial CT images show a large cystic mass (arrow heads) in the left iliac fossa and inguinal area, displacing femoral vessels to medial side (arrow). No contrast enhancement is seen within the mass. (**h**), (**i**) Coronal and (**j**) sagittal CT images demonstrate the extension of the mass (arrow heads). The cystic mass appears to have eroded adjacent cortical bone (long arrows) of preexisting osteolysis in the left iliac bone and acetabulum. (**g**) T1 TSE axial and (**k**) T2 STIR coronal MR images show a large hemorrhagic mass with dark signal intensity wall on both images (arrow head). A mixture of low to high signal intensity on both images suggests repeated bleeding

(WAIOT) definition. The WAIOT definition includes only two imaging techniques, bone scan and WBC scan, respectively, as a rule-out and rule-in test to define PJI [10].

TPBS has high sensitivity but low specificity for diagnosing certain disease including PJI. However, if TPBS is negative in all three phases, infection can be ruled out considering the high negative predictive value (NPV) [11].

WBC scan—if necessary, combined with a bone marrow scan—has very high specificity for identifying PJI and is the most reliable imaging tool. The reported accuracy of the combined WBC scan and bone marrow scan ranges from 83% to 98% for both hip and knee prosthesis infections [12]. Most of the largest researches show a high NPV for WBC scan, ranging from 92% to 100% [13]. SPECT/CT using ^{99m}Tc-HMPAO-WBC without performing bone marrow scan can be the most valuable imaging technique in diagnosing PJI [14]. As with TPBS, PJI can be excluded from diagnosis if the WBC scan is negative.

Case 11.3

Two years after the patient of Case 11.1 and 11.2 undergoing excision of CEH and revision of the left acetabular cup, he visited again the outpatient clinic because of pain and discharge in the right proximal thigh for a month. Right hip revision surgery was performed due to loosening 10 years ago. He had a draining sinus in the skin of anterolateral proximal thigh (Fig. 11.3a). He had already been taking antibiotics at another clinic for 10 days. Radiograph showed no significant abnormal findings (Fig. 11.3b). TPBS showed distinctly increased vascular and blood pool in the right anterolateral thigh (Fig. 11.3d, e) and increased uptake around greater trochanter reattachment device (GTRD), zone 1 and 7 of the right femur on delayed phase (Fig. 11.3f). CT showed a complicated fluid collection from the anterolateral side of the right hip, which drain to the skin (Fig. 11.3c). It was not difficult to diagnose PJI clinically because there was turbid discharge through the skin sinus tract. He had extensive and meticulous debridement of infected soft tissue and irrigation, and then an antibiotic impregnated cement spacer was placed in its place (Fig. 11.3g). Surgeons confirmed during surgery that the draining sinus in the skin was communicated to the hip joint. Microbial cultures of synovium and periprosthestic soft tissue collected during surgery and preoperatively were all negative, and pathologic report revealed inflamed granulation tissue with abscess and necrosis. After 7 weeks, he underwent surgery to remove the antibiotic spacer and additional debridement through irrigation, but exchange of prosthesis was not performed considering the patient's various circumstances.

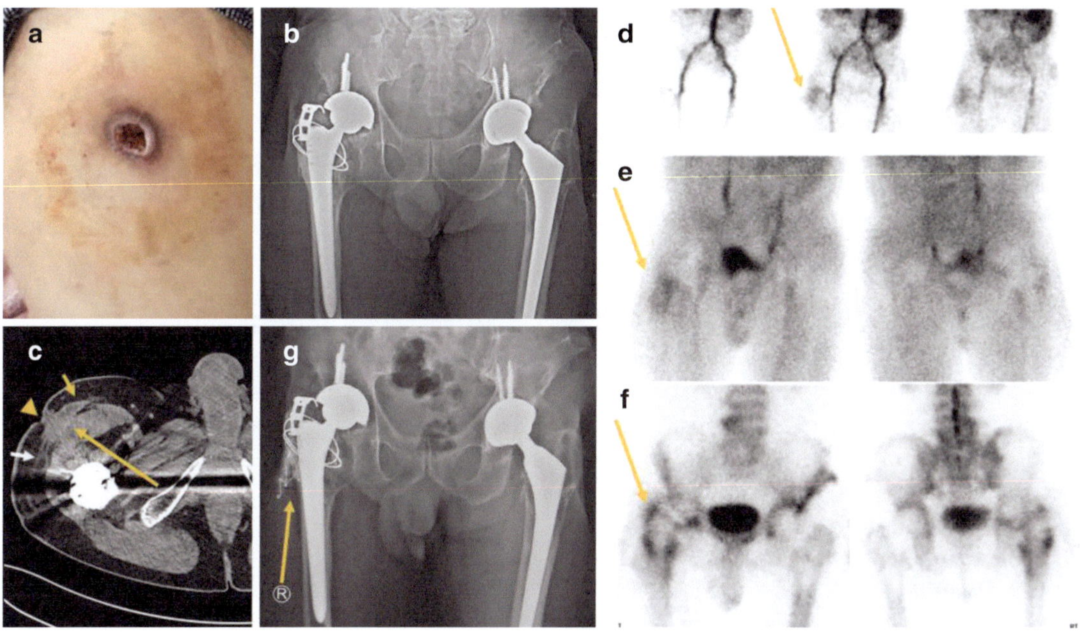

Fig. 11.3 (**a**) Sinus tract on anterolateral skin of right proximal thigh. (**b**) Radiograph shows a thin radiolucency in zones 1 and 7 and periosteal bone formation in zones 1, 2, 5, and 6 of right femur without longstanding change (serial radiographs not shown). (**c**) Enhanced axial CT shows fluid collection (long arrow) with a skin sinus tract (arrow head) in anterolateral thigh and surrounding subcutaneous infiltration (short white arrow). There is peripheral rim enhancement (short arrow) in the fluid collection. (**d**), (**e**) Localized increased uptake (arrow) in anterolateral proximal thigh on both vascular and blood pool phase of bone scan, which may be corresponding to the fluid collection area on CT. (**f**) Increased uptake (arrow) around GTRD, zones 1 and 7 of the right femur on delayed phase bone scan. (**g**) Radiograph after surgery shows placement of antibiotic spacer (arrow)

11.4 Osteolysis in THA

Osteolysis (OL) is expansile lytic lesion adjacent to one of the implants that is greater than or equal to 1 cm in any one dimension or increasing in size on serial radiographs or CT [2]. OL is usually aseptic and the result of an inflammatory immune response to particulate wear debris [15].

Serial radiographs are most commonly used to identify OL, but radiography has a sensitivity of only 41.5% [16]. CT provides greater sensitivity for OL detection than radiography and is marginally superior to MRI [17]. The sensitivity and specificity for diagnosing acetabular OL by bone scan were 34% and 0%, respectively [18]. The significance of bone scan for diagnosing OL is still uncertain. OL itself does not imply loosening, but OL can predate aseptic loosening. It is often difficult to predict the progression of OL because most cases are asymptomatic. Clinical decision-making regarding asymptomatic OL in patients with otherwise well-functioning THA remains a challenge. If the amount of the remaining bone stock is small, the outcome of revision surgery is likely to be poor. Therefore, regardless of functional failure of THA, the operation may be decided by considering the rate of OL, the amount of the remaining bone stock, and the patient's medical risk.

Case 11.4

A 78-year-old man who underwent bilateral THA visited to the outpatient clinic with intermittent right hip pain. The right one was operated 17 years ago and the left one 13 years ago.

Serial radiographs showed the position of the right femoral head was gradually shifting upper outward (Fig. 11.4a–c), suggesting polyethylene (PE) liner wear. Localized osteolytic lesions in zones I and II of the right acetabulum have newly appeared on latest radiograph (Fig. 11.4c). For femoral component, subsidence of the right femur prosthesis progressed gradually, and radiolucency around the flange of femoral stem was increasing (Fig. 11.4a–c). Pelvic bone CT showed large (5 × 4.6 × 2.6 cm in dimension) osteolysis in zones I–III of the right acetabulum, and the extent of osteolysis was wider than radiograph (Fig. 11.4d). TPBS showed no abnormal uptake in the right hip prosthesis area in all three phases (Fig. 11.4e, f). He underwent revision operation, and loosening of the acetabular cup was confirmed at the time of surgery. Osteolytic bone defect in the acetabulum was filled using allograft bone chips, and acetabular cup and femoral head were exchanged.

11.5 Failure of Impacted Bone Graft in THA

Impaction bone grafting (IBG) is now a routine technique in revision THA for acetabular defects caused by OL or loosing. Bone graft provides a substrate and scaffolding for development of bone structure. Allograft is commonly used, despite of drawbacks such as lack of osteoinductive property, disease transmission, inconsistent incorporation, and immune reactions. Histological studies have shown complete incorporation of allograft cancellous chips was replaced by newly formed trabeculae [19].

Bone allografts have high opacity and attenuation on initial postoperative radiograph and CT, which gradually decrease over time, as graft incorporation progresses. This process can take up to 18 months and CT can better show this process.

TPBS can be used to evaluate the viability of bone graft. Increased flow indicates preserved blood supply to graft region along with increased blood pooling, and delayed image reveals increased uptake ascertaining the integrity and viability of the bone allograft. However, these findings can be seen in various diseases. SPECT/CT can be useful in the assessment of graft viability in THA because CT can increase the specificity.

Case 11.5

A 81-year-old woman who underwent revision THA of right hip 9 years ago was referred to the clinic to evaluate the worsening right hip pain for 1 month.

On radiograph, one of the screws inserted into the acetabular cup came out to the level of femur neck, and the density of acetabulum around the cup appeared to be rather high (Fig. 11.5a). CT showed high attenuation area that looked like

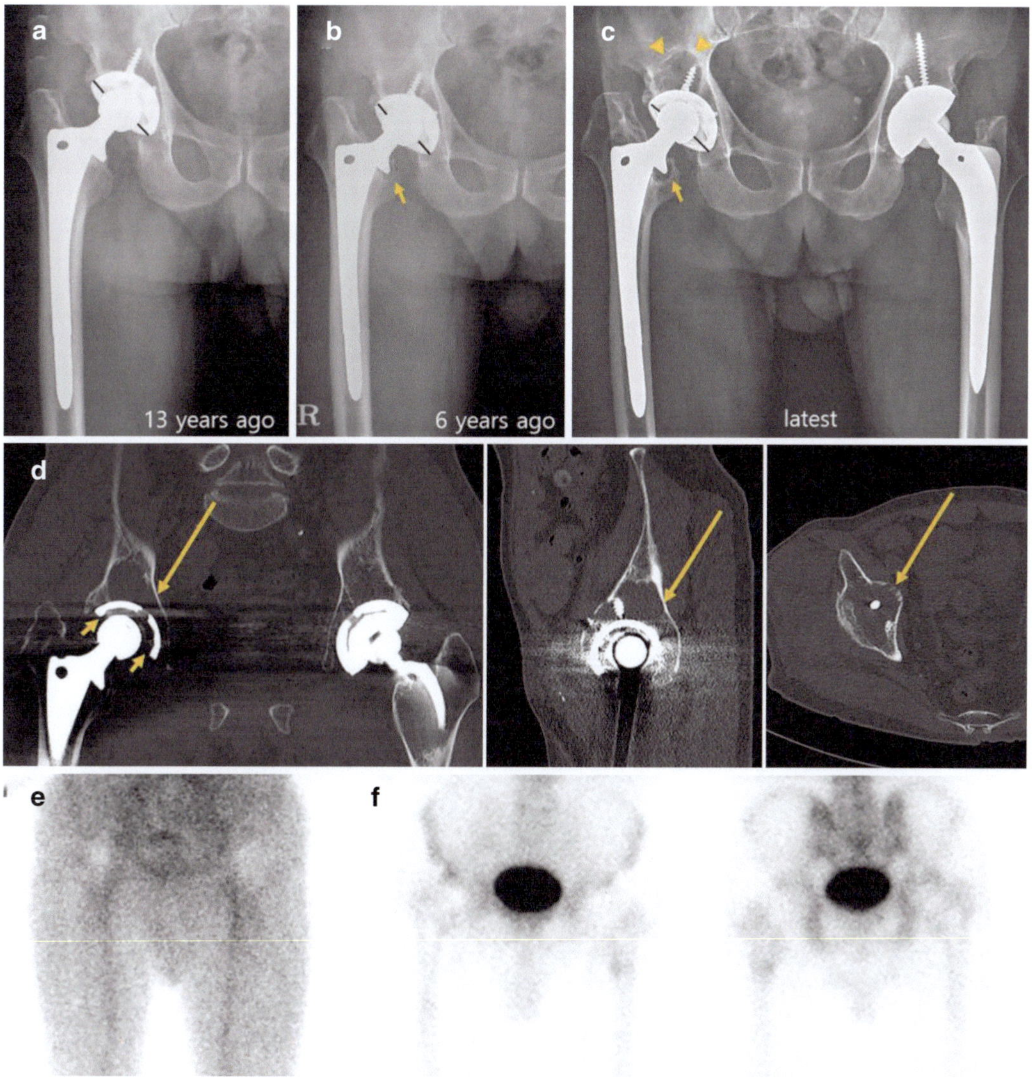

Fig. 11.4 (**a**–**c**) Serial radiographs show (1) wear of PE liner; see the length of black bars, (2) gradual progression of subsidence of right femoral stem, (3) radiolucency around flange of the femoral stem (short arrow), (4) an osteolytic lesion above acetabular cup (arrow heads). (**d**) Coronal, sagittal, and axial CT show a large osteolysis (arrows) in zones I–III of right acetabulum. Note wear of PE liner on coronal image (short arrow). (**e**), (**f**) There is no abnormal uptake in right hip region on blood pool and delayed image of bone scan

mosaic fragments in the acetabulum around the cup (Fig. 11.5c–e). Bone scan showed slightly increased uptake approximating to the acetabular cup (Fig. 11.6b). SPECT/CT showed slightly increased uptake in IBG area of the acetabulum (Fig. 11.5f–h).

Although there was no clear evidence to consider the cause of the pain in clinical and imaging investigation, she finally underwent re-revision surgery because she complained of very severe hip pain. There was no loosening of the acetabular cup at the time of surgery, but the bone graft fragments filled in the acetabulum during revision 9 years ago remained unincorporated into the host bone (Fig. 11.5i). After removing all the bone fragments, new implants were placed.

Radiotracer uptake in bone graft is accepted as an evidence of bone viability and patency of microvascular anastomosis. It is hard to explain why this happened and what is the relation between failure of incorporation of bone graft and worsening hip pain in this patient.

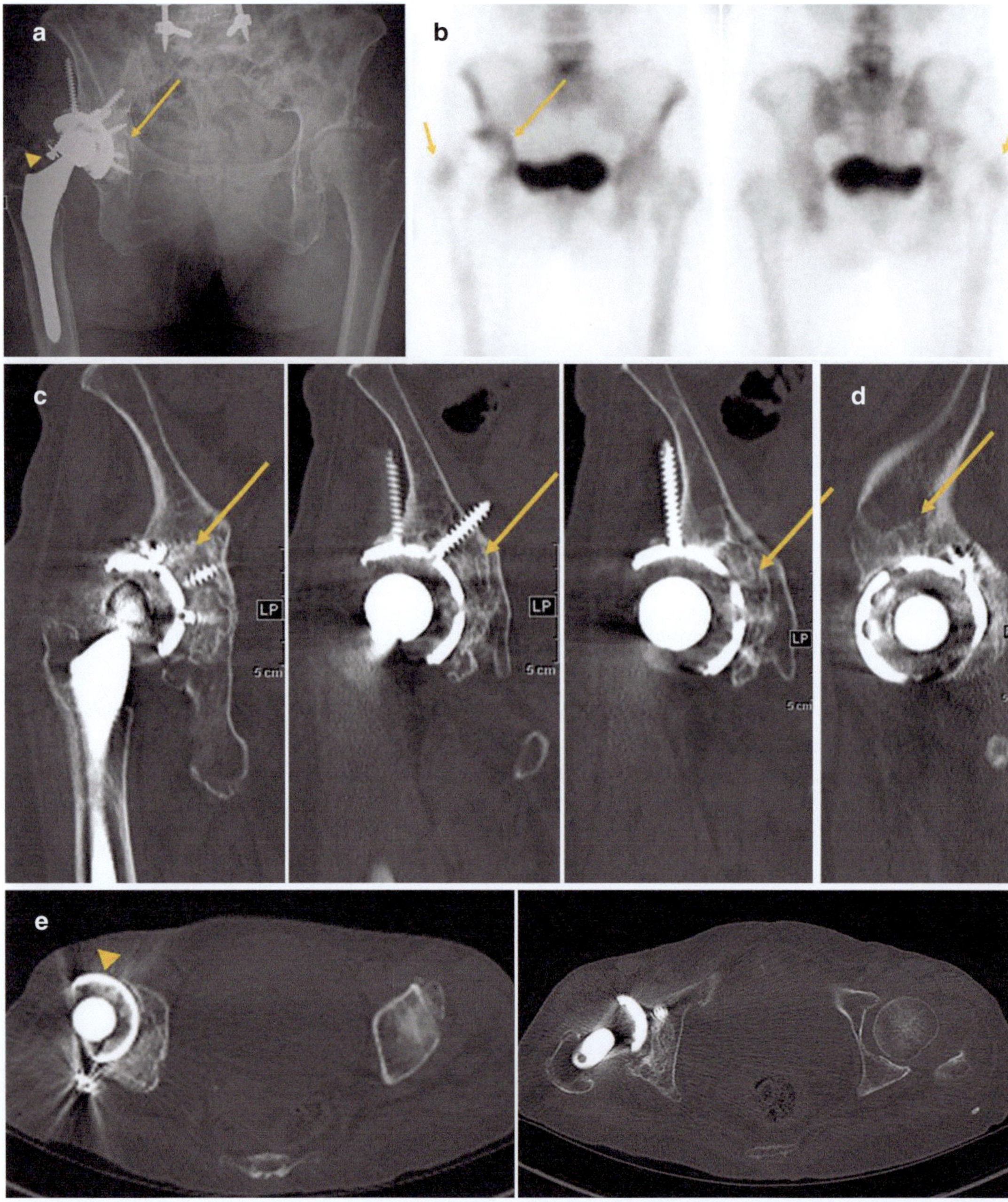

Fig. 11.5 (**a**) Radiograph shows an acetabular screw prolapse (arrow head) and high attenuation (arrow) around the acetabular cup. (**b**) Bone scan shows slightly increased uptake approximating to the acetabular cup (arrow) and greater trochanter (short arrow, shown as osteolysis on radiograph). (**c**), (**d**) Coronal and sagittal CT images show well high attenuation area that looks like mosaic fragments (arrows) in acetabulum around the cup, which has proved to bone graft fragments filled during previous surgery. (**e**) In addition, axial CT image shows acetabular component retroversion (arrow). (**f**) Bone SPECT, (**g**) CT, and (**h**) fused SPECT/CT images show slightly increased uptake in IBG area of the acetabulum. (**i**) There are few traces of bone ingrowth on outer surface of retrieved cup (short arrow). Removed bone fragments maintain their shape one by one (long arrow)

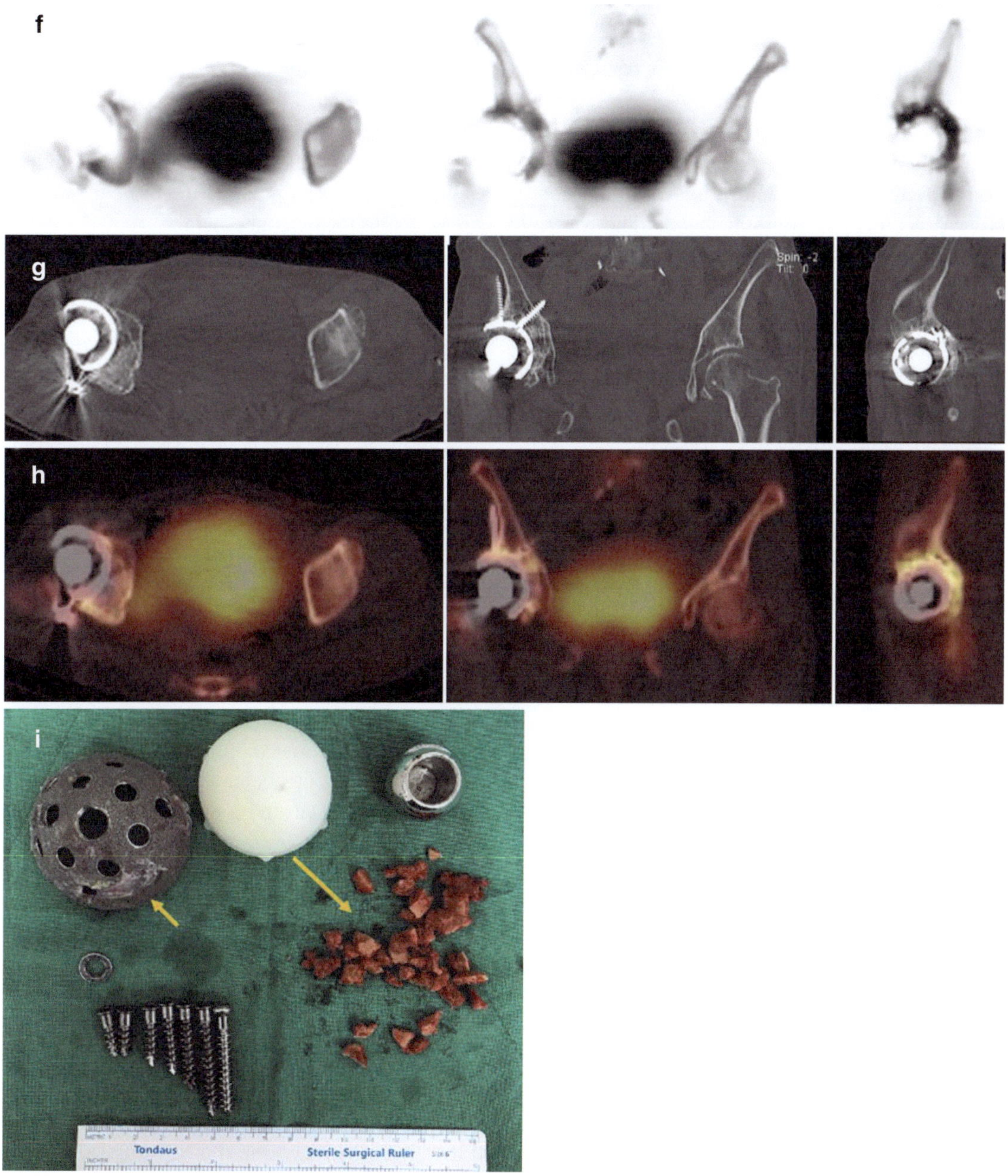

Fig. 11.5 (continued)

11.6 Avascular Necrosis of Femoral Head After Internal Fixation of Femoral Neck Fractures

One of the main complications after internal fixation of femoral neck fracture is avascular necrosis (AVN) of the femoral head. The overall incidence of AVN after internal fixation of femoral neck fracture is 15–25%, and about 20% of these patients required further surgical treatment. Disruption of the blood supply to the femoral head at the time of injury is considered primary mechanism responsible for AVN of the femoral head following femoral neck fracture.

MRI is the most useful imaging modality in detecting early stage of AVN of the femoral head; however, the diagnostic value of MRI in patients undergoing internal fixation has a limitation due to susceptibility artifact from metallic implant.

Bone scan has advantages in this respect and has been widely used in diagnosing early AVN because the blood supply is one of the major factors affecting bone uptake of bone radiotracer. By applying SPECT to bone scan and adding a CT image with SPECT, diagnostic ability in the detection of AVN has improved [20]. The performance of bone SPECT/CT for predicting development of AVN depends on the time point of imaging after surgical fixation because revascularization occurs; therefore, bone SPECT/CT can be performed at least 3 months after surgery of femoral neck fracture to reliably predict the possibility of AVN [21].

Case 11.6

A 60-year-old woman 5 months after undergoing multiple pinning for fracture of right femur neck was considering joint replacement surgery for the fused left hip joint. She took radiography, bone scan, and SPECT/CT for preoperative evaluation. Radiograph showed complete union of fracture of the right femur neck with multiple pinning still in place (Fig. 11.6b). Bone scan showed marked lumbar scoliosis and left hip flexion deformity due to fused hip joint. Moderately increased linear uptake was observed in the right femoral neck, which may be suspected for delayed healing, and abnormal uptake in the right femoral head was not evident (Fig. 11.6a). However, SPECT and SPECT/CT revealed a relatively large size of photon defect in most of anterior half of the right femur head with surrounding irregular band-like uptake (Fig. 11.6c–e), which is reasonable for osteonecrosis.

In this case, it was difficult to diagnose with planar images alone, but it was possible to diagnose by obtaining SPECT/CT. Since the location of the photon defect was in anterior half of the femoral head, it is thought that the lesion was masked by radioactivity of posterior half of the head and distorted pelvic position. The increased uptake in the femur neck area on planar image (Fig. 11.6a) represents reactive margin of AVN, not delayed healing of the fracture.

11.7 Fracture-Related Infection

Fracture-related infection (FRI) is a serious complication in orthopedic surgery leading to poor bone healing and loss of function. In the case of open fractures, it has been reported that the incidence of FRI can reach up to 30%.

The radiologic signs, suggesting FRI, are as follows: bone lysis (fracture site, around the implant), implant loosening, sequestration, nonunion, and periosteal bone formation at localizations other than the fracture site.

Bone scan (including triple phase) has a high sensitivity (89–100%) but low specificity (0%–10%) for diagnosing FRI, so it is not recommended in the assessment of FRI. WBC scan is the most reliable imaging tool for orthopedic infection. Due to the physiological bone marrow uptake and the lack of detailed anatomical information, it is often difficult to distinguish between the infection-induced accumulation of labeled leukocytes and the marrow accumulation of these cells. Additional bone marrow scan is sometimes needed to solve this problem. However, recent hybrid SPECT/CT imaging allows for better anatomic details without an additional bone marrow scan. WBC SPECT/CT showed a high diagnostic accuracy (92%) for detecting an FRI in the peripheral skeleton [22].

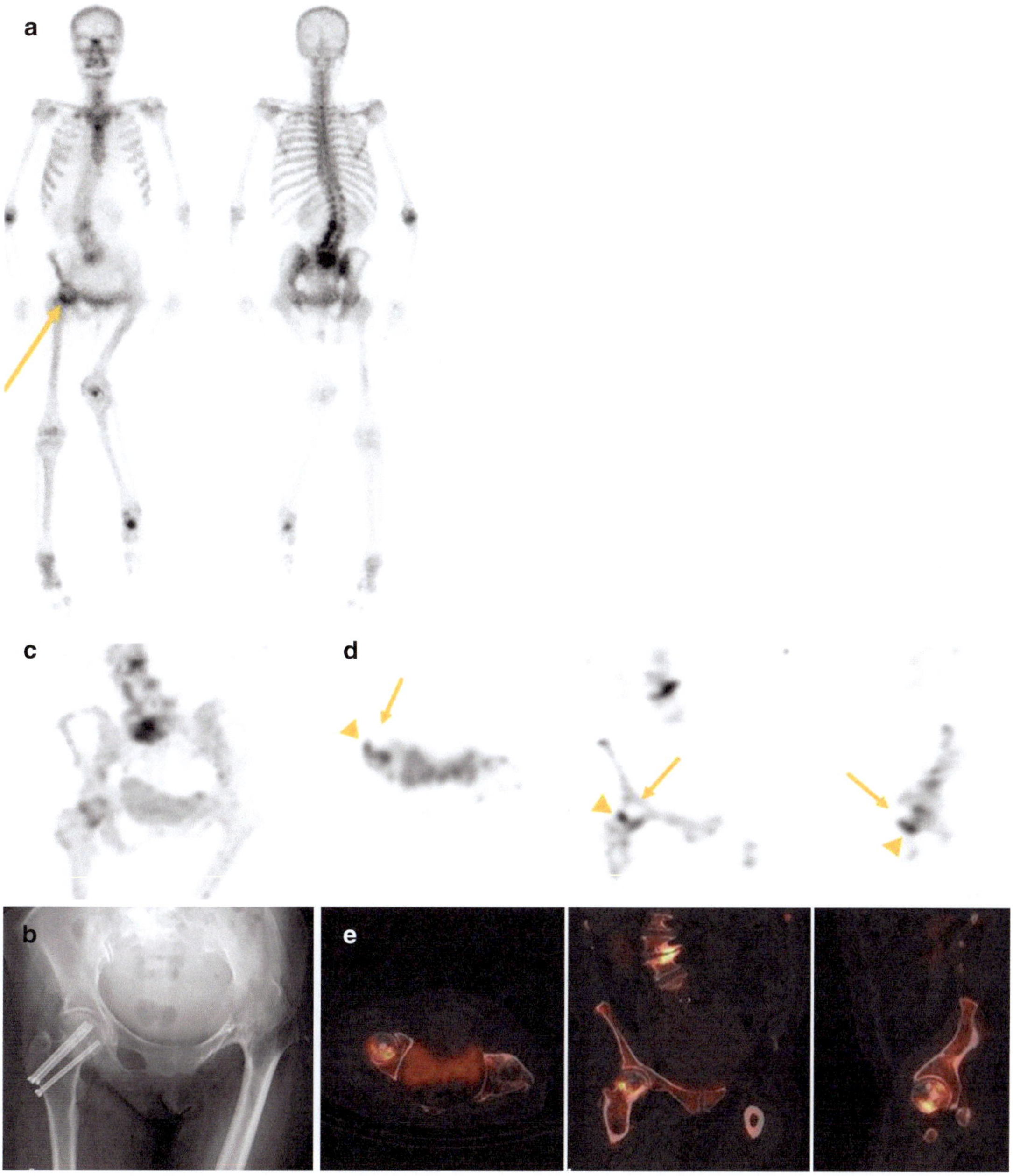

Fig. 11.6 (**a**) Whole-body bone scan shows moderately increased linear uptake (arrow) in right femur neck but no abnormal uptake in right head portion. (**b**) Radiograph shows healed fracture in right femur neck with multiple pinning status. (**c**) MIP image of bone SPECT, (**d**) bone SPECT, and (**e**) fused SPECT/CT images show a large photon defect (arrow) in most of anterior half of right femur head with surrounding irregular band-like radiotracer uptake (arrow head), suggesting reactive margin of osteonecrosis

Case 11.7

A 65-year-old man with hip pain visited to the clinic 4 months after undergoing open reduction and internal fixation due to subtrochanteric fracture of left femur. Radiograph showed non-union of the fracture site and loosening of the inserted screw (Fig. 11.7c). ^{99m}Tc-Hexamethlypropylene amine oxime (HMPAO)-labeled WBC whole-body imaging obtained on 4 h showed multifocal foci of leukocyte uptake in the left upper thigh

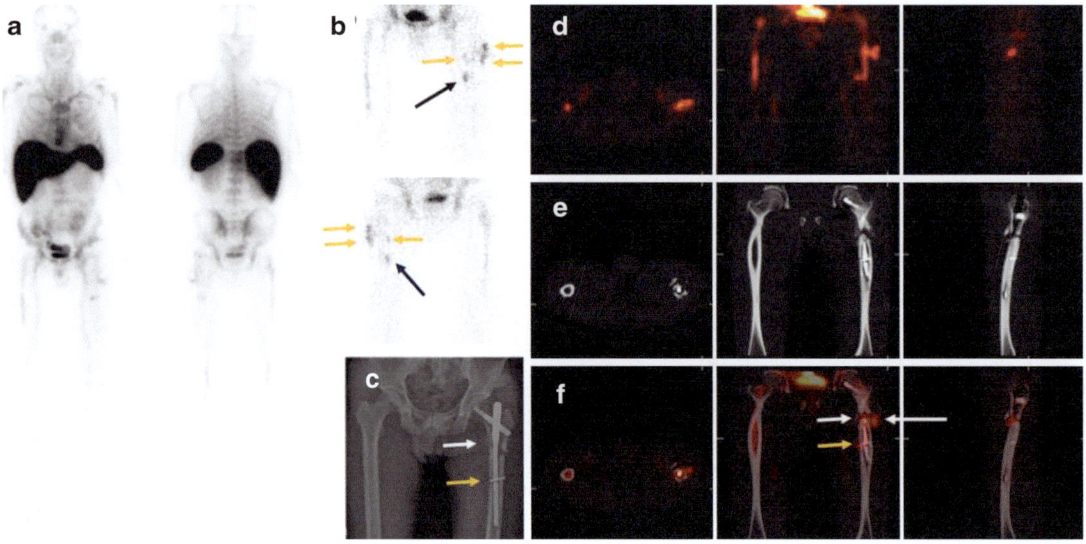

Fig. 11.7 (**a**) ^{99m}Tc-HMPAO whole-body planar images show multifocal foci of leukocyte uptake in the left upper thigh. (**b**) Delayed planar images more clearly show the uptakes (black arrow) seen in early whole-body image and additional foci (yellow arrows) of leukocyte uptakes in the left upper thigh. (**c**) Radiograph shows non-union of the fracture site (white arrow) and loosening of the inserted screw (yellow arrow). (**d–f**) SPECT, CT, and fused SPECT/CT images show accurate localization of leukocyte uptake; the infected non-union site (white arrow), contiguous perifemoral soft tissue abscess (long white arrow), anteromedial aspect of the infected loosening of screw (yellow arrow)

instead of less visible physiologic bone marrow activity in the femur (Fig. 11.7a). Delayed regional planar image obtained on 21 h revealed more clearly the uptakes seen in early image and additional foci of leukocyte uptakes (Fig. 11.7b). ^{99m}Tc-HMPAO SPECT/CT obtained on 4 h showed precise localization of leukocyte uptake in the infected non-union site, contiguous perifemoral soft tissue abscess at lateral aspect of the non-union site, and anteromedial aspect of the infected loosening of screw (Fig. 11.7d–f). In this case, although radiograph shows helpful findings such as non-union and implant loosening suggesting infection (Fig. 11.7c), these are not specific for infection. However, WBC scan and SPECT/CT provide very specific information leading to confirmatory diagnosis.

11.8 Subchondral Insufficiency Fracture of Femur Head

Subchondral insufficiency fracture of femur head (SIFFH) is known as a rare condition and caused by normal or physiological stress without antecedent trauma and usually occurs in elderly patients with poor bone quality. However, it has been reported in patients who were treated with corticosteroids for rheumatoid arthritis and organ (kidney, liver) transplantation.

SIFFH presents acute hip pain and can cause femoral head collapse leading to osteoarthritis, like osteonecrosis. For these reasons, it is often important to differentiate it from osteonecrosis. A majority has symptom resolution with non-operative management, and those that worsened, approximately 35%, are typically managed with surgical treatment, i.e. THA.

MRI is most commonly used for the diagnosis of SIFFH [23]. The characteristic findings such as low signal intensity band-like lesion representing subchondral fracture and bone marrow edema patterns are distinct from those of osteonecrosis.

Radiography is usually normal until head collapse occurs, and CT will be helpful in finding subchondral radiolucent line (crescent sign). Regarding bone scan, several cases of increased uptake of femoral head have been reported.

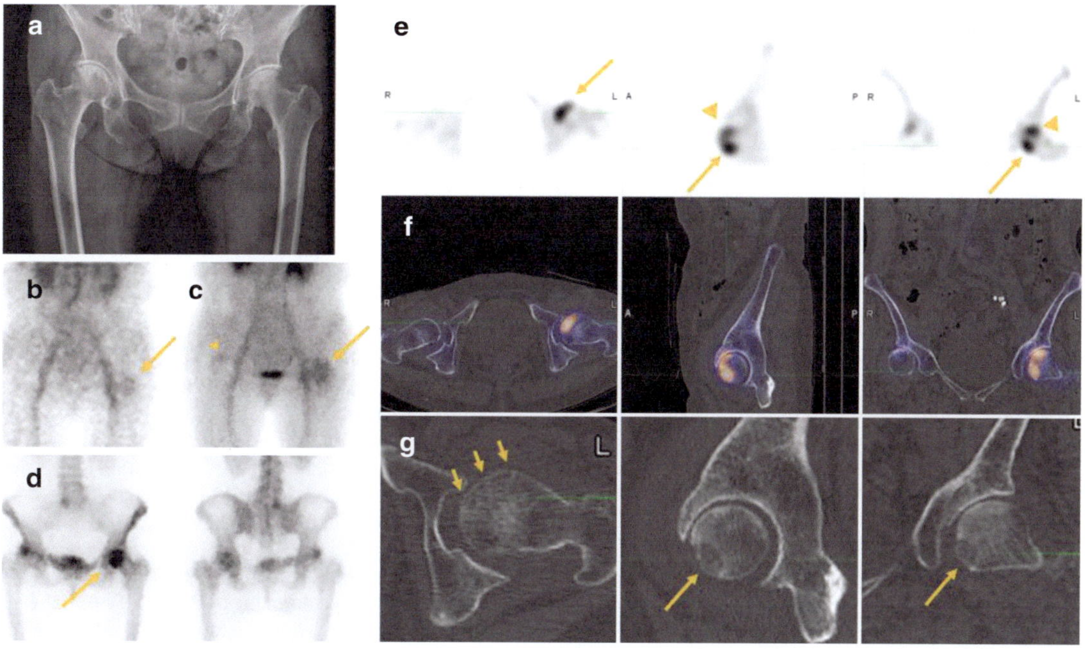

Fig. 11.8 (**a**) Radiograph shows osteoarthritis in the right hip and no remarkable finding in the left hip region. (**b**), (**c**) Increased uptake in the left femur head region (arrow) on both vascular and blood pool images of bone scan. Mild focal uptake of the right hip joint area in blood pool image is seen (arrow head). (**d**) Delayed anterior and posterior bone scan images show increased uptake in the left femur head (arrow on anterior image) and both hip joints. (**e**), (**f**) On SPECT and SPECT/CT, increased uptake with subchondral fracture is observed in the left femur head (arrow in **e** [SPECT image]) and osteoarthritis (arrow head in **e** [SPECT image]. (**g**) Magnified CT images of the same section show subchondral radiolucency parallel to articular surface (short arrow on axial image, long arrow on sagittal and coronal image), consistent with subchondral fracture

Case 11.8

An 81-year-old woman presented with left hip pain for 2 months. She had no recent trauma history. Radiograph showed no abnormal finding in the left hip and mild osteoarthritic change in the right hip (Fig. 11.8a). TPBS showed increased vascular and blood pool activity in large area of the left femur head region (Fig. 11.8b, c). Delayed image of TPBS showed moderately increased uptake in the left femur head, mainly anterior portion (Fig. 11.8d). SPECT and SPECT/CT showed increased uptake (Fig. 11.8e, f) associated with subchondral radiolucent line (radiographic crescent sign), parallel to articular surface, in anteromedial portion of the left femur head on CT (Fig. 11.8g). This is consistent with subchondral insufficiency fracture.

In patients with acute hip pain who have no antecedent trauma, SIFFH should be included in the differential diagnosis when images of all phases of TPBS show increased uptake in the femoral head. Additional SPECT/CT can be helpful to detect the subchondral fracture.

Teaching Points

- You should consider the following when reading bone scan of patients who have undergone THA: (1) It is to know the normal findings according to the time window after surgery. Bone scan may be falsely positive up to 2 years after hip joint replacement. (2) It is essential to check serial radiographs (beginning with the most recent) and patient's clinical symptoms.
- When a cystic mass is seen in the replaced hip joint area, CEH may be added to differential diagnosis, in addition to ALTR, benign and malignant tumor, and deep infection.
- Bone SPECT/CT can be useful in the assessment of painful hip with/without surgery because CT can increase the specificity.

- WBC SPECT/CT without performing bone marrow scan can be the most valuable imaging technique in diagnosing PJI and FRI.

References

1. Herberts P, Malchau H. Long-term registration has improved the quality of hip replacement: a review of the Swedish THR Register comparing 160,000 cases. Acta Orthop Scand. 2000;71:111–21. https://doi.org/10.1080/000164700317413067.
2. Healy WL, Iorio R, Clair AJ, Pellegrini VD, Della Valle CJ, Berend KR. Complications of total hip arthroplasty: standardized list, definitions, and stratification developed by the hip society. Clin Orthop Relat Res. 2016;474:357–64. https://doi.org/10.1007/s11999-015-4341-7.
3. DeLee JG, Charnley J. Radiological demarcation of cemented sockets in total hip replacement. Clin Orthop Relat Res. 1976;121:20–32.
4. Gruen TA, McNeice GM, Amstutz HC. "Modes of failure" of cemented stem-type femoral components: a radiographic analysis of loosening. Clin Orthop Relat Res. 1979;141:17–27.
5. Temmerman OPP, Raijmakers PGHM, Deville WL, Berkhof J, Hooft L, Heyligers IC. The use of plain radiography, subtraction arthrography, nuclear arthrography, and bone scintigraphy in the diagnosis of a loose acetabular component of a total hip prosthesis: a systematic review. J Arthroplasty. 2007;22:818–27. https://doi.org/10.1016/j.arth.2006.08.004.
6. Temmerman OPP, Raijmakers PGHM, Berkhof J, Hoekstra OS, GJJ T, Heyligers IC. Accuracy of diagnostic imaging techniques in the diagnosis of aseptic loosening of the femoral component of a hip prosthesis: a meta-analysis. J Bone Joint Surg Br. 2005;87:781–5. https://doi.org/10.1302/0301-620X.87B6.15625.
7. Reid JD, Kommareddi S, Lankerani M, Park MC. Chronic expanding hematomas. A clinicopathologic entity. JAMA. 1980;244:2441–2.
8. Goddard MS, Vakil JJ, McCarthy EF, Khanuja HS. Chronic expanding hematoma of the lateral thigh and massive bony destruction after a failed total hip arthroplasty. J Arthroplasty. 2011;26:338.e13–5. https://doi.org/10.1016/j.arth.2009.11.015.
9. Ando W, Yamamoto K, Koyama T, Hashimoto Y, Yasui H, Tsujimoto T, et al. Chronic expanding hematoma after metal-on-metal total hip arthroplasty. Orthopedics. 2017;40:e1103–6. https://doi.org/10.3928/01477447-20170619-04.
10. Bozhkova S, Suardi V, Sharma HK, Tsuchiya H, Del Sel H, Hafez MA, et al. The W.A.I.O.T. definition of peri-prosthetic joint infection: a multi-center, retrospective validation study. J Clin Med. 2020;9:1965. https://doi.org/10.3390/jcm9061965.
11. Signore A, Sconfienza LM, Borens O, Glaudemans AWJM, Cassar-Pullicino V, Trampuz A, et al. Consensus document for the diagnosis of prosthetic joint infections: a joint paper by the EANM, EBJIS, and ESR (with ESCMID endorsement). Eur J Nucl Med Mol Imaging. 2019;46:971–88. https://doi.org/10.1007/s00259-019-4263-9.
12. Gemmel F, Van den Wyngaert H, Love C, Welling MM, Gemmel P, Palestro CJ. Prosthetic joint infections: radionuclide state-of-the-art imaging. Eur J Nucl Med Mol Imaging. 2012;39:892–909. https://doi.org/10.1007/s00259-012-2062-7.
13. Erba PA, Glaudemans AWJM, Veltman NC, Sollini M, Pacilio M, Galli F, et al. Image acquisition and interpretation criteria for 99mTc-HMPAO-labelled white blood cell scintigraphy: results of a multicentre study. Eur J Nucl Med Mol Imaging. 2014;41:615–23. https://doi.org/10.1007/s00259-013-2631-4.
14. Kim HO, Na SJ, Oh SJ, Jung BS, Lee S, Chang JS, et al. Usefulness of adding SPECT/CT to 99mTc-hexamethylpropylene amine oxime (HMPAO)-labeled leukocyte imaging for diagnosing prosthetic joint infections. J Comput Assist Tomogr. 2014;38:313–9. https://doi.org/10.1097/RCT.0000000000000011.
15. Hallab NJ, Jacobs JJ. Biologic effects of implant debris. Bull NYU Hosp Jt Dis. 2009;67:182–8.
16. Claus AM, Engh CA, Sychterz CJ, Xenos JS, Orishimo KF, Engh CA. Radiographic definition of pelvic osteolysis following total hip arthroplasty. J Bone Joint Surg Am. 2003;85:1519–26. https://doi.org/10.2106/00004623-200308000-00013.
17. Walde TA, Weiland DE, Leung SB, Kitamura N, Sychterz CJ, Engh CA, et al. Comparison of CT, MRI, and radiographs in assessing pelvic osteolysis: a cadaveric study. Clin Orthop Relat Res. 2005;437:138–44. https://doi.org/10.1097/01.blo.0000164028.14504.46.
18. Geerdink CH, Grimm B, Rahmy AIA, Vencken W, Heyligers IC, Tonino AJ. Correlation of Technetium-99m scintigraphy, progressive acetabular osteolysis and acetabular component loosening in total hip arthroplasty. Hip Int. 2010;20:460–5. https://doi.org/10.1177/112070001002000408.
19. Butscheidt S, Moritz M, Gehrke T, Püschel K, Amling M, Hahn M, et al. Incorporation and remodeling of structural allografts in acetabular reconstruction: multiscale, micro-morphological analysis of 13 pelvic explants. J Bone Joint Surg Am. 2018;100:1406–15. https://doi.org/10.2106/JBJS.17.01636.
20. Han S, Oh M, Yoon S, Kim J, Kim J, Chang J, et al. Risk stratification for avascular necrosis of the femoral head after internal fixation of femoral neck fractures by post-operative bone SPECT/CT. Nucl Med Mol Imaging. 2017;51:49–57. https://doi.org/10.1007/s13139-016-0443-8.
21. Kim JW, Ryu J, Baek S, Byun S, Chang JS. The timing of bone SPECT to predict osteonecrosis after internal fixation of femur neck fractures. J Orthop Sci

Off J Japan Orthop Assoc. 2017;22:457–62. https://doi.org/10.1016/j.jos.2016.12.014.

22. Govaert GAM, Bosch P, Ijpma FFA, Glauche J, Jutte PC, Lemans JVC, et al. High diagnostic accuracy of white blood cell scintigraphy for fracture related infections: Results of a large retrospective single-center study. Injury. 2018;49:1085–90. https://doi.org/10.1016/j.injury.2018.03.018.
23. Cabarrus MC, Ambekar A, Lu Y, Link TM. MRI and CT of insufficiency fractures of the pelvis and the proximal femur. AJR Am J Roentgenol. 2008;191:995–1001. https://doi.org/10.2214/AJR.07.3714.

Knee Prostheses

12

Yoo Sung Song

Abstract

Knee surgeries can be classified as joint-preserving surgeries such as osteotomy, ligament reconstruction, meniscus repair, and cartilage repair, and joint-replacing arthroplasties such as unicondylar knee arthroplasty (KA), patellofemoral joint arthroplasty, and total knee arthroplasty. While the incidence of knee surgeries has been increasing worldwide, substantial portion of patients experience failure. In Korea, over 70,000 cases of primary knee arthroplasties were done in 2019, with over 5000 cases of revision arthroplasties. The complicated knee anatomy and various etiologies of arthroplasty failure interfere with the accurate assessment of post-operative complications.

There are many knee prosthesis-related complications such as periprosthetic infection, aseptic loosening, polyethylene wear, osteolysis, metallosis, instability, and periprosthetic fracture. Distinguishing the periprosthetic uptake patterns on bone scans aids the differential diagnosis.

Keywords

Aseptic loosening · Bone SPECT/CT · Knee arthroplasty · Knee prosthesis · Periprosthetic fracture · Periprosthetic infection · Polyethylene wear

12.1 Assessment of Knee Operations

Uptake on single-photon emission computerized tomography and conventional computerized tomography (SPECT/CT) has been known to correlate with the degree of arthritis. Due to its unique features, SPECT/CT allows early detection of osteoarthritis by showing the loading on different compartments of the knee. Also, the operation results may be assessed by evaluating the change of tracer uptakes according to the realignment of mechanical stress.

Case 12.1 Post-operative Evaluation

A 59-year-old woman presented to the outpatient clinic due to bilateral knee pain. The impression was degenerative arthritis in both knee joints, with varus deformities. Radiographs showed joint space narrowing at bilateral joint spaces with varus alignments. Patient was planned for sequential high tibial open wedge osteotomy for bilateral knee joints, starting from the right knee joint. SPECT/CT images

Y. S. Song (✉)
Department of Nuclear Medicine, Seoul National University Bundang Hospital, Seongnam-si, Gyeonggi-do, Republic of Korea
e-mail: syoosung@snubh.org

S.-O. Yang et al. (eds.), *Atlas of Nuclear Medicine in Musculoskeletal System*,
https://doi.org/10.1007/978-981-19-2677-8_12

were acquired on post-operative day 1, immediately after right high tibial osteotomy. Images showed increased uptake in the right patellofemoral compartment and bilateral medial compartments. Two months after right high tibial osteotomy, the patient underwent left high tibial osteotomy. Serial SPECT/CT images were acquired 3 months after left high tibial osteotomy. The increased uptakes in the medial compartments on previous SPECT/CT showed significant improvement, implying redistribution of the mechanical load. Left knee showed post-operation-related uptakes in the osteotomy site (Fig. 12.1).

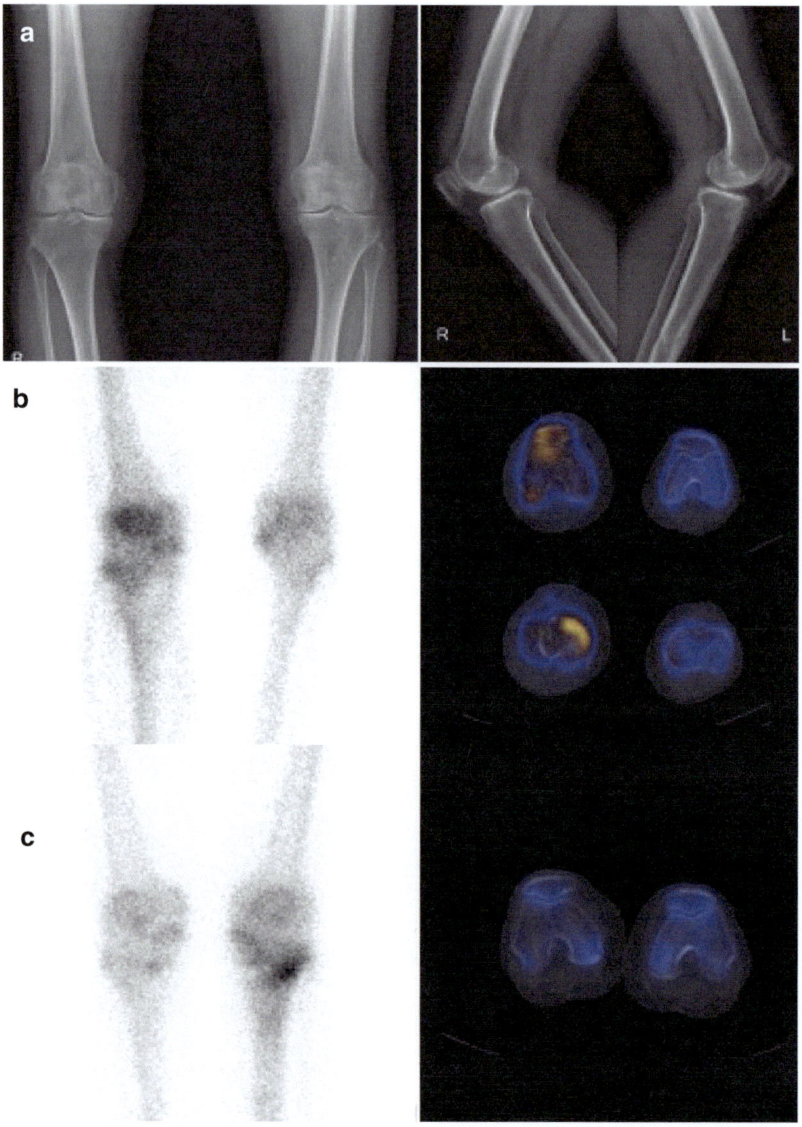

Fig. 12.1 (**a**) Preoperative radiograph, joint space narrowing at bilateral joint spaces with varus alignments. (**b**) Preoperative bone scan and SPECT/CT images, showing increased uptake in bilateral medial compartments and right patellofemoral compartment, consistent with degenerative arthritis findings. (**c**) Patient received right and left tibial wedge osteotomy serially. SPECT/CT was taken 12 months after right knee surgery, which was 2 months after left knee surgery. Uptakes of the right medial compartments have improved. Post-operative uptakes in the left wedge resection site are observed

12.2 Periprosthetic Infection

Acute periprosthetic infection occurs in about 2% of the patients who undergoes KA [1]. However, radiography has limited value in the diagnosis of infection, since findings vary from complete normal to total bone destruction [2]. Three-phase bone scans were reported to have a specificity of 56% and a sensitivity of 93% in the diagnosis of periprosthetic infection [3]. Lack of increased uptake in the blood flow phase and the blood pool phase is an important finding to exclude periprosthetic infection.

Case 12.2 Periprosthetic Infection
A 67-year-old woman presented to the outpatient clinic due to recently developed left knee pain. The patient had received bilateral total knee replacement arthroplasty (TKRA) 3 years ago. Serum ESR rates (34 mm/h) and CRP levels (7.47 mg/L) were elevated, with high WBC counts (13.0×10^9/L). Radiographs showed no abnormal post-operative findings. Bone scan and SPECT/CT images revealed diffuse increased uptake in the left tibial periprosthetic area.

Patient underwent revision surgery for all components of the left TKRA. During implant removal, there were severe bone defects in the tibial compartment, with pus discharge and yellowish soft tissue inflammation (Fig. 12.2).

Case 12.3 Periprosthetic Infection
A 76-year-old man presented to the outpatient clinic due to left knee pain that developed 2 months ago. Patient received bilateral TKRA 10 years ago. Radiographs showed radiolucent osteolysis in the left femoral compartment, with anterior cortex scalloping. Femoral loosening was suspected, and the patient underwent bone SPECT/CT. Bone SPECT/CT revealed diffuse increased uptake in the osteolytic lesion of the femoral compartment, with also diffuse increased uptake in the periprosthetic area of the tibial compartment. Patient underwent total replacement of the previous knee arthroplasty. Surgical findings revealed serous colored joint fluids, with bone defects in the periprosthetic area. There was a pus-filled cavity in the metaphyseal area of the femur (Fig. 12.3).

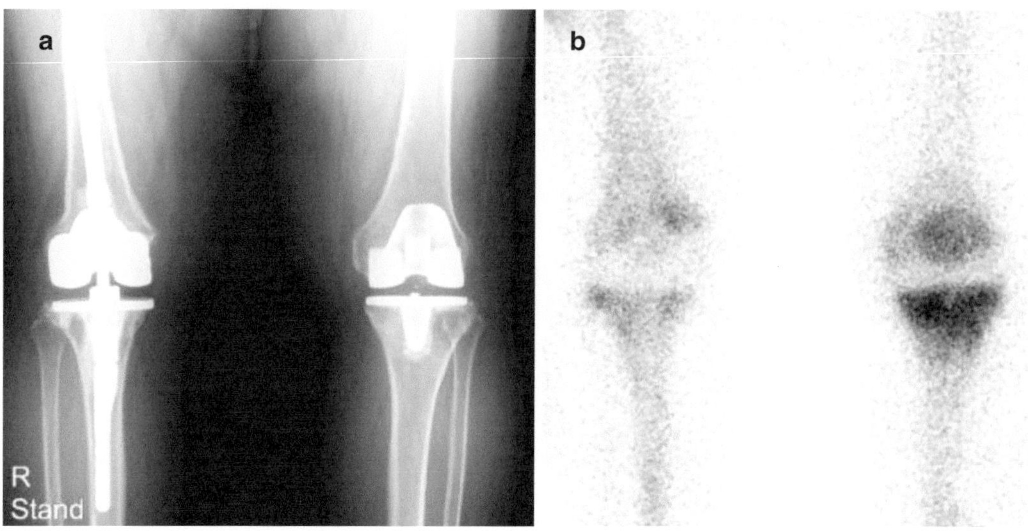

Fig. 12.2 (**a**) Anteroposterior radiograph view of the knee shows no significant abnormal findings. (**b**) Planar bone scan shows diffuse increased uptake in the left periprosthetic area, in the weight-bearing tibial aspect. (**c**) Bone SPECT/CT images also show diffuse increased uptake in the left tibial periprosthetic area, mainly in the anterior aspect seen on the sagittal view

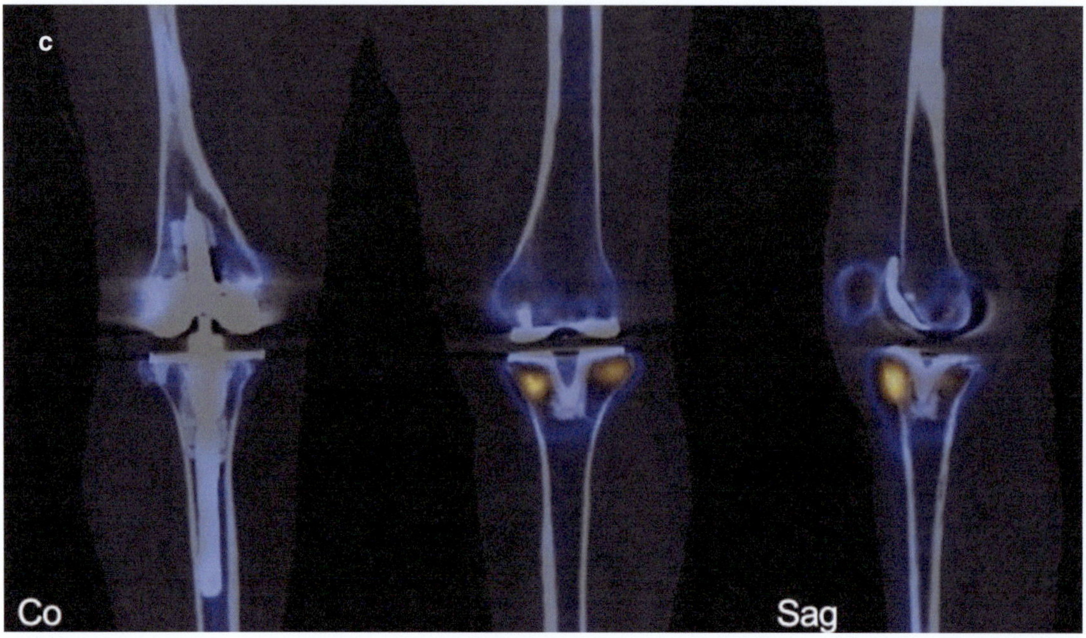

Fig. 12.2 (continued)

Fig. 12.3 (**a**) Osteolysis of the femoral compartment is suspected in the radiograph (red arrowhead). (**b**) Diffuse increased uptake of the left femoral compartment and periprosthetic area of the tibial compartment is observed in the planar bone scan. (**c**) Diffuse rim uptake around the osteolytic lesion of the femoral compartment is seen on SPECT/CT

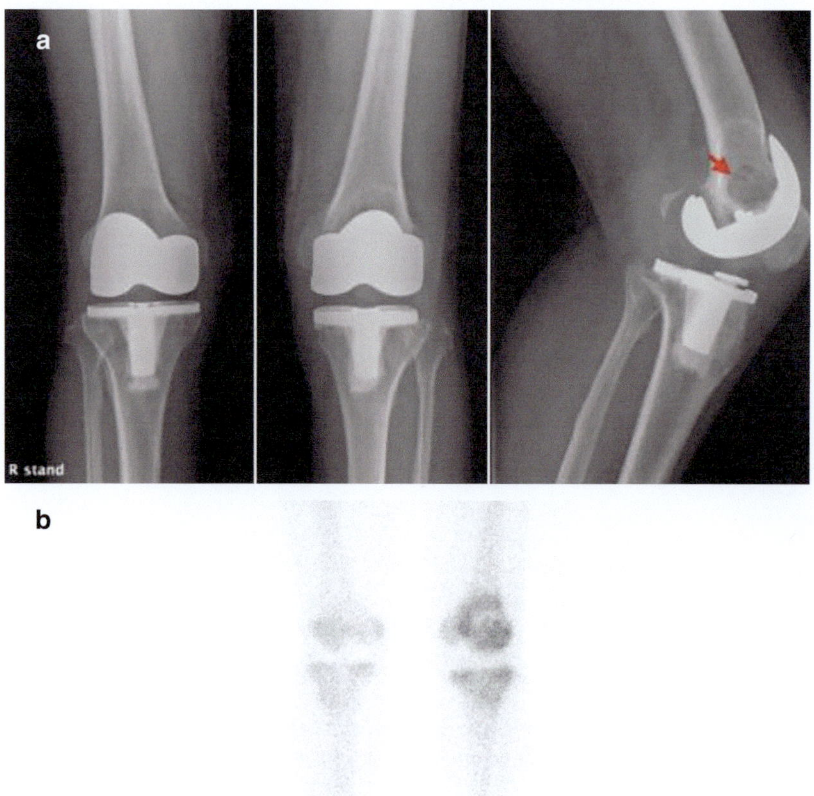

Fig. 12.3 (continued)

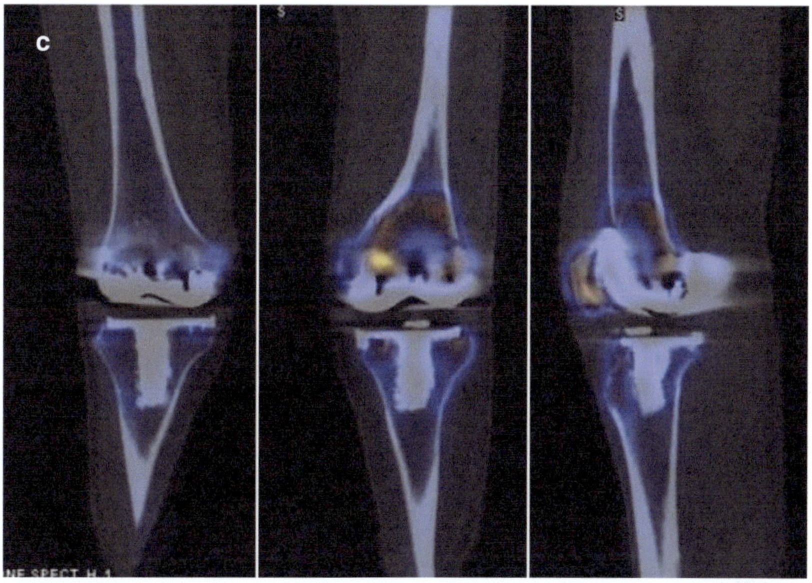

12.3 Aseptic Loosening

Aseptic loosening is the most common cause of late KA failure. It may be caused by metallic particle debris or repetitive mechanical stress. Typical radiographic findings show periprosthetic radiolucency, increasing in width on sequential follow-up. However, evaluating the width has its limitations due to standardizing proper position, rotation, and knee alignment during image acquisition [4]. Three-phase bone scans alone cannot differentiate between infection and aseptic loosening, since all phases may show increased uptakes. Also, interpretation of bone scans may be difficult in patients with suspected loosening, due to the variable periprosthetic uptake related to the post-operative physiological response.

Case 12.4 Prosthetic Loosening
A 74-year-old woman presented to the outpatient clinic due to left knee pain that developed 1 year ago. Patient received bilateral TKRA 8 years ago. Radiographs showed periprosthetic lucency under the medial and lateral tibial baseplate in the left knee, indicative of loosening. Bone SPECT/CT revealed increased uptake in the left femur medial condyle around the periprosthetic area. Patient received total replacement of knee arthroplasty for the left knee. Surgical findings revealed complete detachment of the femoral component with migration and collapse of the medial femoral condyle (Fig. 12.4).

12.4 Polyethylene Wear

Polyethylene wear is also a common complication, due to the friction of metal compartment to the polyethylene or delamination of the polyethylene surface. Radiographic findings show joint space loss, usually in the medial and lateral compartments. Polyethylene wear may also occur in the patellar compartment, which is better visualized in the axial radiographs compared to the lateral radiographs. Polyethylene wear-induced osteolysis may occur, resulting in aseptic loosening. However, the usefulness of bone scan in polyethylene wear is to evaluate the presence of consequent aseptic loosening.

Case 12.5 Polyethylene Wear
A 76-year-old woman presented to the outpatient clinic due to bilateral knee pain that developed 3 years ago. Patient received bilateral TKRA 15 years ago. Radiographs showed osteolysis at bilateral posterior flanges. Varus alignments with left joint space narrowing were observed. Bone

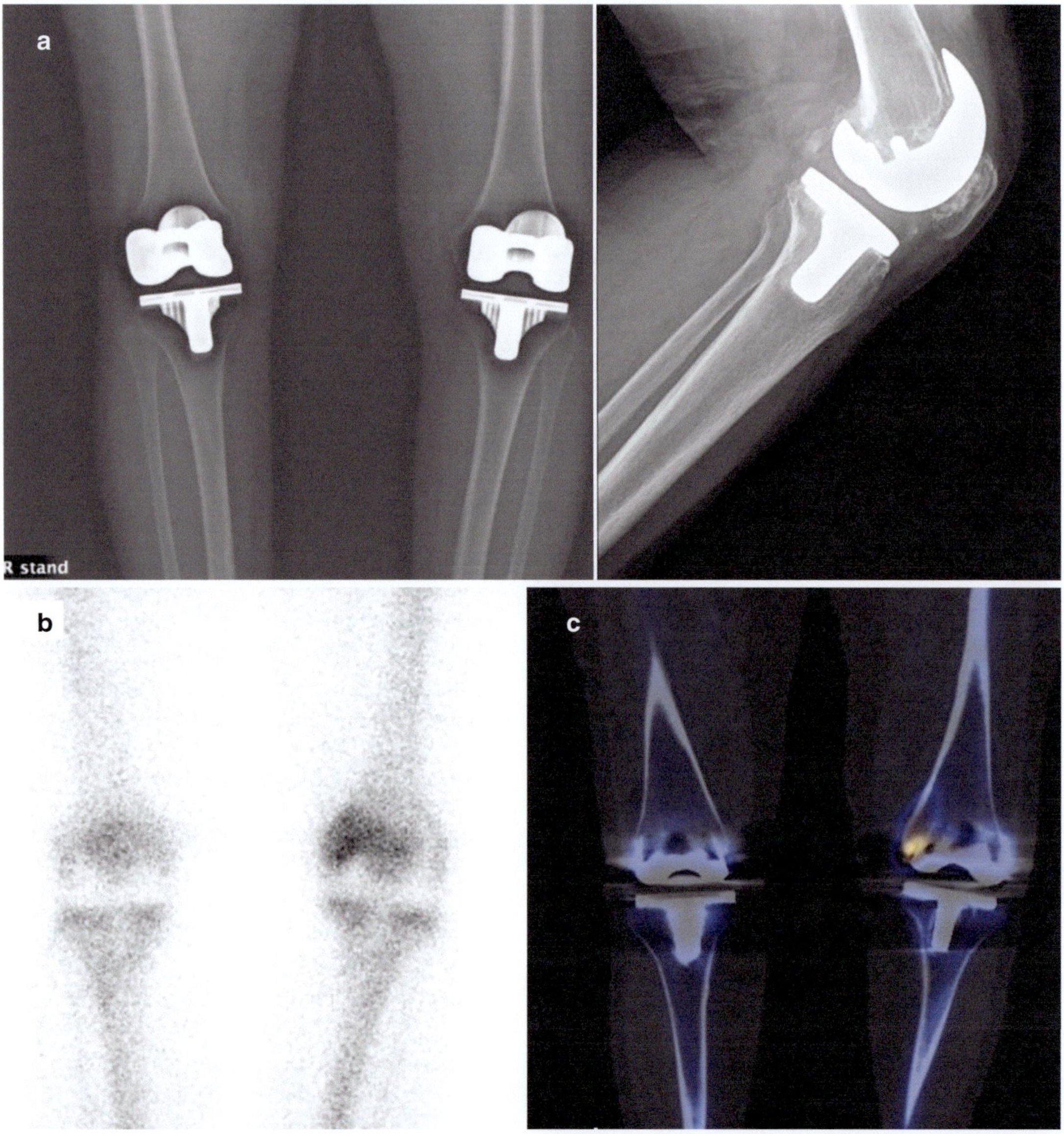

Fig. 12.4 (**a**) Radiolucency is suspected in the tibial base plate of the left knee, but no significant abnormalities in the femoral compartment. (**b**) Planar bone scan and (**c**) SPECT/CT image reveal diffuse increased uptake in the left femur medial condyle around the periprosthetic area

SPECT/CT revealed increased uptake in bilateral medial compartments of the tibia. Patient received revision surgery of the previous knee arthroplasty. There was no gross evidence of infection on surgical findings, but evident wearing and loosening. Bone defects were found at both tibia and femur, at the metal augmentation side (Fig. 12.5).

12.5 Periprosthetic Fracture

Periprosthetic fractures may occur in both TKA and high tibial osteotomy surgeries. Metal components of the prosthesis are stress focusing factors, frequently being the starting point of the fracture line. Fractures are classified in reference to the anatomical components [5, 6]. TKA-related periprosthetic fractures may

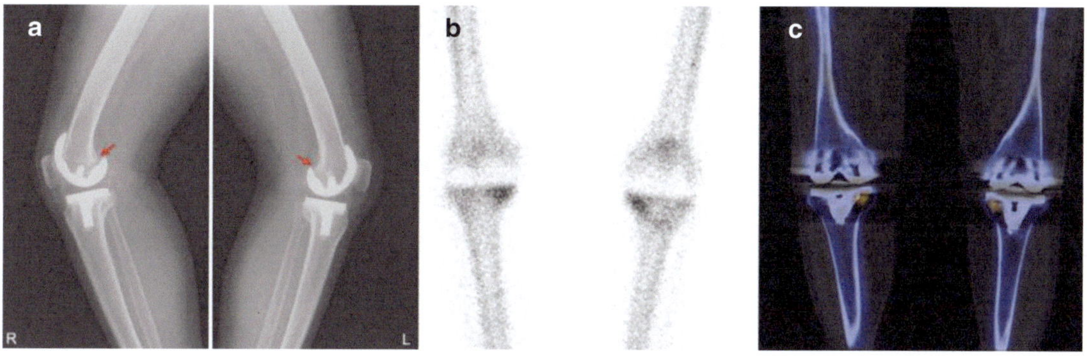

Fig. 12.5 (**a**) Osteolysis is observed in the posterior flanges of both knees (red arrowheads). (**b**) Planar scan reveals diffuse increased uptakes in both medial compartments, tibial aspects. (**c**) SPECT/CT shows diffuse periprosthetic uptakes in both knees, suggesting loosening more likely than periprosthetic inflammation

involve the distal femur, proximal tibia, or the patella. Distal femur fractures may be related with mismatch of metallic component and the femoral cortex or constrained components. Tibial fractures may be related to loosening or malposition of components. Patellar fractures may be related to osteonecrosis, asymmetric resection, or metal backing on the patella. Fracture after wedge osteotomy may result in nonunion or delayed union, bringing recurrent varus deformity.

Case 12.6 Periprosthetic Fracture

A 53-year-old man presented to the outpatient clinic due to left knee pain. The impression was degenerative arthritis, with varus deformity. Radiographs showed joint space narrowing at the medial compartment of left knee, with varus alignments, and the patient received high tibial closed wedge osteotomy for the left knee joint. One month after surgery, patient complained of sudden knee pain after walking. Radiograph revealed fracture in the tibia posteromedial cortex, with collapse. Patient received open reduction and internal fixation for the tibial fracture, with plate and screw fixation of the medial border. Follow-up SPECT/CT images after 3 months showed improvement of the previous degenerative change in the medial compartment and the healing status of the tibial fracture (Fig. 12.6).

12.6 Metallosis

Metal debris may be released into the knee joint, by gross polyethylene failure. This induces foreign body reaction resulting in inflammation and staining of the joint capsule, cavity, or extra-articular tissues. Eventually, metallosis may also be associated with periprosthetic osteolysis and loosening. Radiographs may show focal metal densities, with increased periprosthetic soft tissue densities. Bone scans are not usually used for the diagnosis of metallosis but, instead, may detect accompanied loosening.

Case 12.7 Metallosis

A 74-year-old woman presented to the outpatient clinical due to right knee pain. She had received bilateral TKRA 9 years ago. She was diagnosed of loosening of the right femoral compartment and underwent revision surgery for the right knee. On surgery, there were no gross evidence of infection, but frail and grey-colored granulation tissues were found in between the prosthesis and femoral compartment, due to metallosis. Diffuse bone defects were found in both tibial and femoral compartments. Previous prostheses were removed completely, and revision surgery was done (Fig. 12.7).

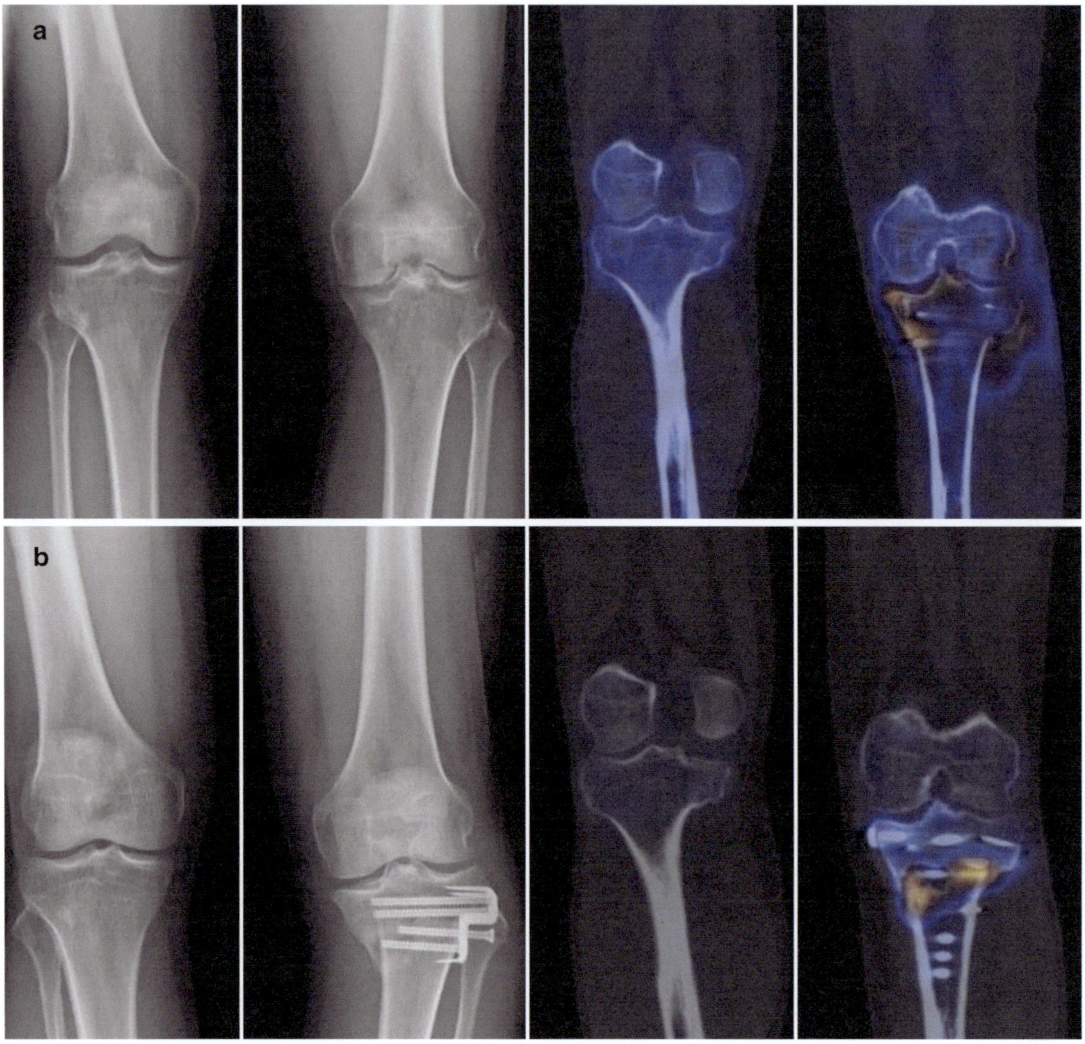

Fig. 12.6 (**a**) Preoperative radiographs and bone SPECT/CT images. Joint space narrowing of the left knee with increased uptake in the medial tibial plateau. (**b**) 1 month after lateral closed wedge osteotomy, the medial tibia has collapsed. Increased uptake along the fracture line in the tibial cortex is observed

12.7 Instability

Instability is the excessive displacement of the articular elements, in which most cases require revision surgeries [7]. Instability following TKA can be divided into different types, as extension, flexion, and genu recurvatum [8]. Causes include ligament imbalance, component misalignment, component failure, bone loss, etc. Bone scans aid the diagnosis by detecting asymmetric stress and excluding other causes of knee pain.

Case 12.8 Instability
A 60-year-old woman visited to the hospital for right knee pain. She was diagnosed of degenerative arthritis and TKRA. One year after surgery, she complained of severe right knee pain, with soft tissue edema. She was diagnosed of flexion insta-

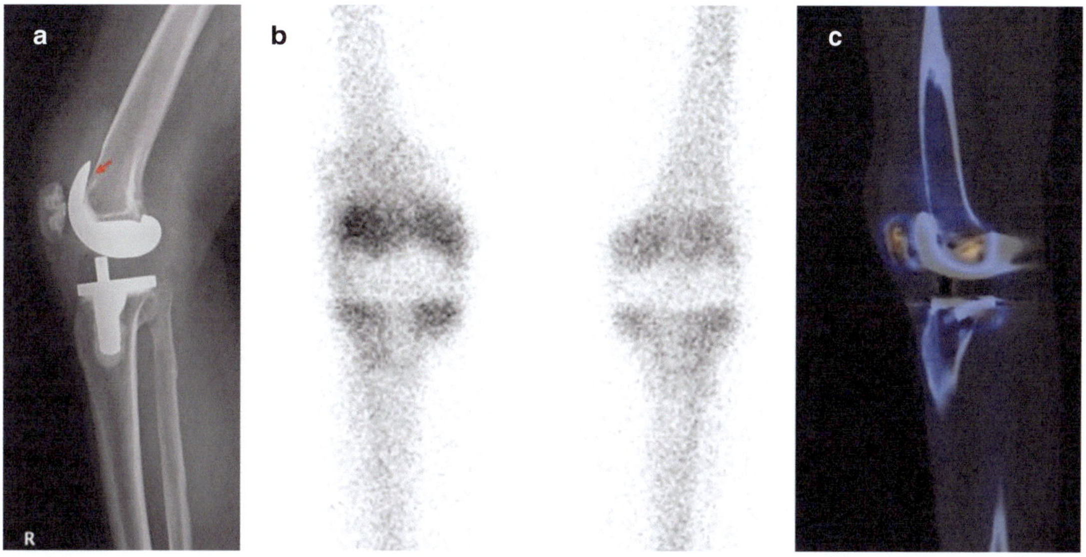

Fig. 12.7 (**a**) Lateral knee radiograph before TKRA revision surgery. There is right knee joint effusion with loosening around the right femoral component anterior flange (red arrow). (**b**) Planar scan and (**c**) SPECT/CT image show diffuse increased uptake around the prostheses, indicating loosening and need for revision surgery. Metallic debris is not suggested on neither images and only could be seen in the surgical field

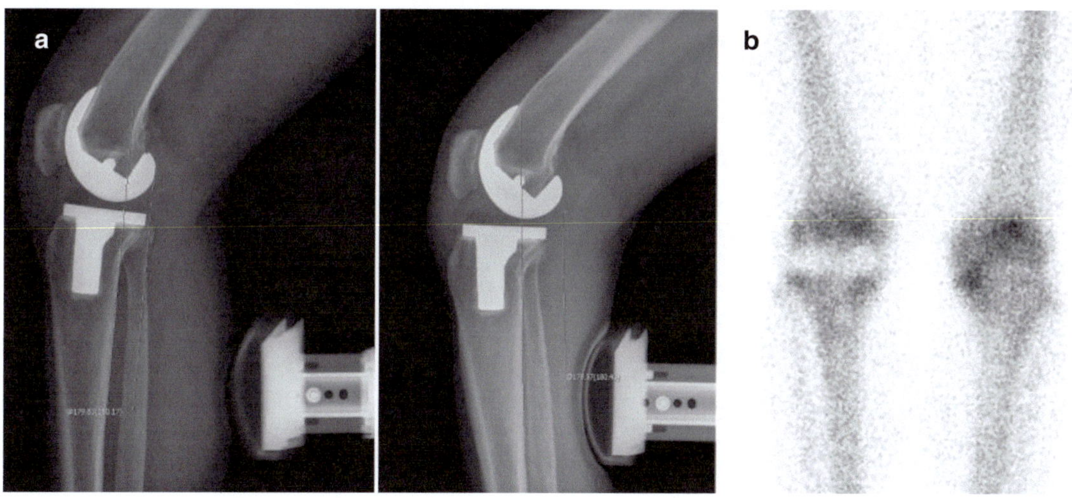

Fig. 12.8 There are no unusual findings in the radiographs, but anterior translation of the tibia is observed on the anterior drawer test (**a**). Bone scan shows diffuse increased uptake in both femoral and tibial components, indicating loosening (**b**)

bility and mediolateral instability. Therefore, the patient received revision of the right TKRA. On surgical findings, there were no gross evidence of infection, with only mild wearing and synovitis. Previous prostheses were removed completely, and revision surgery was done (Fig. 12.8).

Teaching Points

- Complications of prosthesis-related knee surgeries include periprosthetic infection, aseptic loosening, polyethylene wear, metallosis, instability, and periprosthetic fracture.
- Periprosthetic uptake patterns on bone scans aid the differential diagnosis.

References

1. Gonzalez MH, Mekhail AO. The failed total knee arthroplasty: evaluation and etiology. J Am Acad Orthop Surg. 2004;12(6):436–46.
2. Mulcahy H, Chew FS. Current concepts in knee replacement: complications. AJR Am J Roentgenol. 2014;202(1):W76–86.
3. Verberne SJ, et al. What is the accuracy of nuclear imaging in the assessment of periprosthetic knee infection? A meta-analysis. Clin Orthop Relat Res. 2017;475(5):1395–410.
4. Fehring TK, McAvoy G. Fluoroscopic evaluation of the painful total knee arthroplasty. Clin Orthop Relat Res. 1996;331:226–33.
5. Felix NA, Stuart MJ, Hanssen AD. Periprosthetic fractures of the tibia associated with total knee arthroplasty. Clin Orthop Relat Res. 1997;345:113–24.
6. Takeuchi R, et al. Fractures around the lateral cortical hinge after a medial opening-wedge high tibial osteotomy: a new classification of lateral hinge fracture. Arthroscopy. 2012;28(1):85–94.
7. Rodriguez-Merchan EC. Instability following total knee arthroplasty. HSS J. 2011;7(3):273–8.
8. Parratte S, Pagnano MW. Instability after total knee arthroplasty. Instr Course Lect. 2008;57:295–304.

13 Ankle and Shoulder

So Won Oh and Jee Won Chai

Abstract

The ankle and shoulder are major joints that are responsible for the active movements of the body; thus, various orthopedic disorders occur in association with overuse, strain, trauma, etc. Unlike the knee or hip, degenerative arthritis infrequently involves the ankle and shoulder, and other pathological conditions such as dislocation or trauma to these joints can cause serious disabilities and discomfort in daily activities. Plain radiography, CT, and MRI are the main diagnostic tools for musculoskeletal disorders, since they could provide clues to understand the pathophysiology by means of excellent anatomical information. Bone scintigraphy is a highly sensitive diagnostic tool for evaluating blood flow and bone remodeling activity. Bone SPECT/CT has recently gained attention as a helpful modality for understanding orthopedic disorders by combining functional information and precise anatomical localization. Among various pathological disorders of the two joints, only a few clinically significant diseases of the ankle and shoulder are briefly introduced, including the foot.

Keywords

Ankle and foot · Shoulder · Bone SPECT/CT

13.1 Ankle Osteoarthritis

13.1.1 Etiology and Clinical Significance

The ankle is affected by osteoarthritis (OA) in approximately 1% of the world's adult population, which results in pain, dysfunction, and impaired mobility [1]. The ankle is an uncommon site for OA compared with other sites such as the knee, hand, and hip, as it is strongly contained in ligaments and tendons. On the contrary, the ankle is particularly prone to injury because of its flexibility in movement. Irreversible cartilage damage may occur at the time of injury, and articular incongruity and instability can lead to chronic cartilage overloading. Thus, ankle OA is usually a consequence of significant trauma or the cumulative effects of repeated minor physical insults. In this regard, patients with post-traumatic OA are generally younger than those with primary OA [2].

S. W. Oh (✉)
Department of Nuclear Medicine, Seoul National University Boramae Medical Center, Seoul, Republic of Korea

J. W. Chai
Department of Radiology, Seoul National University Boramae Medical Center, Seoul, Republic of Korea

S.-O. Yang et al. (eds.), *Atlas of Nuclear Medicine in Musculoskeletal System*,
https://doi.org/10.1007/978-981-19-2677-8_13

13.1.2 Imaging

Ankle OA generally refers to the degeneration of the talocrural joint between the talus, tibia, and fibula, which is known as the true ankle joint. The subtalar joint, however, is often considered the second part of the ankle joint, because it contributes to ankle motion and shares biomechanical and pathomechanical factors of ankle instability [3].

Radiography is the diagnostic tool of choice for the evaluation of OA despite the advent of new imaging techniques. Typical radiographic findings of OA include joint space narrowing, subchondral sclerosis, and osteophytosis. Weight-bearing mortise and lateral views of the ankle are needed for the optimal visualization of OA features [4].

MRI is a very helpful diagnostic tool for the evaluation of soft tissues in joints, such as cartilage and tendons. Although MRI is still less accessible than radiography, it provides insights and clues to pathomechanics in relation to the development of ankle OA, based on the excellent spatial resolution and three-dimensional information.

Case 13.1

A 69-year-old man presented to the outpatient clinic with right ankle pain that developed 3 days prior. He denied any preceding traumatic injury to the ankle. The radiographs showed bilateral pes planus and severe OA in the right talocrural joint. Bone SPECT/CT showed increased uptake in the anterior aspect of the right talocrural joint. Primary ankle OA was diagnosed based on the clinical symptoms and radiographic findings (Fig. 13.1).

Case 13.2

A 54-year-old man presented to the outpatient clinic with pain in the lateral aspect of the right ankle, and tenderness was elicited in the right lateral gutter area. He had an ankle injury when he was 25 years old. Bone SPECT/CT showed diffusely increased radiotracer uptake along the right subtalar joint. Post-traumatic OA of the subtalar joint was diagnosed, and medical treatment with anti-inflammatory drugs was prescribed (Fig. 13.2).

13.2 Osteochondral Lesion of the Talus

13.2.1 Etiology and Clinical Significance

Osteochondral lesions of the talus (OLT) cover a wide spectrum of pathologies, including subchondral contusion, osteochondritis dissecans, osteochondral fracture, and OA resulting from long-standing disease [5]. OLT clinically causes ankle pain with a succession of nonspecific signs such as pain without the exact localization necessarily related to the lesion, blocking, click, instability, and joint swelling. OLT mainly occurs in active patients in relation to trauma, but the physiopathology and natural course of OLT are still being debated. The location of the OLT is considered to be associated with the mechanism of the injury and direction of the applied force (Fig. 13.3).

13.2.2 Imaging

OLT may be visualized as an area of detached bone surrounded by radiolucency, but it may not appear on plain radiographs in the early stage. Routine radiography often fails to detect OLT, particularly when placed posteriorly [6]. Thus, cross-sectional imaging such as CT or MRI could be helpful in patients with prolonged symptoms to detect OLT and exclude other ankle and foot pathologies.

Case 13.3

A 59-year-old woman was referred to the orthopedic clinic to rule out osteochondritis dissecans of the left ankle. The pain persisted for more than 10 years. Radiography revealed an osteochondral

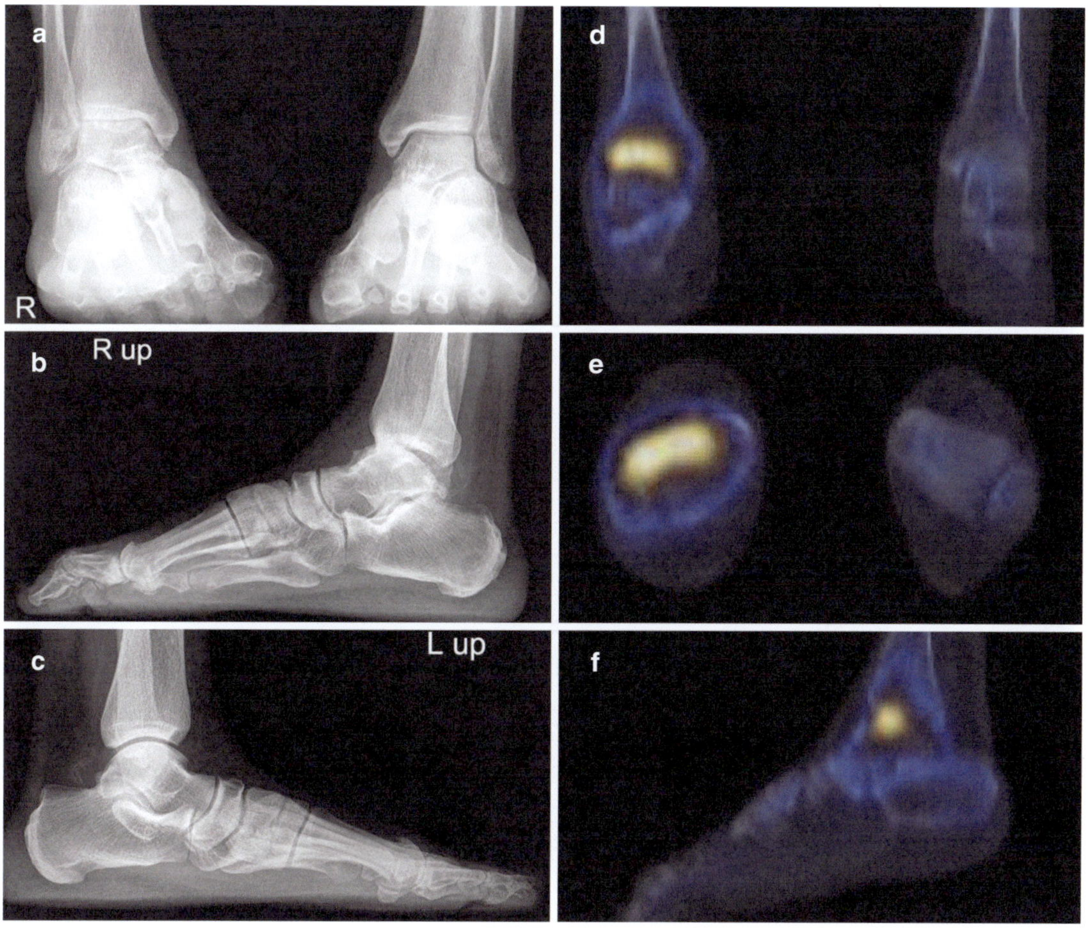

Fig. 13.1 The ankle mortise view shows severe osteoarthritis in the right talocrural joint; the joint space is diffusely narrowed, and subchondral sclerosis is visualized in the anterior tibial plafond and talar dome area (**a**). The lateral ankle views show anterior subluxation of the right ankle joint (**b**), compared with the normal position of the left ankle joint (**c**). Bone SPECT/CT shows increased uptake in the anterior aspect of the right talocrural joint, with joint space narrowing and osteophytosis (**d**–**f**)

lesion in the left talar dome area. MRI showed a multiloculated cystic lesion surrounded by bone marrow edema in the medial area of the left talar dome. Bone SPECT/CT showed a cystic lesion that was matched with focal increased uptake in the medial aspect of the left talar dome. Aching pain subsided after administration of anti-analgesic medication under the diagnosis of OLT. Surgical curettage of the osteochondral cyst can be considered in cases where the symptoms persist (Fig. 13.4).

13.3 Anterior Ankle Impingement Syndrome

Impingement refers to a clinical syndrome with pain or restricted joint motion induced by an abnormal entrapment or contact of structures. Anterior ankle impingement (AAI) syndrome, also known as "footballer's ankle," results from compression of anterior osteophytes of the dorsal talar neck and distal tibia during dorsiflexion of the foot [7]. Repetitive repair following injury

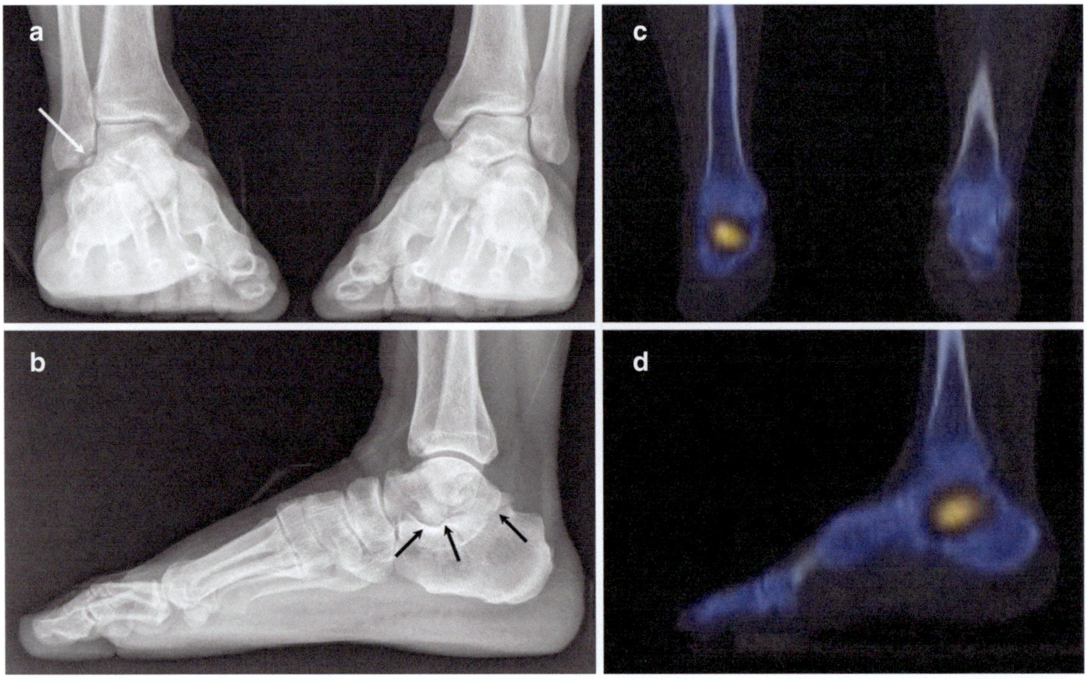

Fig. 13.2 The mortise view shows no abnormal findings except os subfibulare at the right lateral malleolus (white arrow) (**a**). The lateral view of right ankle showed diffuse narrowing of the subtalar joint space and subchondral sclerosis (black arrows) (**b**). Bone SPECT/CT demonstrates diffusely increased radiotracer uptake along the right subtalar joint (**c**, **d**)

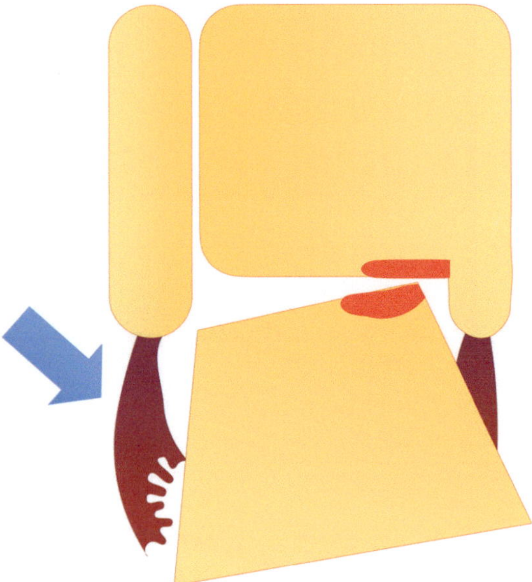

Fig. 13.3 Sprain of the lateral collateral ligament (arrow) may transmit the force diagonally, which can cause injury to the talar dome and/or kissing tibial lesion. In consequence, medial-sided osteochondral lesions of the talus involving both articular cartilage and subchondral bone of the talar dome may develop in association with the lateral collateral ligament injury

leads to the formation of osteophytes that may cause contact between opposing bone or entrap soft tissue with consequent narrowing of the anterior joint space. In this regard, AAI may occur due to repetitive impaction injury to the anterior chondral margin from hyper-dorsiflexion or direct impact from an external object, such as a soccer ball [8]. Patients with AAI typically complain of chronic ankle pain with a history of recurrent ankle sprain accompanied by a decrease in the overall ankle range of motion, mostly affecting dorsiflexion.

13.3.1 Imaging

Radiography can visualize bony osteophytes of the ankle well. However, plain radiography or CT may not be valuable for the evaluation of soft tissue impingement. MRI can accurately detect bony osteophytes as well as soft tissue lesions, such as synovitis, tenosynovitis, and concomitant chondral injury. In addition, MR arthrography is

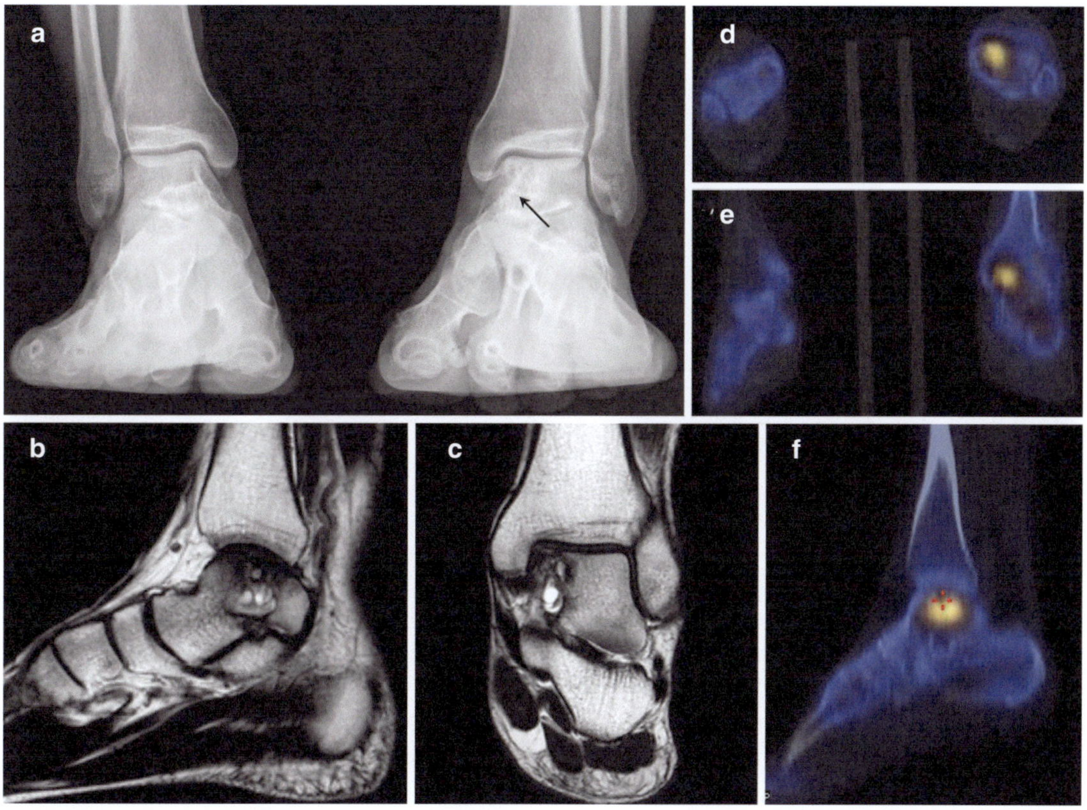

Fig. 13.4 The mortise view shows a small radiolucent lesion (black arrow) in the medial aspect of the left talar dome (**a**). Left ankle MRI shows a non-displaced osteochondral lesion with cystic change and irregular cartilage defect and thinning at the medial talar dome (**b**, **c**). Bone SPECT/CT shows focal increased uptake in the medial aspect of the left talar dome area (**d**–**f**)

highly accurate in the assessment of soft impingement when clinical signs of AAI are overt. Ultrasonography has also gained popularity as a reliable and inexpensive modality for evaluating impingement lesions.

Case 13.4

A 22-year-old soldier complained of right ankle pain that developed 2 weeks prior and was aggravated during dorsiflexion. He had undergone arthroscopic surgery for the treatment of an osteochondral lesion of the talus 6 years prior. Bone scintigraphy of the right foot revealed diffusely increased tracer uptake in the right tibial plafond. Right ankle MR showed diffuse bone marrow edema in the tibial plafond. Based on clinical examination and imaging, AAI syndrome was diagnosed (Fig. 13.5).

13.4 Plantar Fasciitis

13.4.1 Etiology and Clinical Significance

Plantar fasciitis is the most common cause of heel pain and is more common in runners. Although the name itself implies inflammation, it is currently considered that degeneration of the plantar fascia related to repetitive micro-tears of the fascia is the main cause that lacks an inflammatory reaction [9]. Plantar fasciitis causes stabbing pain in the heel pad that usually occurs after a period of rest and eases while walking. Causes of plantar fasciitis are considered multifactorial, with abnormal biomechanics and delayed healing as likely contributors.

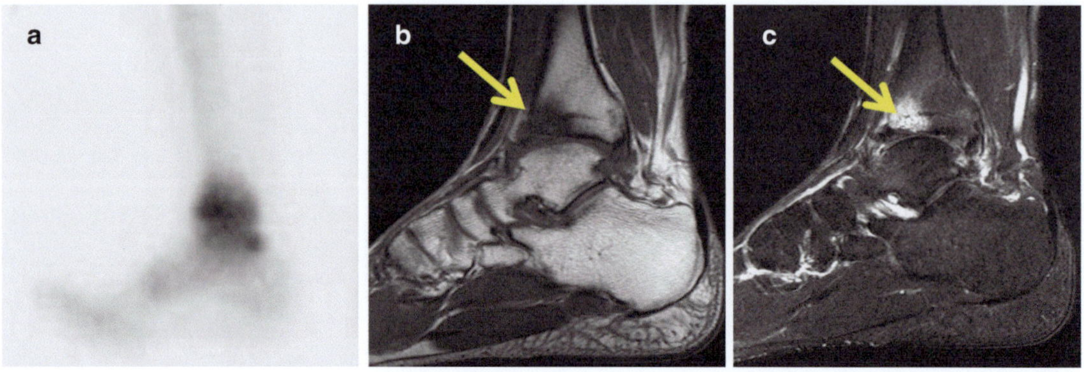

Fig. 13.5 Bone scintigraphy of the right foot shows diffusely increased tracer uptake in the right tibia plafond (**a**). Right ankle MRI shows diffuse bone marrow edema (yellow arrows) in the tibial plafond (**b**, **c**)

13.4.2 Imaging

The diagnosis of plantar fasciitis is clinically made, although imaging can confirm the diagnosis or rule out other causes of heel pain. Almost half of the patients with plantar fasciitis have heel spurs, but they are incidental and nonspecific to clinical symptoms. Ultrasonography can show thickening and low echogenicity of the plantar fascia. The differential diagnosis of heel pain can be Achilles' tendonitis, retrocalcaneal bursitis, subtalar joint abnormalities, and fractures of the calcaneus. The management of plantar fasciitis is typically conservative, because pain is self-limiting and resolves within a year.

Case 13.5

A 45-year-old man visited the orthopedic clinic due to sudden onset of stabbing pain on the left heel pad. He had been followed up for the treatment of ankylosing spondylitis at the Department of Rheumatology. Under the impression of enthesopathy of the left hill pad, imaging workups, including ultrasonography, plain radiography, and bone SPECT/CT, were performed. Ultrasonography showed thickening and low echoic change of the left plantar fascia at the calcaneal insertion site, but there were no abnormal findings in the Achilles tendon. Plantar fasciitis was diagnosed based on clinical examination and imaging (Fig. 13.6).

13.5 Accessory Ossicles

13.5.1 Etiology and Clinical Significance

Accessory ossicles around the foot and ankle are common developmental variations that occur due to the failure of union of secondary ossification centers. These ossicles are mostly detected incidentally and usually remain asymptomatic, but they can become painful in relation to fractures, dislocations, etc. Thus, the prevalence of ossicles varies, and the true prevalence of ossicles is unknown. The most common accessory ossicles in the foot are the os trigonum, os peroneum, and os naviculare [10]. Among them, the os navicular often receives attention when it presents with clinical symptoms.

Os naviculare, known as accessory navicular, usually co-exist with pes planus, which is often associated with painful conditions and bursa formation, especially in young athletes. Type 2 os naviculare is the most common type, and the most common presenting symptom is medial foot pain that is aggravated by walking or running. In addition, type 1 and 2 os naviculare can cause posterior tibial tendinopathy due to the insertion site of the tibialis posterior tendon on the accessory navicular bone.

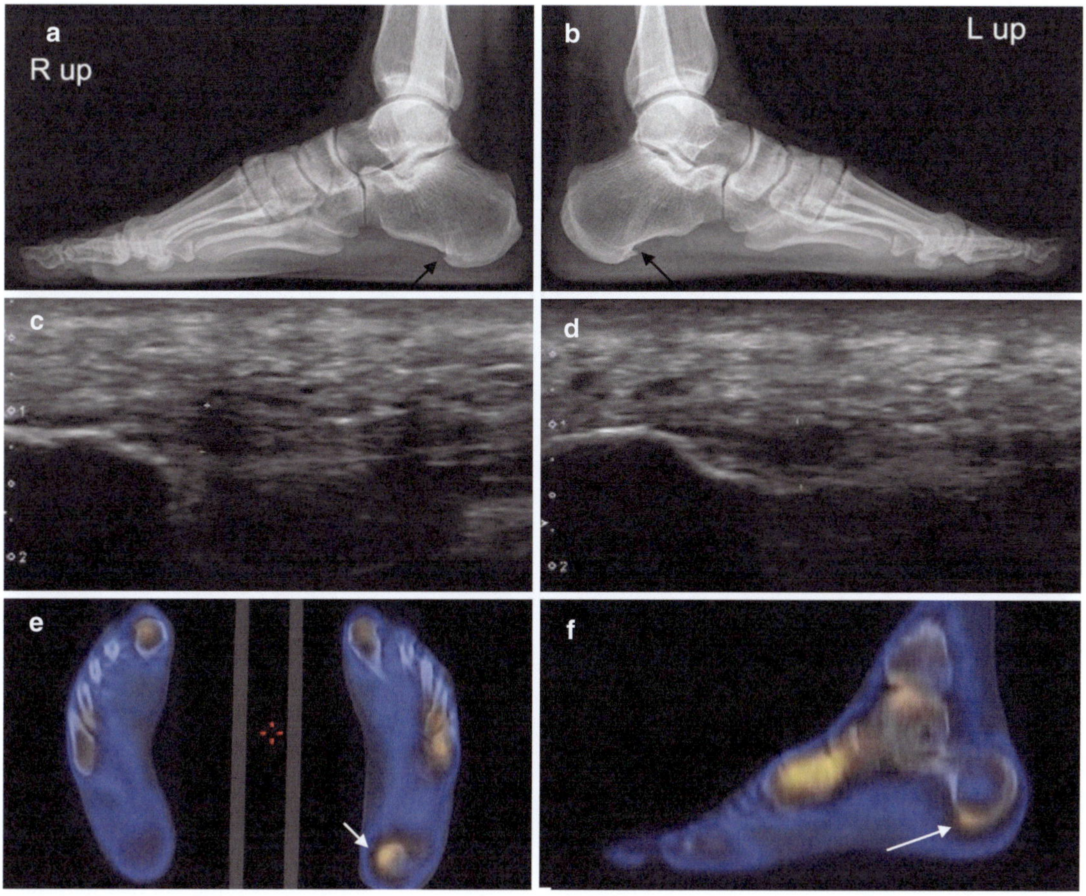

Fig. 13.6 The lateral ankle views show plantar calcaneal spurs (black arrows) at both sides (**a**, **b**). Ultrasonography shows thickening of the planar fascia at both sides. The plantar fascia is slightly thicker (4.6 mm) in the left side (**d**), compared with the right side (3.2 mm) (**c**). Bone SPECT/CT shows matched increased uptake (white arrows) at the left calcaneal spur only (**e**, **f**)

13.5.2 Imaging

Radiography can show ossicles in the foot, but it is difficult to prove a causal relationship with pathological conditions and the presence of the ossicles. MRI could be useful to identify symptomatic accessory ossicles, which can accompany bone or soft tissue changes in and around the os, and exclude other causes of foot pain, such as tumors or fractures [11]. When acute pain develops in this region, bone scintigraphy may help differentiate accessory ossicles from an acute injury.

Case 13.6
A 19-year-old man visited the outpatient clinic because of bilateral ankle pain that developed 2 weeks prior. The time to walk or stand had increased since he started working as a kitchen assistant 3 months ago. Radiography revealed bilateral type 2 accessory navicular bones. Bone SPECT/CT showed focal increased uptake at the right accessory navicular bone. Pre-hallux syndrome was diagnosed, and supportive management, including anti-inflammatory agents, was prescribed (Fig. 13.7).

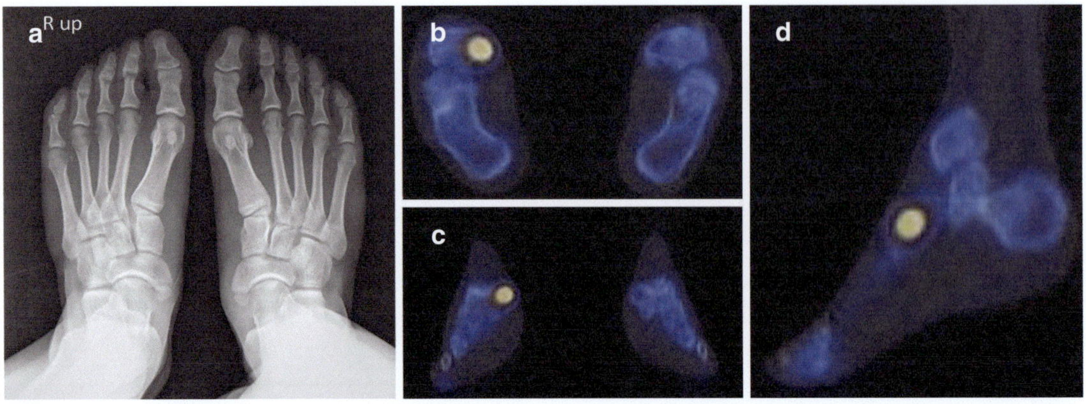

Fig. 13.7 The standing foot radiograph shows type 2 accessory navicular bones of both feet (**a**). Bone SPECT/CT shows focally increased radiotracer uptake at the right accessory navicular bone (**b**–**d**)

13.6 Mid-foot Sprain

13.6.1 Etiology and Clinical Significance

The mid-foot joint complex, known as the Lisfranc joint, has a specialized bony and ligamentous structure that provides stability by holding the metatarsals. A twisting fall can break or dislocate these bones out of place, resulting in Lisfranc injuries, because there is no connective tissue holding the first metatarsal to the second metatarsal. A Lisfranc injury is commonly seen in football and soccer players, but it is often mistaken for a simple sprain, especially if the injury is a result of a straightforward twist and fall. It is a severe injury that may take many months to heal and may require surgery for treatment.

13.6.2 Imaging

Variable clinical presentations and radiographic findings make Lisfranc ligament injuries difficult to detect, especially in cases of incomplete or subtle injuries. CT and MRI usage has increased over the last decade, while conventional radiography is often inaccurate in reliably detecting Lisfranc injuries. Ultrasonography has become popular for the assessment of Lisfranc injuries because of its noninvasive nature and ability to measure dynamic changes under loading [12]; however, it is limited by the depth of penetration and resolution, with heterogeneous evidence regarding the accuracy of the various measurement techniques.

Case 13.7

A 24-year-old man visited the outpatient clinic because of right mid-foot pain. He had an injury while stepping on the right foot during a soccer game 3 months prior. He had been treated with splint application and pain medication, but pain was redeveloped on the right mid-foot in a soccer game a week prior. Lisfranc injury was diagnosed based on clinical history and imaging findings (Fig. 13.8).

13.7 Shoulder Dislocation

13.7.1 Etiology and Clinical Significance

A Hill–Sachs defect is a compression fracture of the posterolateral humeral head, and a Bankart lesion is an injury at the anteroinferior aspect of the glenoid labral complex. Both lesions are associated with anterior shoulder dislocation, which typically occurs with the shoulder in

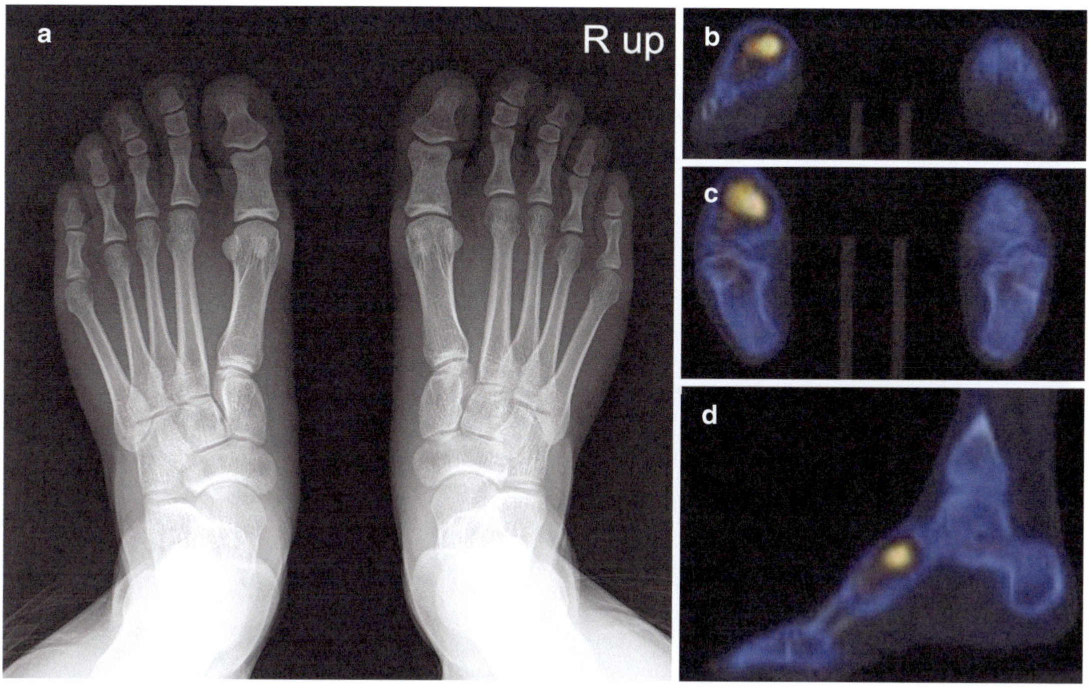

Fig. 13.8 The standing foot radiograph shows no abnormality in the right foot (**a**). Bone SPECT/CT shows increased uptake between the right medial cuneiform and the second metatarsal bone base (**b** coronal; **c** transverse; **d** sagittal)

abduction and external rotation. The biomechanical association between these lesions and anterior shoulder instability is evident, but the etiologies of both lesions have not been clearly established [13]. The prevalence of both lesions is closely related and likely to be high in patients with recurrent anterior shoulder instability, although the true incidence of both lesions remains unknown. The choice of management depends on the clinical significance of the lesions, particularly with respect to anterior shoulder instability. For bony Bankart, immediate and appropriate treatment is required to prevent glenoid bone loss. Bankart repair is the most common surgical treatment for traumatic anterior shoulder instability.

13.7.2 Imaging

Wedge-shaped defects may be visualized in the posterolateral aspect of the humeral head on the anteroposterior radiograph with internal rotation, but they could be missed in the early stages or in cases of small size defects such as glenoid rim fractures. Thus, CT and MRI are recommended as superior imaging options for evaluating glenoid bone loss and identifying small defects. MR arthrography may provide information on the glenoid and/or humeral head defect, but it is an invasive procedure that requires puncture of the joint synovium. When a Hill–Sachs defect is identified, the anterior glenoid should be carefully assessed to defect a Bankart lesion.

Case 13.8

A 37-year-old man visited the emergency room (ER) due to left anterior shoulder dislocation 3 weeks prior. Shoulder dislocation occurred after he fell to the ground drunk with the outstretched arm on the day of his visit to the ER. He complained of severe pain accompanied by tenderness of the left shoulder, but he denied a previous history of shoulder dislocation. He was sent home after the application of the abduction brace followed by manual reduction. A week later, the left shoulder dislocation redeveloped while he hit the left shoulder on the armrest during a car accident. Imaging studies including radiography, three-dimensional CT, and bone SPECT/CT were performed, and a Hill–Sachs lesion with a bony Bankart lesion was diagnosed. He was admitted to the Department of Orthopedics for arthroscopic repair of bony Bankart lesion (Figs. 13.9 and 13.10).

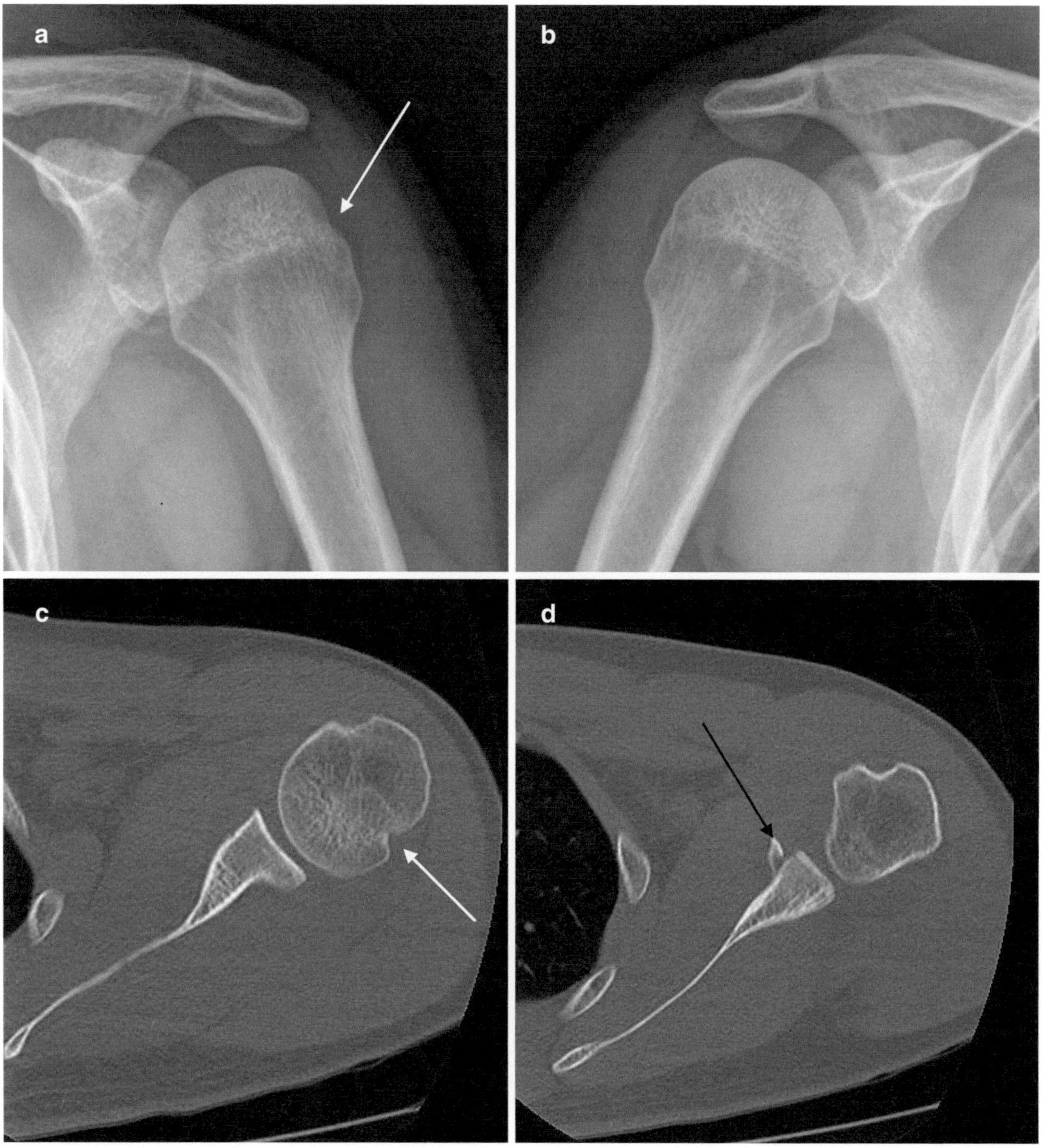

Fig. 13.9 A wedge-shaped defect is demonstrated at the left posterosuperior humeral head on the internal rotation view (**a**), compared with the normal-looking right side (**b**). CT also shows a wedge-shaped depression in the posterolateral aspect of the left humeral head (**c**) and bony Bankart lesion as a fracture at the left glenoid anteroinferior area (**d**). White arrows indicate a Hill–Sachs lesion, and a black arrow shows a bony Bankart lesion

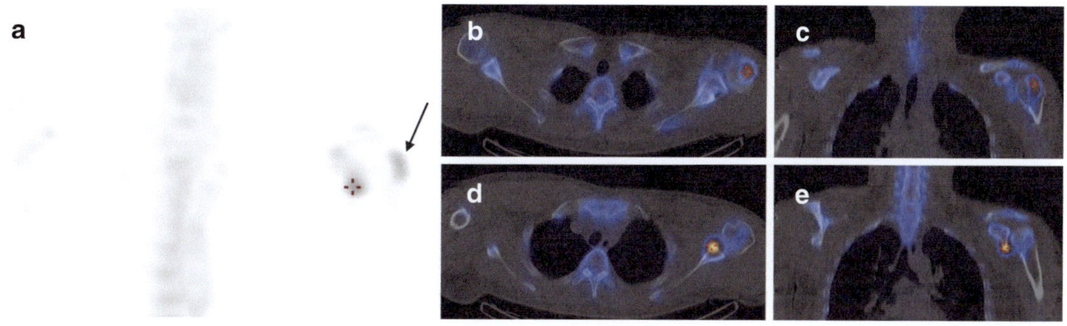

Fig. 13.10 The maximal intensity projection image of bone SPECT shows two foci of an increased uptake in the left shoulder; a black arrow points the left humeral head, lateral aspect, and a star indicates the left scapular glenoid inferior area (**a**). Focal increased uptakes are matched with a Hill–Sachs lesion in the posterolateral aspect of the left humeral head (**b**, **c**) and a bony Bankart lesion in the left glenoid anteroinferior area (**d**, **e**)

13.8 Rotator Cuff Tear

13.8.1 Etiology and Clinical Significance

The shoulder has the highest mobility, but the least intrinsic stability of all joints in the human body. The glenohumeral (GH) joint lacks intrinsic osseous constraints, which are compensated for by many static stabilizers, such as the labrum, joint capsule, and GH ligaments. The rotator cuff, which consists of the supraspinatus, infraspinatus, teres minor, and subscapularis muscles, plays a crucial role in maintaining the dynamic stability of the naturally unstable GH joint. Rotator cuff tears (RCTs) commonly occur when the tendons pull away from the bones in active situations, such as baseball or tennis. RCTs are very common injuries, but the true prevalence is unknown; asymptomatic cuff abnormalities are noted in 30% of patients aged >60 years and 62% of those aged >80 years [14].

13.8.2 Imaging

Plain radiographs are usually normal in acute stages and may show radiographic abnormalities when chronic RCTs develop arthropathy. The multiplanar imaging capabilities of MRI combined with its excellent soft tissue contrast make it ideal for imaging the rotator cuff. MRI can be used to evaluate the integrity of the cuff overall or determine whether an existing tear is repaired when other findings are ambiguous. Ultrasonography is an alternative modality for evaluating the rotator cuff, which can provide images with high image contrast without the use of ionizing radiation. The diagnostic accuracy of shoulder ultrasonography for RCTs can reach as high as 91% and 100% for partial- and full-thickness tears, respectively [15].

Case 13.9

A 50-year-old man visited the outpatient clinic because of left upper arm pain that developed 3 months prior. Plain radiographs showed no abnormal bony abnormality in the left shoulder, but shoulder ultrasonography showed a near-full-thickness tear at the far anterior portion of the left supraspinatus tendon. Pain persisted after taking analgesic medication, and further evaluation including MR arthrography and bone SPECT/CT was performed for the arthroscopic repair of RCT (Fig. 13.11).

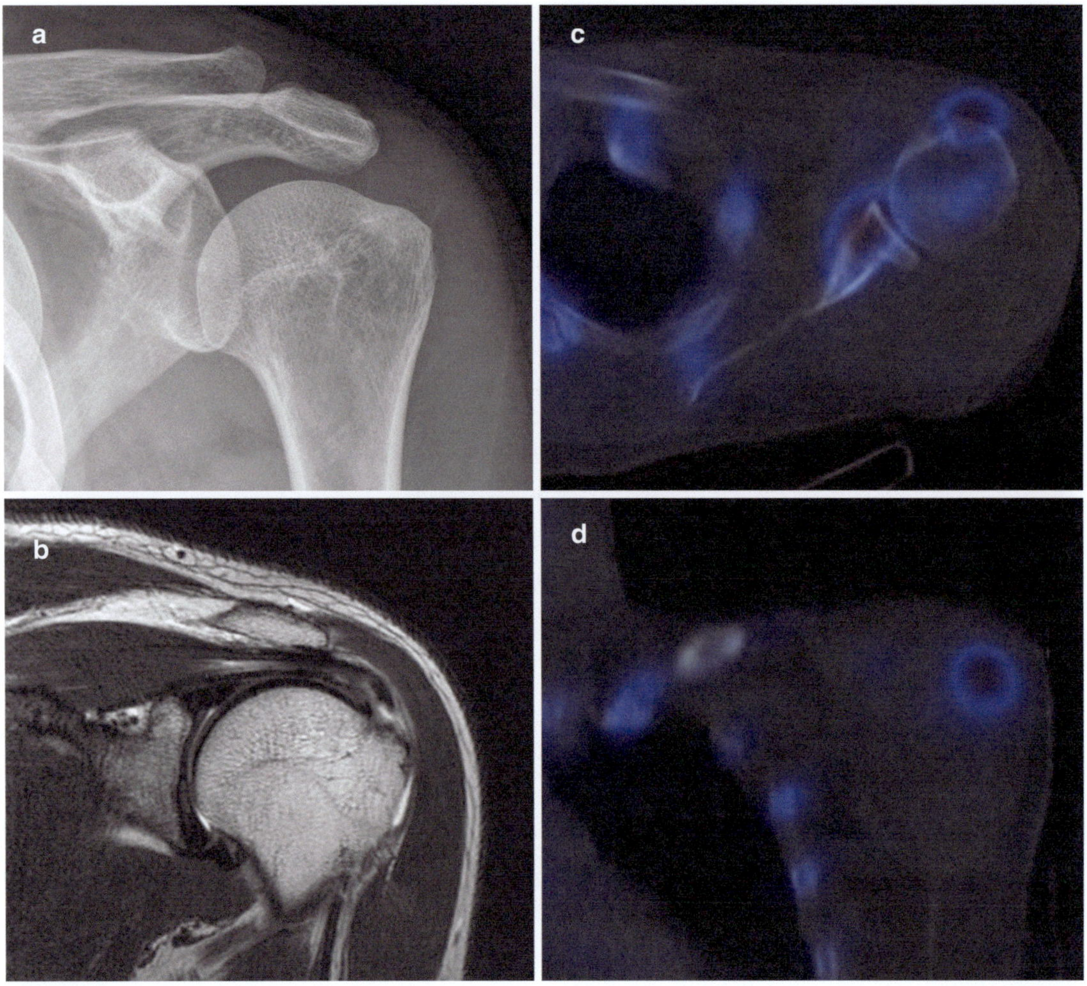

Fig. 13.11 The radiograph shows no abnormal bony abnormality in the left shoulder (**a**). MR arthrography shows high-grade bursal surface partial thickness tear at the anterior to mid portion of the supraspinatus tendon (SST) (**b**). Bone SPECT/CT shows focal uptake in the anterior aspect of the left humeral head that is the insertion site of SST (**c**, **d**)

Teaching Points

- The ankle and shoulder are major joints that are responsible for the active movements of the body; thus, various orthopedic disorders can occur in association with overuse, strain, trauma, etc.
- Cross-sectional images such as CT or MRI are advantageous to evaluate orthopedic disorders involving ankle and shoulder joints owing to high spatial resolution for soft tissue as well as bone and cartilage.
- Bone scintigraphy was not useful in the assessment of the ankle and shoulder joint disorder, but the introduction of SPECT/CT is expected to help understanding pathomechanics related to the development of orthopedic disorders.

References

1. JG P. The epidemiology of osteoarthritis. In: Moskowitz RW, Howell DS, Goldberg VM, Mankin HJ, editors. Osteoarthritis. Diagnosis and treatment. Philadelphia, PA: WB Saunders; 1984. p. 9–27.
2. Barg A, Pagenstert GI, Hugle T, et al. Ankle osteoarthritis: etiology, diagnostics, and classification. Foot Ankle Clin. 2013;18:411–26.
3. Bonnel F, Toullec E, Mabit C, Tourne Y, Sofcot. Chronic ankle instability: biomechanics and pathomechanics of ligaments injury and associated lesions. Orthop Traumatol Surg Res. 2010;96:424–32.
4. Kraus VB, Kilfoil TM, Hash TW 2nd, et al. Atlas of radiographic features of osteoarthritis of the ankle and hindfoot. Osteoarthr Cartil. 2015;23:2059–85.
5. Posadzy M, Desimpel J, Vanhoenacker F. Staging of osteochondral lesions of the talus: MRI and cone beam CT. J Belg Soc Radiol. 2017;101:1.
6. Verhagen RA, Maas M, Dijkgraaf MG, Tol JL, Krips R, van Dijk CN. Prospective study on diagnostic strategies in osteochondral lesions of the talus. Is MRI superior to helical CT? J Bone Joint Surg Br. 2005;87:41–6.
7. Vaseenon T, Amendola A. Update on anterior ankle impingement. Curr Rev Musculoskelet Med. 2012;5:145–50.
8. Lavezry KP, McHale KJ, Rossy WH, Theodore G. Ankle impingement. J Orthop Surg Res. 2016;11:97.
9. Goff JD, Crawford R. Diagnosis and treatment of plantar fasciitis. Am Fam Physician. 2011;84:676–82.
10. Lawson JP. International skeletal society lecture in honor of Howard D. Dorfman. Clinically significant radiologic anatomic variants of the skeleton. AJR Am J Roentgenol. 1994;163:249–55.
11. Choi YS, Lee KT, Kang HS, Kim EK. MR imaging findings of painful type II accessory navicular bone: correlation with surgical and pathologic studies. Korean J Radiol. 2004;5:274–9.
12. Woodward S, Jacobson JA, Femino JE, Morag Y, Fessell DP, Dong Q. Sonographic evaluation of Lisfranc ligament injuries. J Ultrasound Med. 2009;28:351–7.
13. Griffith JF, Antonio GE, Yung PS, et al. Prevalence, pattern, and spectrum of glenoid bone loss in anterior shoulder dislocation: CT analysis of 218 patients. AJR Am J Roentgenol. 2008;190:1247–54.
14. Sambandam SN, Khanna V, Gul A, Mounasamy V. Rotator cuff tears: an evidence based approach. World J Orthop. 2015;6:902–18.
15. Okoroha KR, Fidai MS, Tramer JS, Davis KD, Kolowich PA. Diagnostic accuracy of ultrasound for rotator cuff tears. Ultrasonography. 2019;38:215–20.

Part IV

Metabolic and Endocrine Osseous Disorders

Metabolic Bone Disease

14

Jin-Sook Ryu and Hye Won Chung

Abstract

Metabolic bone disease (MBD) includes a wide range of clinically distinct diseases that cause changes in bone structure, mineralization, and/or mass. MBD can be inherited or acquired. Skeletal dysplasia is a heterogeneous group of genetic disorders caused by defective genes during the bone formation process. These disorders overlap with MBD. In MBD, most pathological processes accelerate osteoblast and osteoclast activity, resulting in increased bone turnover. Although MBD is common, clinical diagnosis based on radiological findings may be challenging. ^{99m}Tc-labeled diphosphonate binding to hydroxyapatite crystals depends on the degree of local bone formation regulated by osteoblastic activity. Bone scan has the advantage of high sensitivity with the capacity to easily image the whole body. Bone scan can provide a functional map of bone turnover, displaying pathology that is global, focal, or multifocal. Understanding the diverse manifestations of MBD using nuclear medicine imaging studies assists in early and specific diagnosis.

In this chapter, we will review the application of nuclear medicine imaging studies in various MBDs that exhibit abnormal bone loss or osteosclerosis. Osteoporosis, the most common MBD, will be dealt with in a separate chapter.

Keywords

Metabolic bone disease · Bone scintigraphy · Osteomalacia · Renal osteodystrophy Paget's disease · Osteopetrosis · Camurati–Engelmann disease

J.-S. Ryu (✉)
Department of Nuclear Medicine, Asan Medical Center, University of Ulsan College of Medicine, Seoul, Republic of Korea
e-mail: jsryu2@amc.seoul.kr

H. W. Chung
Department of Radiology, Asan Medical Center, University of Ulsan College of Medicine, Seoul, Republic of Korea
e-mail: chung@amc.seoul.kr

14.1 Osteomalacia

14.1.1 Etiology and Clinical Significance

Osteomalacia refers to a marked softening of bones caused by impaired mineralization of the osteoid in the cortical and trabecular bones. Two MBDs, osteoporosis and osteomalacia, decrease bone mass. In osteoporosis, there is a decrease in the amount of both mineral and osteoid. However, in osteomalacia, the amount of osteoid (bone formation) is not decreased. Osteomalacia is much less common than osteoporosis. The most common

S.-O. Yang et al. (eds.), *Atlas of Nuclear Medicine in Musculoskeletal System*,
https://doi.org/10.1007/978-981-19-2677-8_14

symptoms of osteomalacia are bone pain, muscle weakness, and waddling gait. If osteomalacia occurs in growing bones prior to the closure of the growth plate, it is termed infantile osteomalacia or rickets. Growing bones fail to mineralize, become soft, and develop deformities [1].

Osteomalacia results from defects in the bone maturation process caused by impaired bone metabolism. These defects are primarily caused by inadequate levels of phosphate, calcium, and vitamin D. Vitamin D deficiency is the most common cause of osteomalacia worldwide. In addition, hereditary disorders of vitamin D metabolism, kidney or liver disease (as these organs are involved in activating vitamin D), small bowel disease, malabsorption, certain drugs, tumors, and many other rare conditions can cause osteomalacia.

14.1.2 Imaging

Radiographs often show generalized osteopenia in patients with osteomalacia. The presence of large quantities of unmineralized osteoid can occasionally be observed as indistinct ill-defined trabecular bone, often giving the impression of a "poor-quality" radiograph [2]. Looser zones, known as pseudo-fractures, are the hallmark signs of osteomalacia. These zones are caused by deposition of unmineralized osteoid at stress sites or along nutrient vessels, which are types of insufficiency fractures. Looser zones are radiolucent bands perpendicular to the cortex, with sclerotic borders, and are often bilateral and symmetrical. The common locations are the inner margin of the femoral neck, pubic rami, ischium, iliac wing, lateral scapula, and ribs. However, they can be easily missed at the early stage. Bone scans are particularly sensitive in terms of identifying pseudo-fractures.

In particular, extensive investigation is required to identify the causes of generalized bone pain in patients with hypophosphatemia. Among the causes, tumor-induced osteomalacia (TIO) is curable. TIO is a paraneoplastic metabolic bone disorder, in which hypophosphatemia and osteomalacia are caused by tumoral production of fibroblast growth factor 23. This process results in the inactivation of the sodium phosphate cotransporter in the proximal renal tubule and renal phosphate wasting [3]. Specifically, for localization of tumors causing osteomalacia, somatostatin receptor imaging such as ^{68}Ga-DOTA-peptide PET/CT can successfully identify the culprit tumor. Many of these tumors are phosphaturic mesenchymal tumors containing somatostatin receptors [4]. Conventional imaging is challenging for visualizing tumors because they are often small and grow slowly. Moreover, these tumors are frequently located in atypical skeletal sites.

Case 14.1
A 40-year-old woman visited an orthopedic clinic with a chief complaint of left hip pain. She was short in stature (height, 131 cm). She was being followed up at a nephrology clinic for bilateral medullary nephrocalcinosis and type I renal tubular acidosis. She had a history of insufficiency fracture at the subtrochanteric area of the left femur 2 years ago. Regarding laboratory values, her blood levels of 25-OH-vitamin D3 (9.4 ng/mL), 1α25-$(OH)_2$-vitamin D3 (8.3 pg/mL), and total calcium (8.5 mg/dL) were decreased. Her osteocalcin level was increased (42.3 ng/mL), and her serum phosphorus and parathyroid hormone levels were within normal limits. Radiographic and whole-body bone scan images were obtained (Fig. 14.1). The patient was diagnosed with vitamin D-deficient osteomalacia with multiple insufficiency fractures and pseudo-fractures.

Case 14.2
A 65-year-old woman was referred to the pain clinic with complaints of multiple atypical body pain. Two years previously, she developed left knee pain without trauma. Despite receiving treatment at orthopedic and neurologic clinics, the pain in her back and flank worsened. She had difficulty in walking due to the severe pain. On screening bone scan, multiple insufficiency fractures were noted in the bilateral ribs, spine, pelvic bones, left proximal femur, and both calcanei, suggesting osteomalacia (Fig. 14.2). Her blood laboratory tests results were normal,

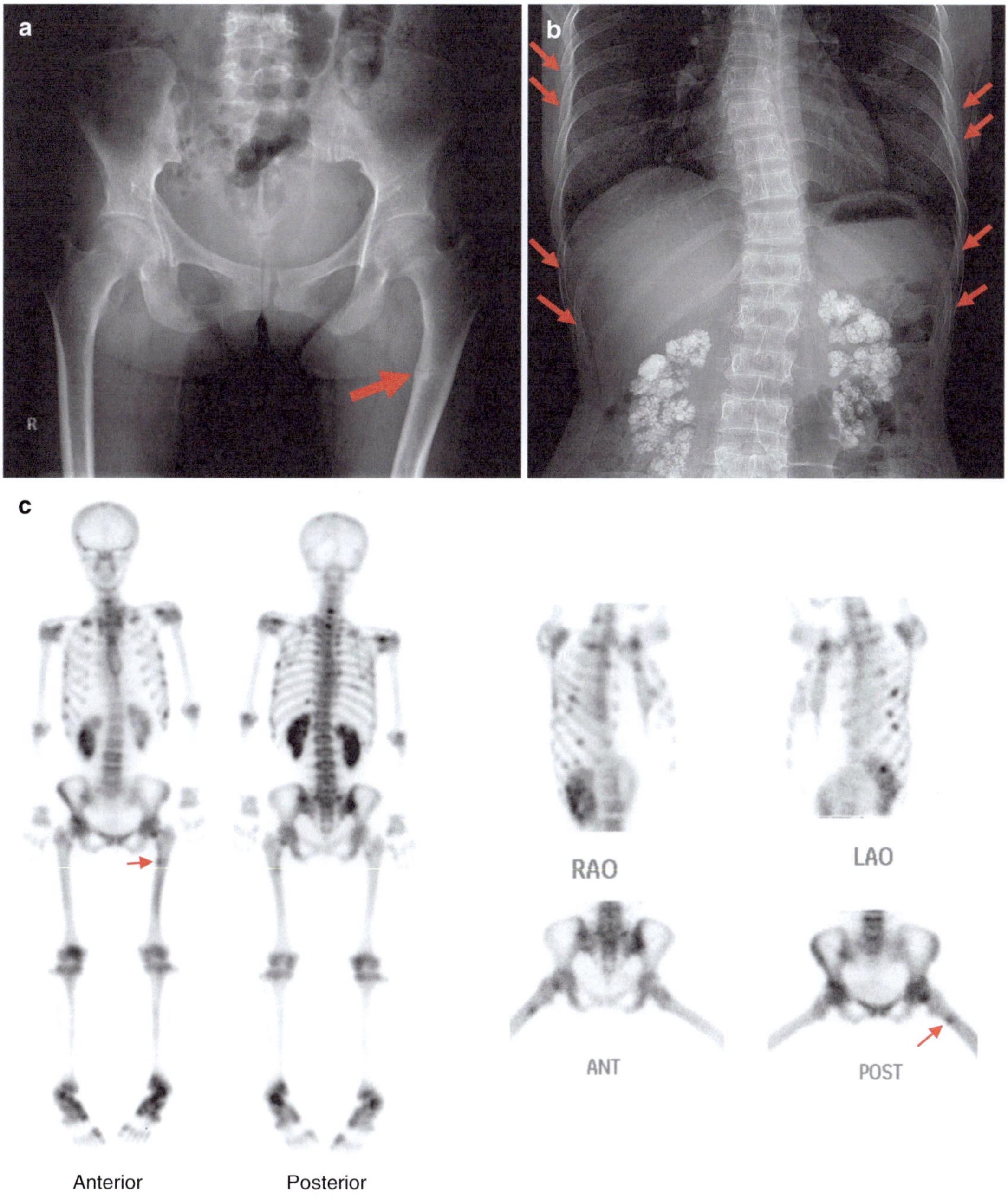

Fig. 14.1 A 40-year-old woman with type I renal tubular acidosis and vitamin D-deficient osteomalacia. The radiograph of the pelvis (**a**) shows insufficiency fracture of the left femur (red arrow). Multiple fractures with callus formation are seen in the bilateral rib cages (red arrows) on the thoracolumbar spine radiograph (**b**). Underlying bone density is decreased, and trabeculae are prominent. Additionally, medullary calcinosis is visualized in both kidneys. Bone scan images (**c**) show multiple foci of focal increased uptakes, suggesting fractures or pseudofractures in the bilateral side of the ribs; C7, T2, and S1 vertebrae; right ilium; left femoral neck; and proximal femur diaphysis (red arrow). Uptakes are also increased diffusely and unevenly in both kidneys

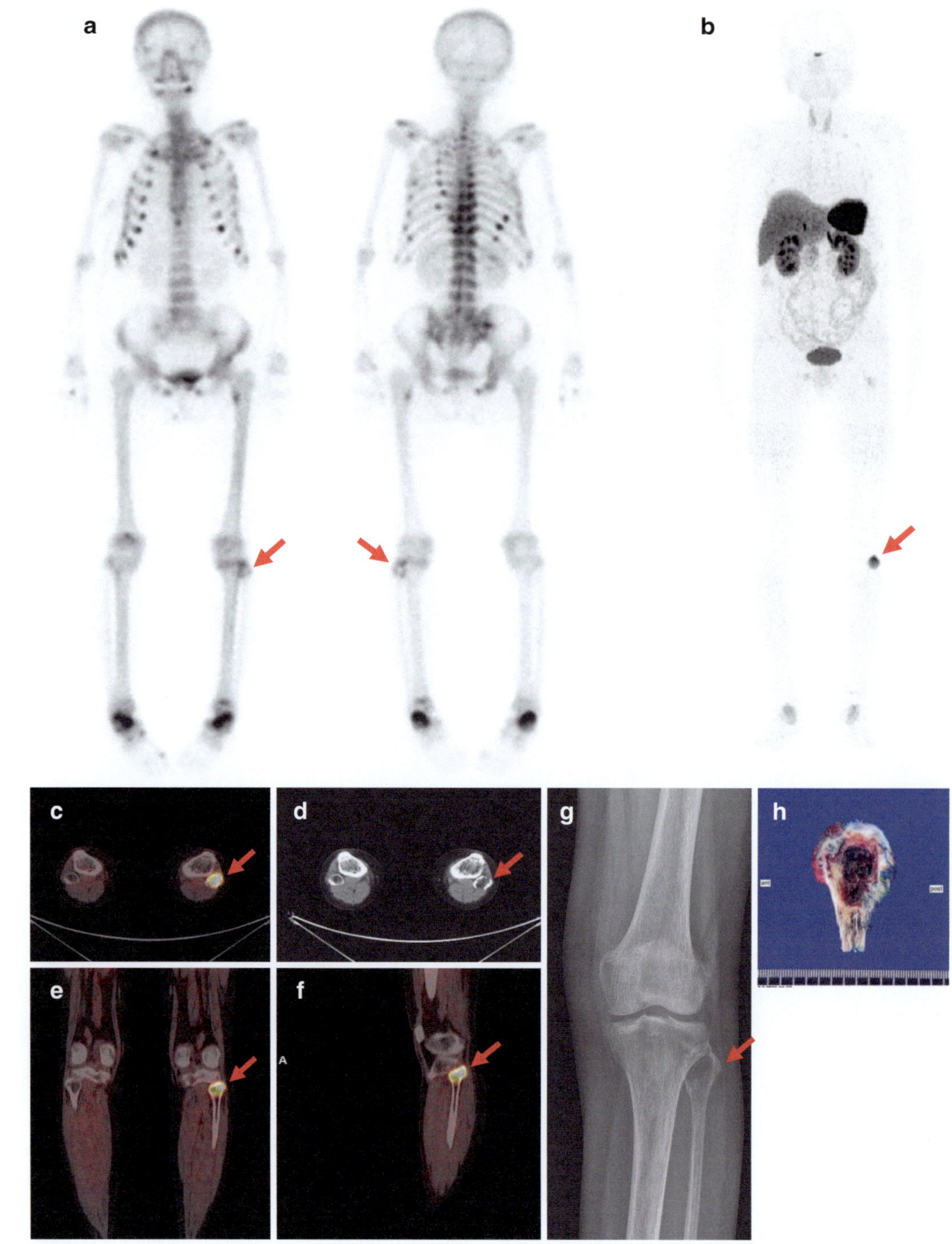

Fig. 14.2 A 65-year-old woman with tumor-induced osteomalacia. Bone scan (**a**) shows multiple focal increased uptakes, suggesting insufficiency fractures in the bilateral ribs, vertebral bodies of the T-L spine, both ilia and pubic rami, medial subtrochanteric cortex of the left proximal femur, left distal tibia, and both calcanei. Mildly increased rim uptake is also observed at the left fibular head (red arrow), which was initially missed. The anterior projection image (**b**) and fusion PET/CT (**c**, **e**, **f**) images of ^{68}Ga-DOTA-TOC PET/CT reveal a focal increased uptake (maximum SUV: 9.9) in the left fibular head (red arrow). On the CT image (**d**) and plain radiograph (**g**), there is an osteolytic bone mass. The cross-sectional image of the surgical specimen (**h**) shows a well-demarcated, ovoid-shaped, solid mass with a focal hemorrhagic focus in the intramedullary portion of the fibular head. This mass was histologically diagnosed as a phosphaturic mesenchymal tumor

except hypophosphatemia (1.3 mg/dL). The patient was referred to the endocrinologic clinic, and further evaluation was performed to search the cause of osteomalacia. Phosphorus supplementation was initiated. ^{68}Ga-DOTA-TOC (edotreotide) PET/CT was performed to identify the culprit tumor that was inducing osteomalacia. An osteolytic bone tumor lesion with high tracer uptake was detected in her left fibular head, suggesting a phosphaturic mesenchymal tumor with overexpression of somatostatin receptor 2. After surgical resection of the tumor, the patients' serum phosphorus level normalized, and her symptoms improved.

Case 14.3

A 46-year-old man visited the orthopedic clinic with a 6-month history of bilateral hip pain. Sequentially, the right hip, left hip, and knee pain occurred without trauma. The patient showed an abnormal antalgic gait. He was a hepatitis B virus carrier and had been prescribed adefovir dipivoxil for 7 years for the treatment of chronic hepatitis B. Five years previously, he was diagnosed with osteoporosis during a routine health checkup. However, no specific treatment was prescribed. On bone densitometry using dual-energy X-ray absorptiometry (DXA), severe osteoporosis of the lumbar spine and femoral neck was shown, with a T-score of −4.1 and −2.9, respectively. Laboratory test results showed that his blood phosphorus level was slightly decreased (2.1 mg/dL) and his alkaline phosphatase was elevated (209 IU/L). Radiography and bone scan with SPECT/CT revealed multiple insufficiency fractures in the spine, bilateral ribs, pelvic bones, both femurs, and left tibia (Fig. 14.3). The patient was diagnosed with drug (adefovir)-induced osteomalacia with secondary multiple insufficiency fractures [5]. The drug was changed to tenofovir alafenamide. Phosphorus, vitamin D supplements, and romosozumab were also initiated, and his symptoms slowly improved.

14.2 Renal Osteodystrophy

14.2.1 Etiology and Clinical Significance

Renal osteodystrophy, also known as uremic osteopathy, refers to skeletal findings observed in patients with chronic kidney disease. The pathophysiology of this condition is complex. Disturbances in vitamin D, phosphate, and calcium metabolism lead to various clinical manifestations. Varying degrees of secondary hyperparathyroidism, osteoporosis, osteomalacia, osteosclerosis, adynamic bone disease, and extraosseous soft tissue calcification are observed. With a decline in renal function, microstructural changes in the bone, vascular system, and soft tissues become macrostructural lesions. These lesions exhibit as low bone mineral density and result in skeletal fractures as well as vascular and soft tissue calcifications [6]. Renal osteodystrophy is usually diagnosed after beginning of treatment for end-stage kidney disease. Amyloid deposition, destructive spondyloarthropathy, osteonecrosis, and musculoskeletal infections may occur as complications of long-term hemodialysis and renal transplantation.

14.2.2 Imaging

Radiographic imaging findings are diverse; thus, radiographs can provide information regarding high bone remodeling and mineralization failure. Osteopenia is often observed at the early stage. In secondary hyperparathyroidism, bone resorption can affect trabecular, endosteal, and cortical bone envelopes or structures close to joints located at the sub-periosteal, sub-ligamentous, and sub-tendinous levels. The characteristic "salt-and-pepper" appearance of the skull and "brown tumors (osteoclastomas)" in the pelvis, long bones, or ribs are rarely encountered currently. A characteristic "rugger-jersey spine (alternating bands of increased density along the endplates

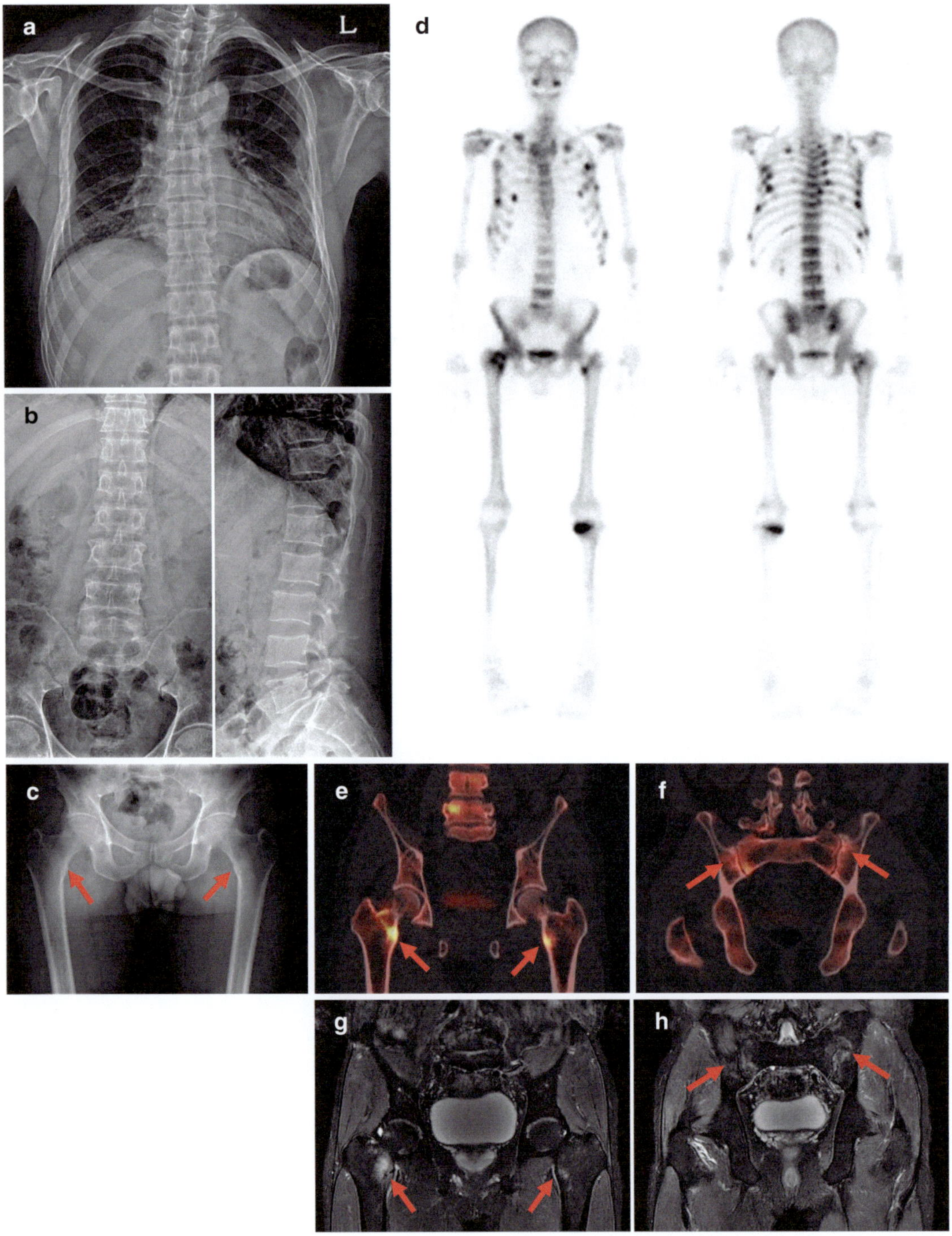

Fig. 14.3 A 46-year-old man with drug (adefovir)-induced osteomalacia. Diffuse osteopenia with multiple bilateral rib fractures, suspicious subchondral bone irregularities at both sacroiliac joints, and subtle sclerotic bone density at the lesser tuberosities of both femurs are noted on radiographs (**a**–**c**). Bone scan (**d**) and SPECT/CT of the pelvis (**e**, **f**) show multiple focal increased uptakes, suggesting insufficiency fractures in the T-L spine, bilateral ribs, right femoral neck, both femoral lesser trochanters, bilateral iliac side of the sacroiliac joints, and left proximal tibia. Pelvic MR images (**g**, **h**) show bone marrow edema with incomplete fracture lines involving the bilateral femoral lesser trochanters and the iliac side of the sacroiliac joints (red arrows)

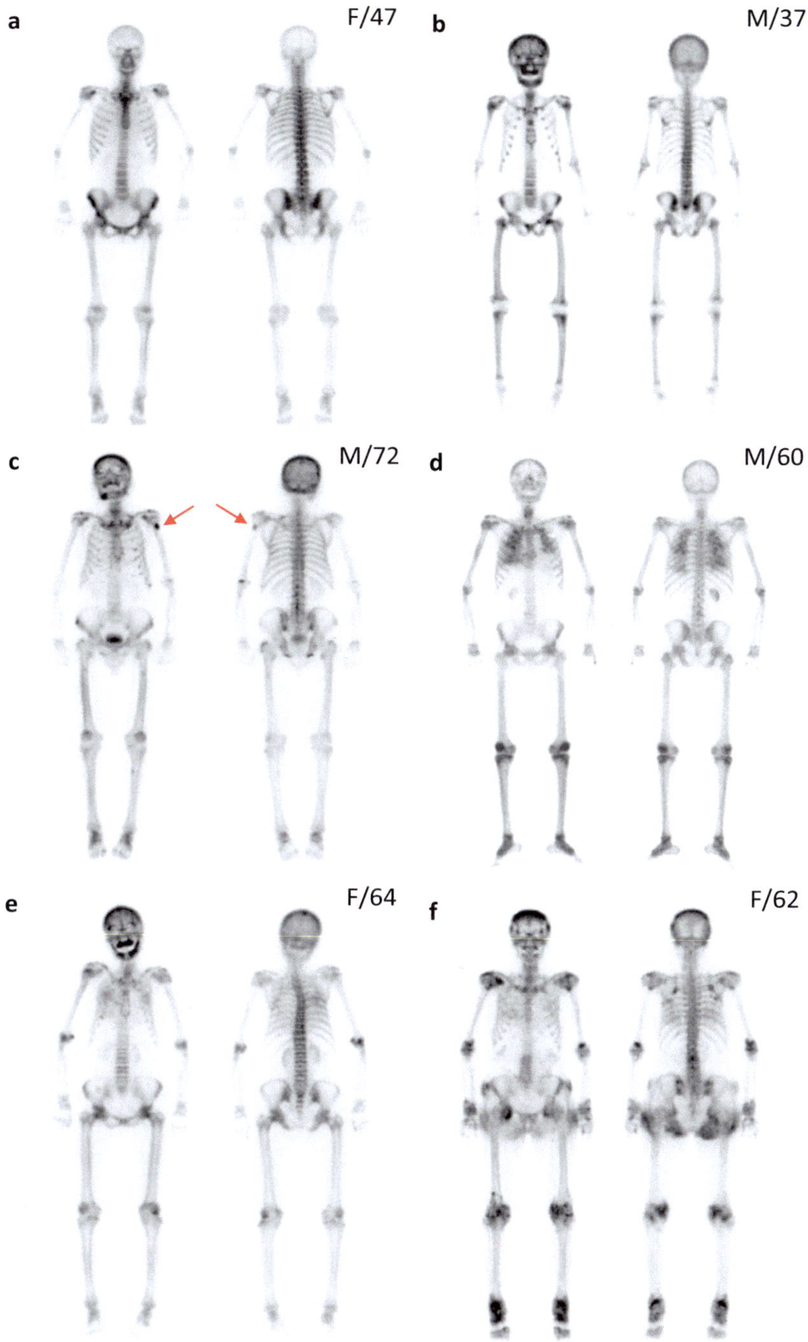

Fig. 14.4 Scintigraphic appearances of renal osteodystrophy in high-turnover disease. The characteristic features are generalized increased uptake with increased contrast between the bone and soft tissue. This leads to "superscan" (**a**–**e**), increased uptake in the long bones, axial skeleton, periarticular bones, calvaria, mandible, costochondral junctions (beading pattern), and sternum with absence of uptake in the kidneys. The more severe forms of hyperparathyroidism are associated with ectopic calcification or tertiary hyperparathyroidism (**b**). Focal skeletal abnormalities may signify associated brown tumors (**c**, left proximal humerus, red arrow). Extra-skeletal uptake is seen in the lungs, stomach, and kidneys (**d**–**f**) because of an increased ratio of serum calcium to phosphate and amyloid deposition (**f**, periarticular and both buttock areas)

and decreased density in the central portion of the vertebral body)" is often detected on lateral lumbar spine radiographs [2]. Osteosclerosis can also occur in conjunction. Osteoblast activation may result in new periosteal bone formation in the long bones and increase cortical thickness. Plain radiographs can also reveal the early features of osteomalacia, pseudo-fractures, or Looser zones prior to fracture occurrence.

Currently, this disease is characterized by three major types—high-turnover disease (most common), low-turnover disease, and mixed disease [7]. Scintigraphy shows a diffusely increased uptake in the skeleton, including the calvaria and mandible, in high-turnover disease type. It accentuates the contrast between the bone and soft tissue with an increased skeletal to renal uptake ratio. Figure 14.4 shows the scintigraphic appearance of renal osteodystrophy in high-turnover disease. Low-turnover disease typically shows a decreased uptake unless it is complicated by a focal pathology. A mixture of these findings is observed in mixed disease.

Case 14.4
A 32-year-old woman was brought to the emergency room due to a sudden, brief seizure-like episode. She had no other specific medical history, except a recent history of back pain and lower extremity weakness. On initial laboratory tests, high blood creatinine (7.5 mg/dL) and phosphorus (5.7 mg/dL) levels, severe hypocalcemia (total calcium 4.9 mg/dL), and anemia (Hb 7.8 g/dL) were noted. Brain MRI revealed normal findings. She was diagnosed with metabolic encephalopathy secondary to severe hypocalcemia and renal failure. After calcium supplementation, her leg weakness improved, and no further seizures occurred. However, low back pain persisted. In the subsequent imaging work-up (Fig. 14.5), renal osteodystrophy and insufficiency fractures were detected. In addition, a markedly high serum parathyroid hormone level (993 pg/mL) was observed.

Case 14.5
A 45-year-old man with end-stage renal disease visited the orthopedic clinic complaining of hip pain that developed 1 month previously. He had been undergoing hemodialysis for 7 years after renal allograft failure. On the imaging work-up with radiography and bone scintigraphy with SPECT/CT, an incomplete fracture of the right femoral neck was noted with underlying renal osteodystrophy findings (Fig. 14.6). Laboratory test findings showed the total calcium level was within the upper normal limit (10.2 mg/dL), with a high phosphorus level (8.4 mg/dL). The serum intact parathyroid hormone level was markedly elevated at 5,280 pg/mL. The patient was diagnosed with tertiary hyperparathyroidism. On parathyroid SPECT/CT with ^{99m}Tc 2-methoxy-isobutyl-isonitrile (MIBI), multiple parathyroid nodules, including an ectopic parathyroid nodule, with increased uptake were detected. Total parathyroidectomy with parathyroid autotransplantation was performed. The postoperative blood parathyroid hormone levels normalized, and the bone pain improved thereafter.

14.3 Paget's Disease

14.3.1 Etiology and Clinical Significance

Paget's disease of the bone, also known as osteitis deformans, is a chronic bone disor-

Fig. 14.5 A 32-year-old woman with renal osteodystrophy secondary to hyperparathyroidism. Bone scan (**a**) shows diffusely increased whole-body skeletal uptakes, especially high uptakes in the skull, sternum, costal ends at bilateral costochondral junctions in a beading pattern, and long bone ends. Bilateral kidney activities are not detectable. These are typical "superscan" findings of renal osteodystrophy. On the pelvic radiograph (**b**) and CT (**c**–**g**) images, generalized osteopenia and subchondral resorption in both sacroiliac joints (**d**) are seen. Associated insufficiency fractures with cortical disruption are noted in the left sacral ala (**e**), anterior column of both acetabula (**f**), and both inferior pubic rami (**g**). On the coronal, T2-weighted STIR MR image, insufficiency fracture reveals irregular hyperintense lesion in the left sacrum (arrow) (**h**). The lateral lumbar radiograph (**i**) and sagittal T2- and T1-weighted MR images (**j**) show "rugger jersey spine" appearance in vertebral bodies along the superior and inferior endplates

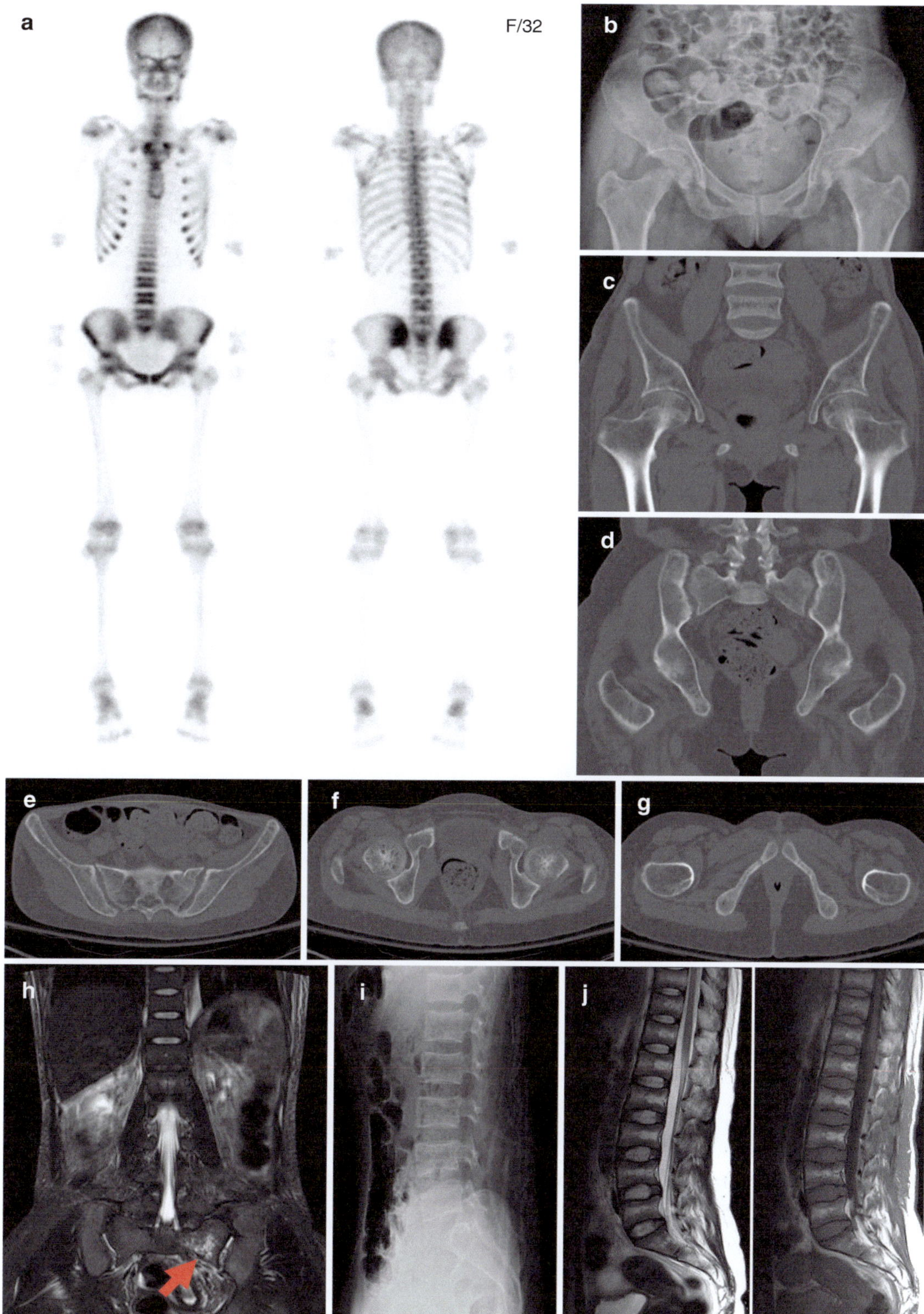
a
F/32
b
c
d
e
f
g
h
i
j

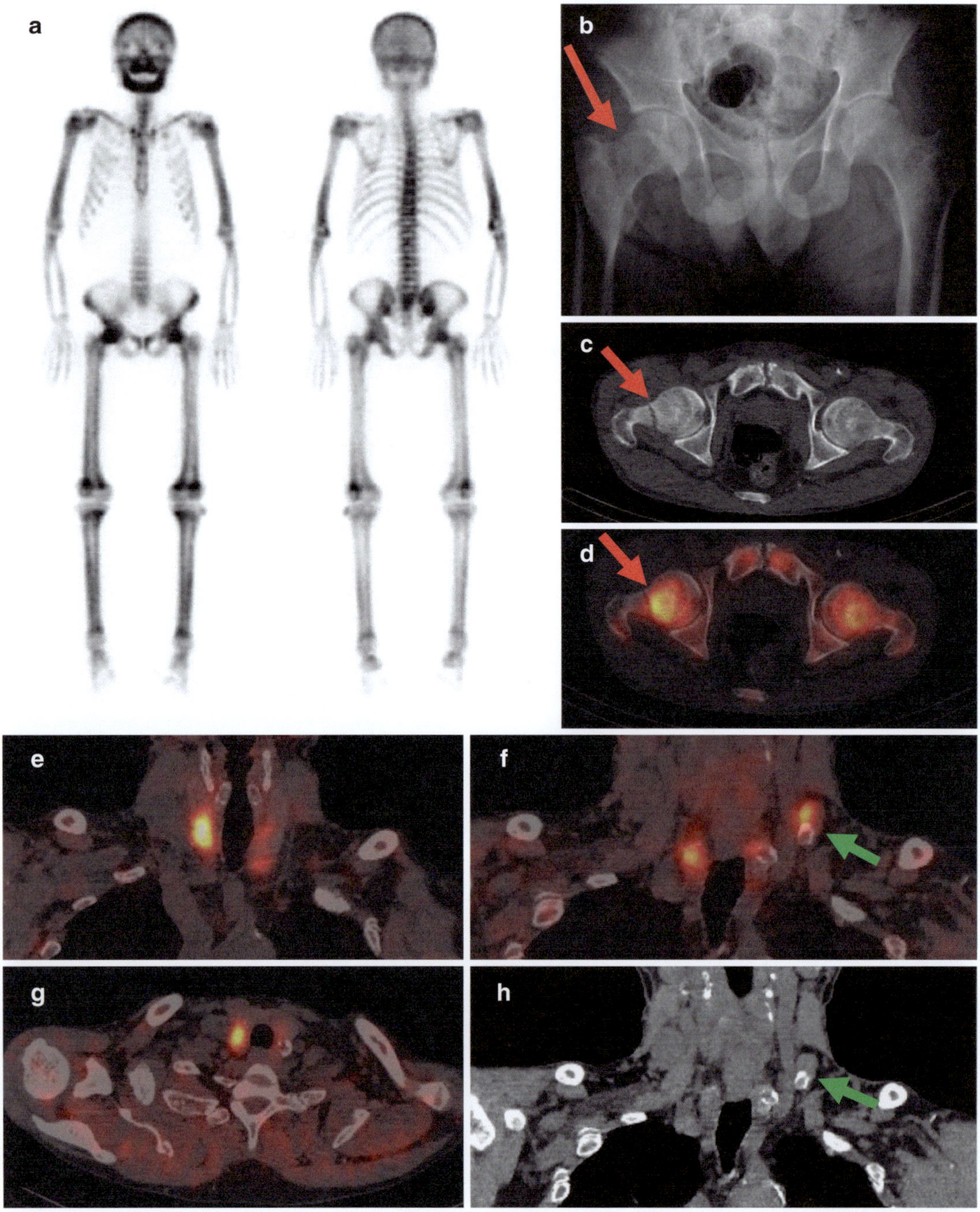

Fig. 14.6 A 45-year-old man with renal osteodystrophy and tertiary hyperparathyroidism. Bone scan (**a**) shows a so-called "superscan" pattern, which denotes generalized increased uptakes in whole-body bone scan, especially in the skull and long bones of the extremities. No kidney uptake is visualized. The plain radiograph (**b**) and SPECT/CT images (**c**, **d**) of the pelvis reveal a linear radiolucent line at the superolateral section of the right femur neck, indicating a pseudo-fracture (red arrow). On 2-h delayed parathyroid SPECT/CT images with ^{99m}Tc-MIBI (**e**–**h**), a total of four nodules with increased focal uptakes are observed at the posteroinferior aspect of the right thyroid lobe lower pole (2.5 cm), posterior aspect of the left thyroid lobe mid portion (1.4 cm), inferior aspect of the left thyroid lobe lower pole (1.5 cm), and ectopic site at the left cervical level IV with calcifications (green arrow)

der characterized by excessive abnormal bone remodeling and deformities. The affected bones show signs of dysregulated bone remodeling, specifically excessive bone breakdown and subsequent disorganized new bone formation. The exact cause of this disease is unknown, although the leading theories suggest that both genetic and acquired factors are involved. Paget's disease may affect any one or multiple bones of the body (most commonly the pelvis, tibia, femur, lumbar vertebrae, and skull). However, the entire skeleton is never involved, and the disease does not spread from bone to bone. The common clinical manifestations are abnormal bone structures, such as localized bone hypertrophy and osteoporosis. These processes lead to bone pain, bone deformity, and fractures. Laboratory findings reveal elevated blood alkaline phosphatase levels due to intense osteoblastic activity.

14.3.2 Imaging

This disease has three phases—early resorptive (incipient active), mixed middle (active), and final (late inactive) sclerotic phases [8]. The diagnosis can typically be made using radiographs, which reveal lytic lesions in early cases and coarsened, expanded bones as the disease progresses to the final phase. Bone scan is highly sensitive and useful for determining the extent and activity of the condition. The bone scan appearance of Paget's disease is striking, with intensely increased tracer localization [9]. Increased uptake is observed in all stages of the untreated disease (Fig. 14.7). Physicians must be aware of the patterns of Paget's disease because it may be found incidentally during screening bone scans for metastatic work-ups as many patients are asymptomatic and/or undiagnosed. If bone scan findings suggest Paget's disease, X-ray of the affected bone(s)

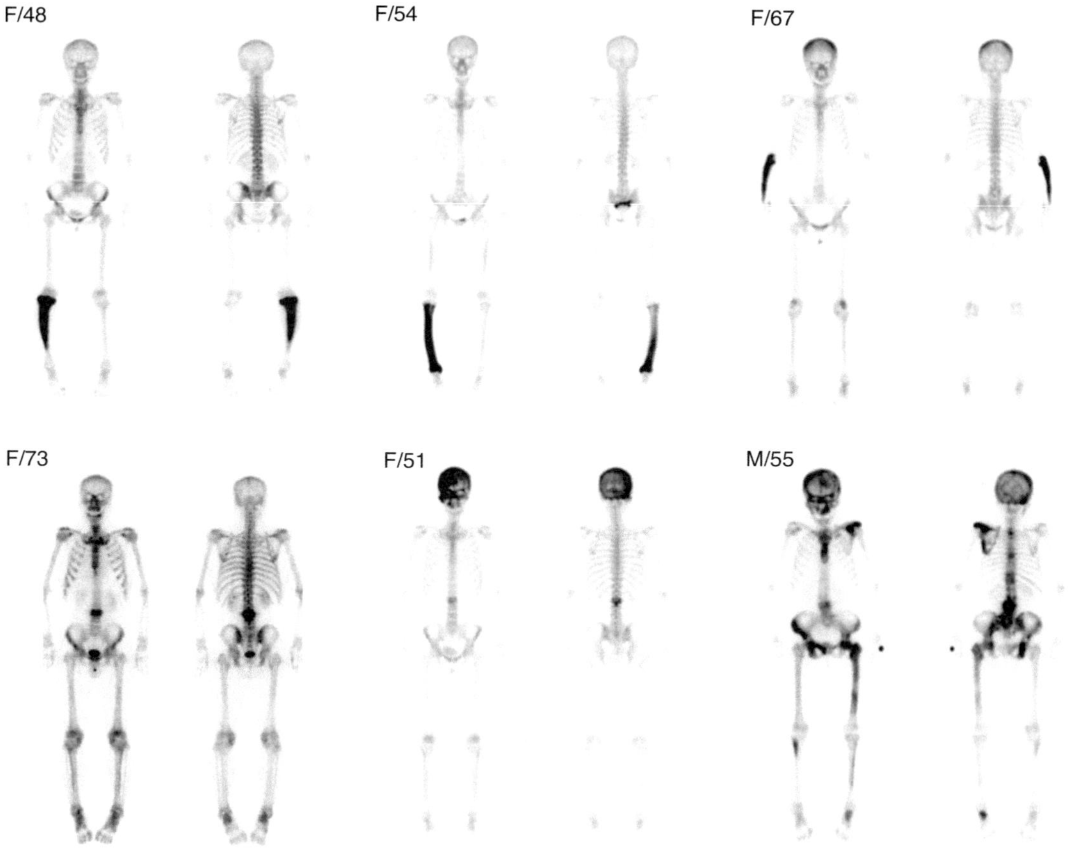

Fig. 14.7 Various scintigraphic appearances of Paget's disease involving one or multiple bones of the body

should be performed to confirm the diagnosis. The uptake intensity of the affected bone on bone scan decreases with effective therapy. After calcitonin or bisphosphonate therapy, bone scans show alterations in the uptake distribution, and the uniform uptake distribution on bone scan may change to a patchy focal uptake [10].

Case 14.6
A 40-year-old man with hepatitis B presented with an increased level of serum alpha-fetoprotein (30.5 ng/mL; normal range, <7.5 ng/mL). Subsequent evaluation revealed a 1-cm arterial-enhancing nodule in the liver at the left lateral segment, suggesting hepatocellular carcinoma on dynamic liver CT. During the preoperative work-up, bone scan revealed a diffusely increased uptake lesion in the right pelvic bone (Fig. 14.8). To exclude bone metastasis, ^{18}F-FDG/CT was performed. The patient underwent left lateral segmentectomy of the liver as the most likely diagnosis was Paget's disease in the right pelvic bone based on imaging findings. After surgery, his alpha-fetoprotein level normalized. At the last postoperative 4-year follow-up, he was stationary without recurrence of tumor.

Case 14.7
A 61-year-old man was diagnosed with prostate cancer during a routine health checkup. He had elevated serum prostate-specific antigen (PSA) level (4.58 ng/mL) and alkaline phosphatase (147 IU/L) levels. In the staging work-up, intensely increased uptake in the left pelvic bone, including the entire left ilium, was detected on whole-body bone scan. He had no bone pain. Compared to the pelvic CT and MRI findings, the presumed diagnosis of the bone lesions was Paget's disease (Fig. 14.9). Subsequently, the patient underwent robot-assisted laparoscopic prostatectomy. During postoperative follow-up, his blood alkaline phosphatase level increased along with an increase in the left iliac bone uptake intensity on bone scan. However, there was no other evidence of cancer recurrence, with an undetectable serum PSA level. After initiating treatment (zoledronic acid injection and oral alendronate/cholecalciferol), his follow-up alkaline phosphatase level was normal, and bone scans showed decreased intensity of the left iliac bone uptake.

Case 14.8
A 76-year-old woman with multiple body aches was referred to our endocrinology clinic. She was diagnosed with Paget's disease 10 years previously after a fracture in her left hip. However, her condition was not managed appropriately. Thus, she developed total hearing loss 1 year ago and developed headache and dizziness developed 5 months later. Her blood alkaline phosphatase level was high at 923 IU/L. A skeletal survey by plain radiography and whole-body bone scan revealed multiple bone involvement, including involvement of the skull, with Paget's disease (Fig. 14.10). Bone densitometry using DXA showed severe osteoporosis of the lumbar spine (0.665 g/cm^2; T-score, −3.7). Treatment was initiated for the management of Paget's disease, followed by imaging and laboratory tests.

14.4 Osteopetrosis

14.4.1 Etiology and Clinical Significance

Osteopetrosis, literally "stone bone," also known as marble bone disease, is a prototype of osteosclerosing dysplasia. It is an extremely rare inherited disorder with both autosomal-dominant and autosomal-recessive subtypes, resulting in defective osteoclasts. Hence, bone resorption fails, but there is continuous bone formation, resulting in excessive bone formation. The bones are also structurally abnormal. This condition makes them prone to fracture and narrowing of the bone marrow space causing a decrease in hematopoiesis and anemia [11].

14.4.2 Imaging

Radiographically, the hallmark of osteopetrosis is increased density within the medullary section of the bone, with relative sparing of the cortices. Erlenmeyer flask deformity (club-like long bones and flaring of ends due to lack of tubulation), "bone-within-bone" appearance, or the "sandwich vertebra" appearance, characterized by dense endplate sclerosis with sharp margins are observed. Bone scans show a diffuse increase in

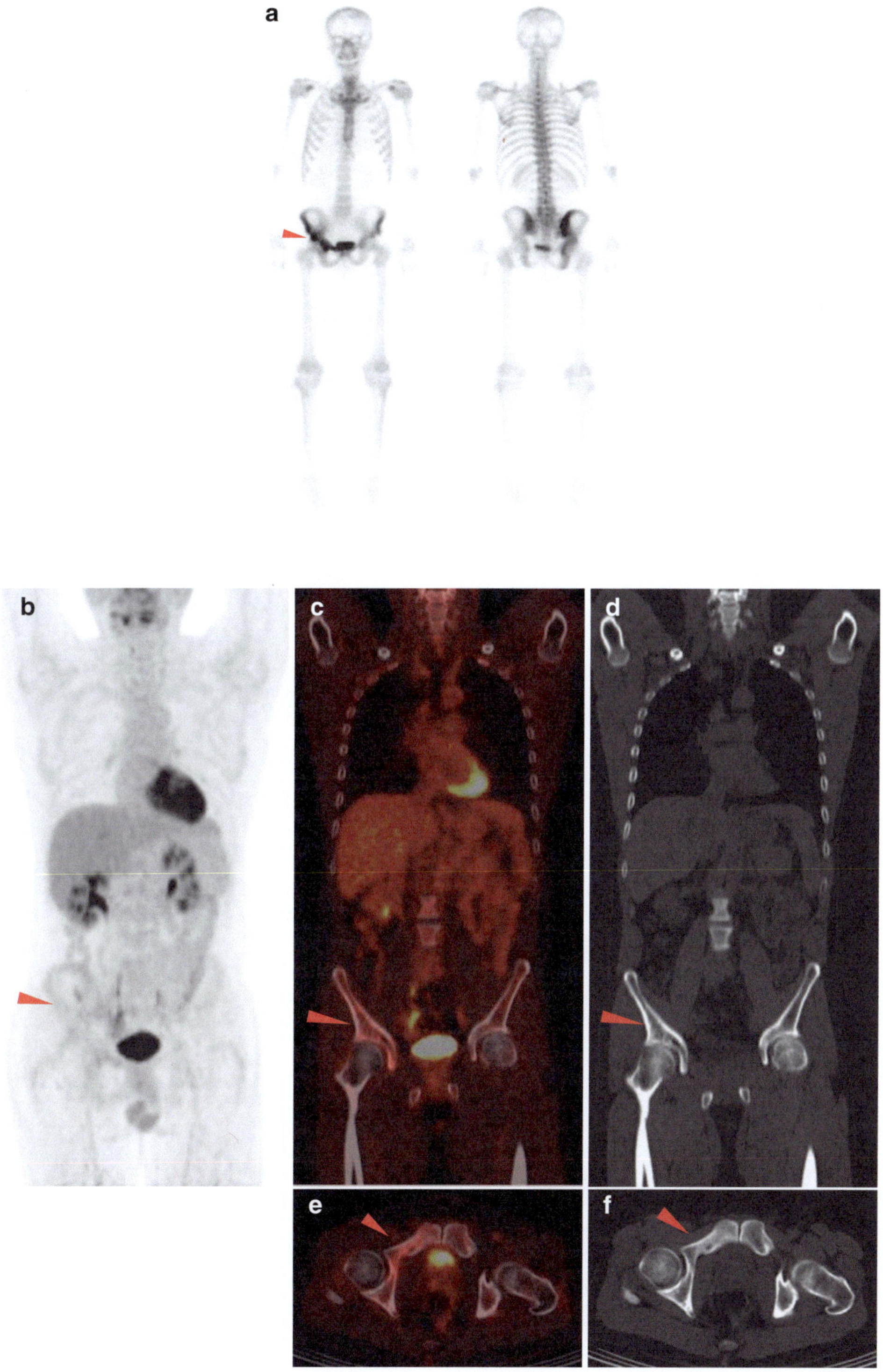

Fig. 14.8 A 40-year-old patient with hepatocellular carcinoma of the left liver lateral segment and Paget's disease in the right pelvic bone. Whole-body bone scan (**a**) shows diffusely increased uptake in the right ilium and superior pubic ramus including the right acetabulum (red arrowhead). The right pelvic bones are mildly hypermetabolic on maximum intensity view (**b**) and fusion PET/CT coronal and transaxial images (**c**, **e**) of the whole-body ^{18}F-FDG/CT, and sclerotic change with preserved internal trabeculation and mild cortical hypertrophy is seen on CT images (**d**, **f**). A liver nodule is not visualized due to isometabolic activity in the normal liver tissue

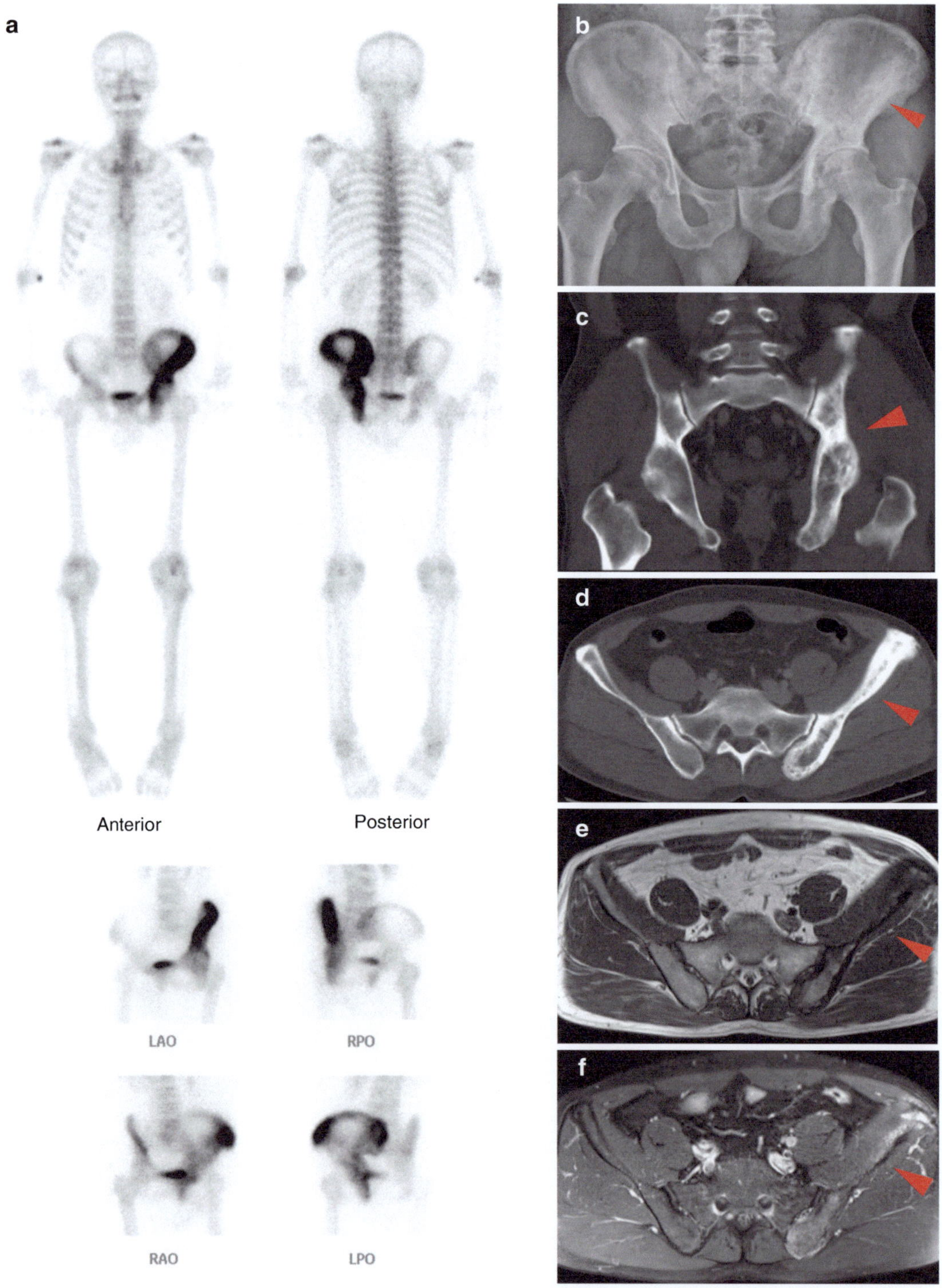

Fig. 14.9 A 61-year-old patient with prostate cancer and Paget's disease in the left iliac bone. Bone scan images (**a**) show diffuse, intensely increased bone uptake in the left ilium. Diffuse osteosclerosis of the left ilium (red arrowhead) is noted on the plain radiograph (**b**) and coronal and axial CT images (**c**, **d**). MR images (**e**, **f**) show cortical thickening and medullary cavity narrowing with heterogeneous contrast enhancement in the left ilium. The serial follow-up bone scan images (**g**) show an abrupt decrease of the left pelvic bone uptake intensity after treatment initiation. Serial plain radiographs (**h**) do not show any change in osteosclerosis during the follow-up period. A decrease in the blood alkaline phosphatase level (**i**) is well correlated with findings of bone scans

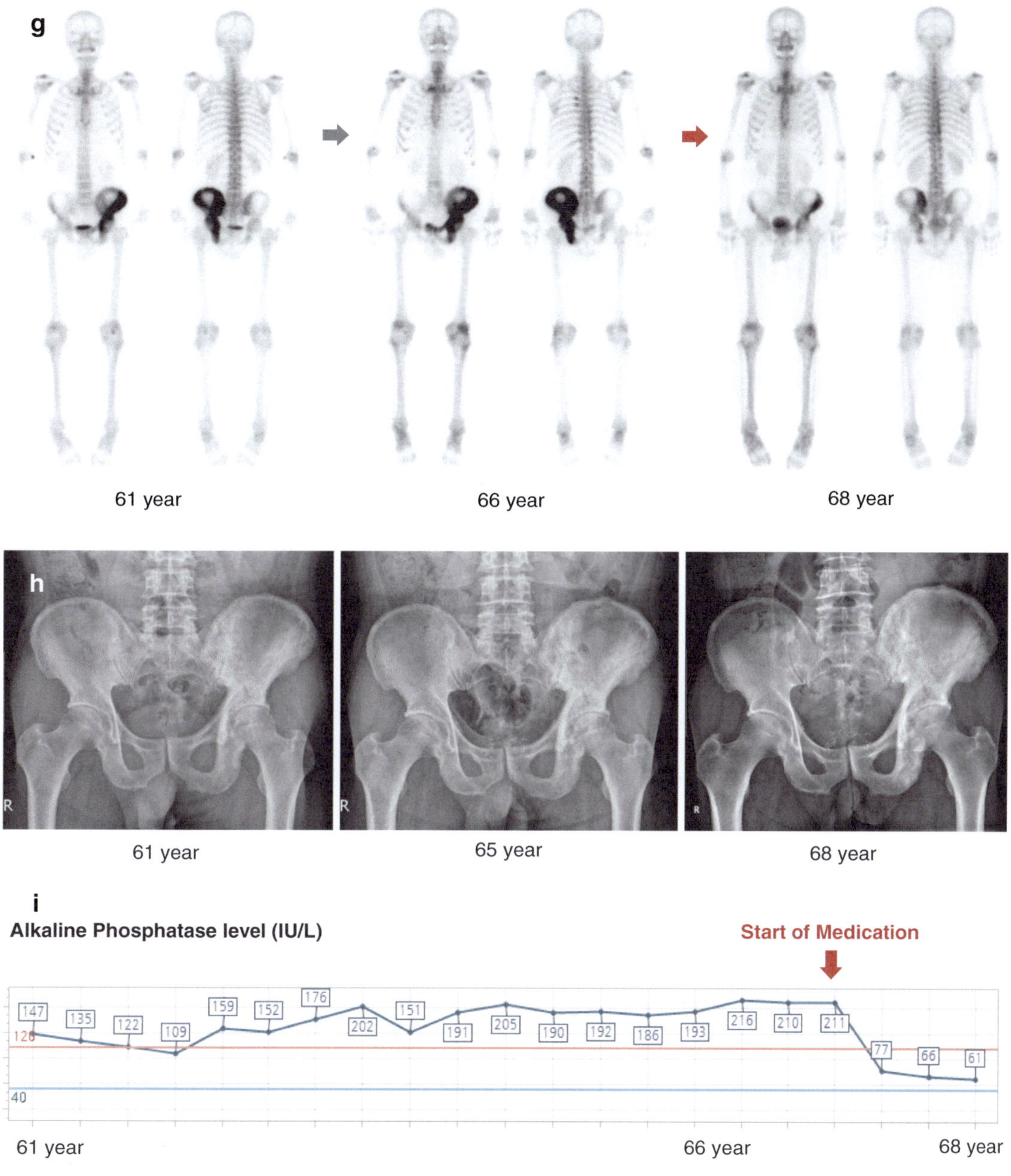

Fig. 14.9 (continued)

skeletal uptake and symmetrically increased focal uptake in the metaphyses and adjacent diaphyses of multiple long bones. These are typical findings in osteopetrosis. Bone scans also contribute to the follow-up of these patients. Bone scans allow longitudinal monitoring of this disease as new asymptomatic bone fractures may be diagnosed. Thus, serial whole-body scans may be useful for both symptomatic and asymptomatic patients with osteopetrosis [11].

Case 14.9

An 18-year-old woman was referred to orthopedic clinic for further evaluation of sclerotic bones, which were observed on chest radiography during a routine school health checkup. Bone scans and skeletal surveys revealed diffusely increased tracer uptake and sclerotic changes in the spine, pelvis, and long bones (Fig. 14.11). Laboratory blood tests findings were normal. The patient was diagnosed with autosomal dominant osteopetro-

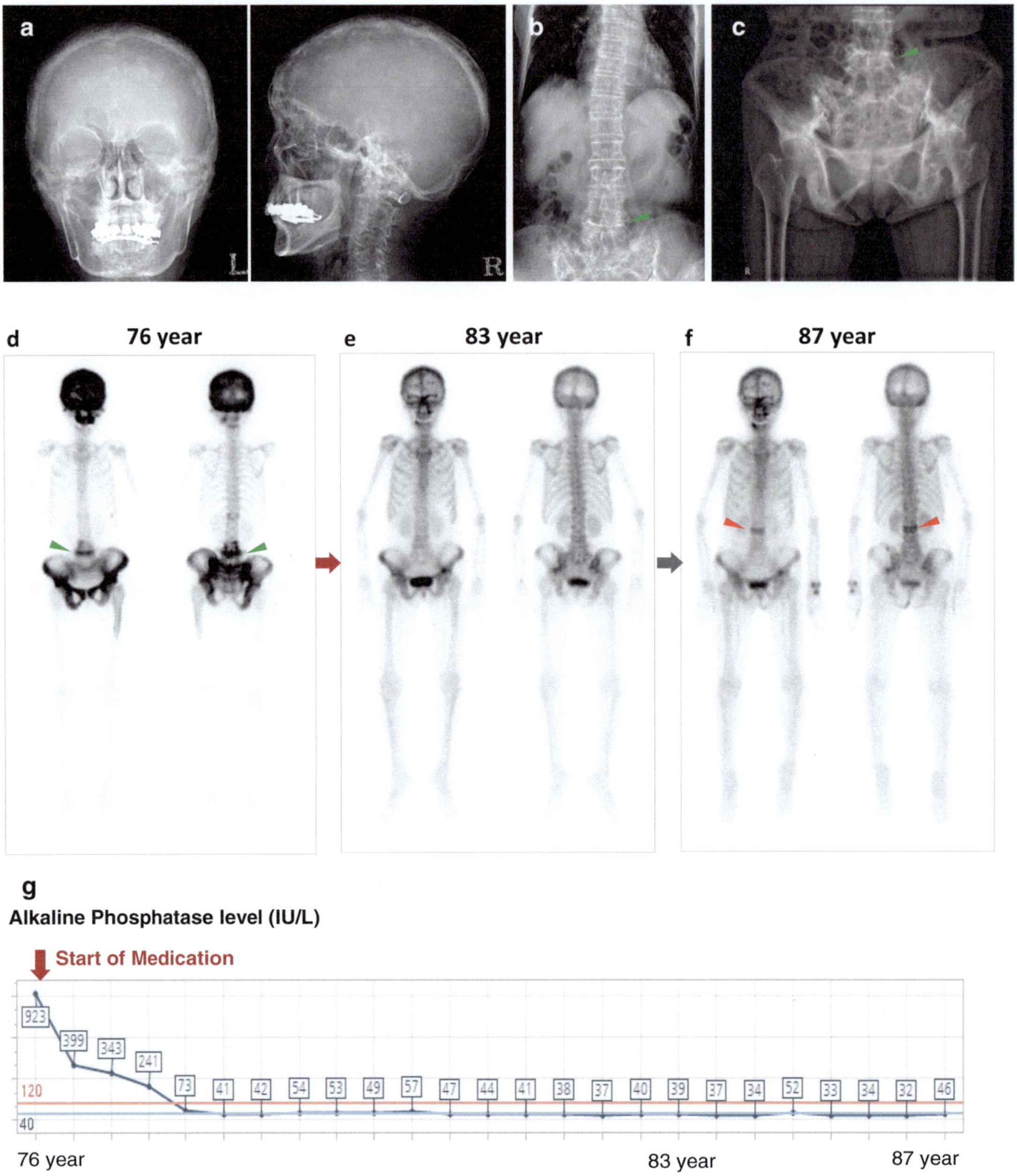

Fig. 14.10 A 76-year-old woman with multiple bone involvement with Paget's disease. Diffuse osteosclerosis is detected in the skull (**a**), bilateral pelvic bones, sacrum, and left proximal femur (**b**, **c**) on radiographs. Compression fracture (green arrowhead) is noted at the L4 body. Initial bone scan (**d**) shows diffuse, intensely increased uptake in the skull, bilateral pelvic bones and sacrum, left proximal femur, and L4 vertebral body. Focal increased uptakes are also noted in the upper C-spine, T12, left seventh rib, and right side L3 body. After treatment initiation, follow-up bone scans (**e**, **f**) show decreased intensity of uptakes in the abovementioned bone lesions. A compression fracture with increased uptake in the L2 vertebral body (red arrowhead) is shown on the last follow-up image (**f**). The graph (**g**) shows the drop in the blood alkaline phosphatase level after treatment initiation

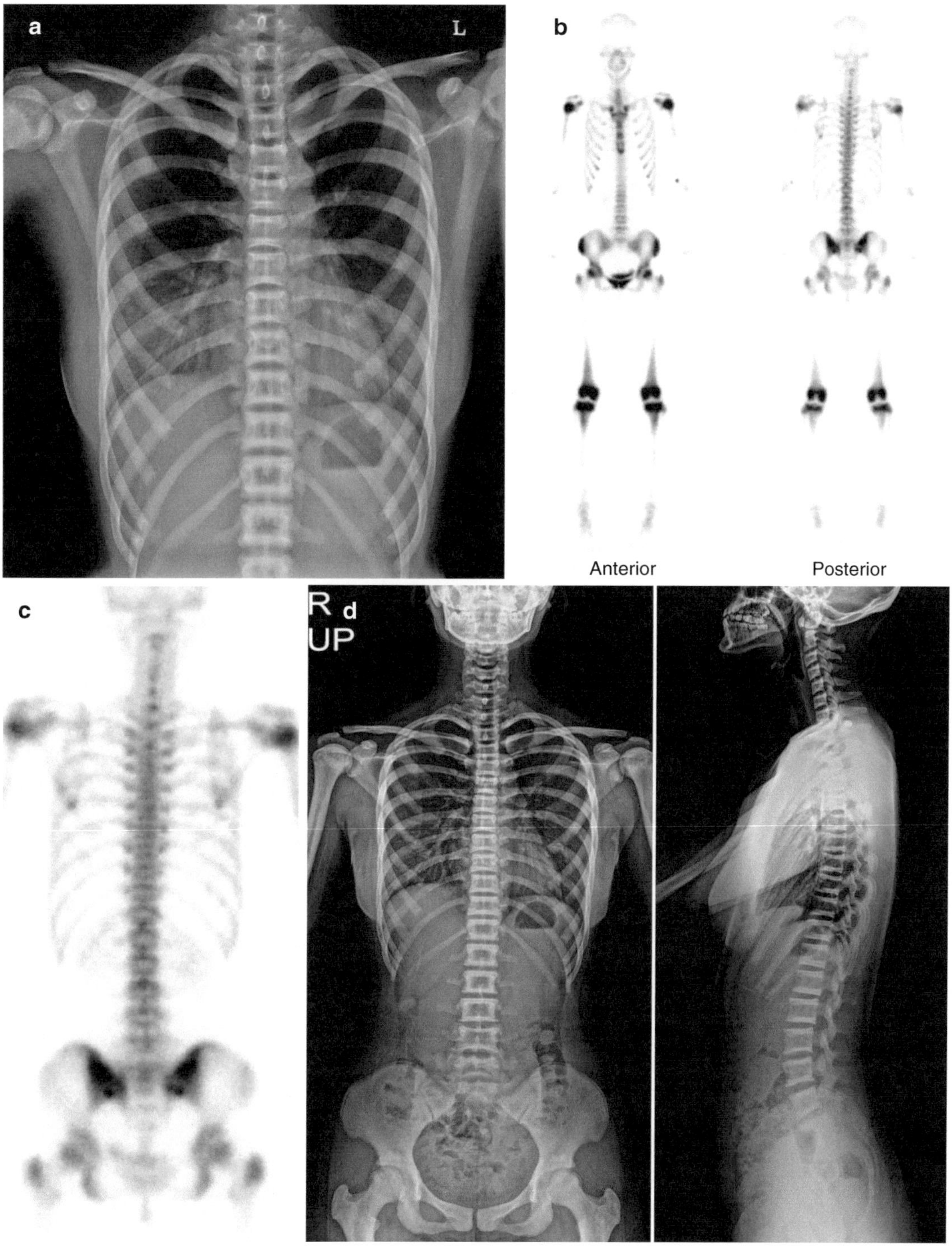

Fig. 14.11 An 18-year-old woman with newly diagnosed osteopetrosis. The chest radiograph (**a**) and anterior and lateral views of the whole spine (**d**) and lower extremities (**f**) show diffusely increased density of all bones. Dense sclerosis of the upper and lower endplates of vertebral bodies with central relatively lucent bone is consistent with a "sandwich vertebrae" or "bone within a bone" appearance. Whole-body bone scan (**b**, **c**, **e**) shows symmetric diffusely increased uptakes along the cortex of the spine, sternum, both pelvic bones, and long bones of both the upper and lower extremities. This is especially prominent at the proximal ends of the humeri and tibiae along with the proximal and distal ends of the femora. These imaging findings are typical features of osteopetrosis

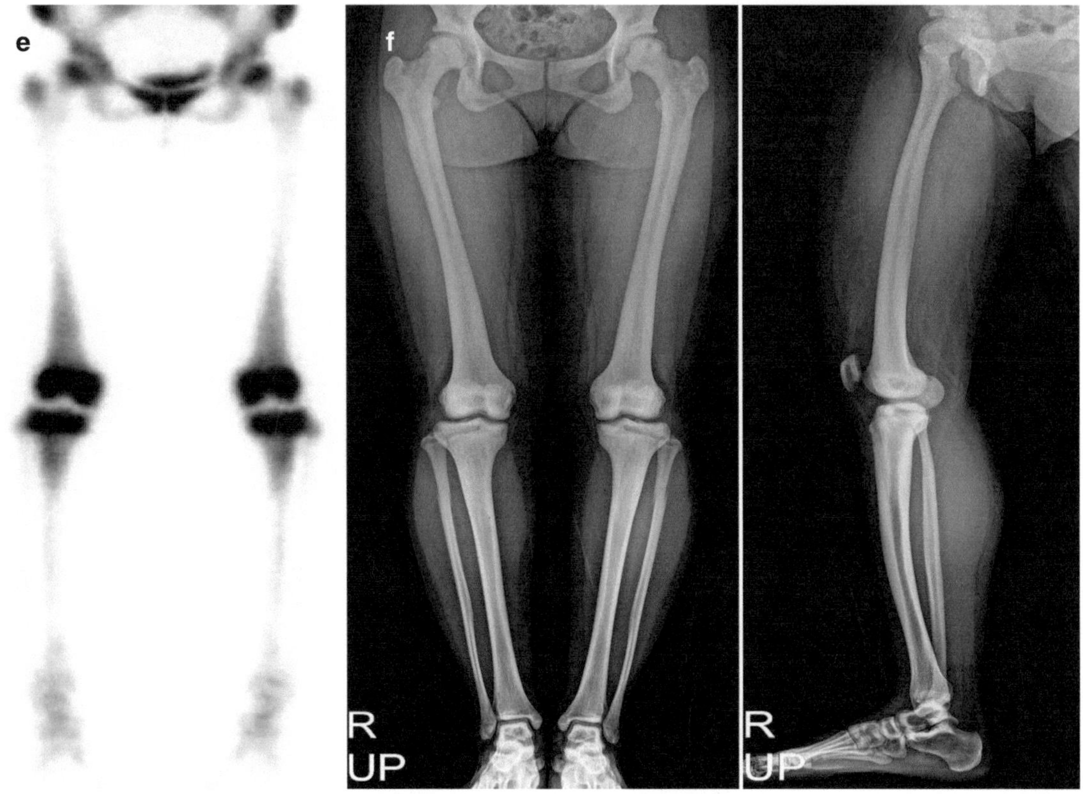

Fig. 14.11 (continued)

sis type 2 with a heterozygous mutation in the CLCN7 gene, detected using diagnostic exome sequencing.

Case 14.10

A 39-year-old woman with a history of left hip pain for several years visited the orthopedic surgery clinic. She requested an opinion regarding hip surgery. Ten years prior, she was diagnosed with osteopetrosis and was taking medication. The patient underwent bone marrow transplantation for hematologic failure. Further imaging studies (Fig. 14.12) were performed for presurgical assessment.

14.5 Camurati–Engelmann Disease

14.5.1 Etiology and Clinical Significance

Camurati–Engelmann disease, also known as progressive diaphyseal dysplasia, is a rare autosomal dominant form of sclerosing bone dysplasia. It begins in childhood (predominantly before the age of <30 years) and follows a progressive course. In most cases, it results from a defect in the transforming growth factor β1 (TGF β1) gene, which causes osteoblastic overactivity

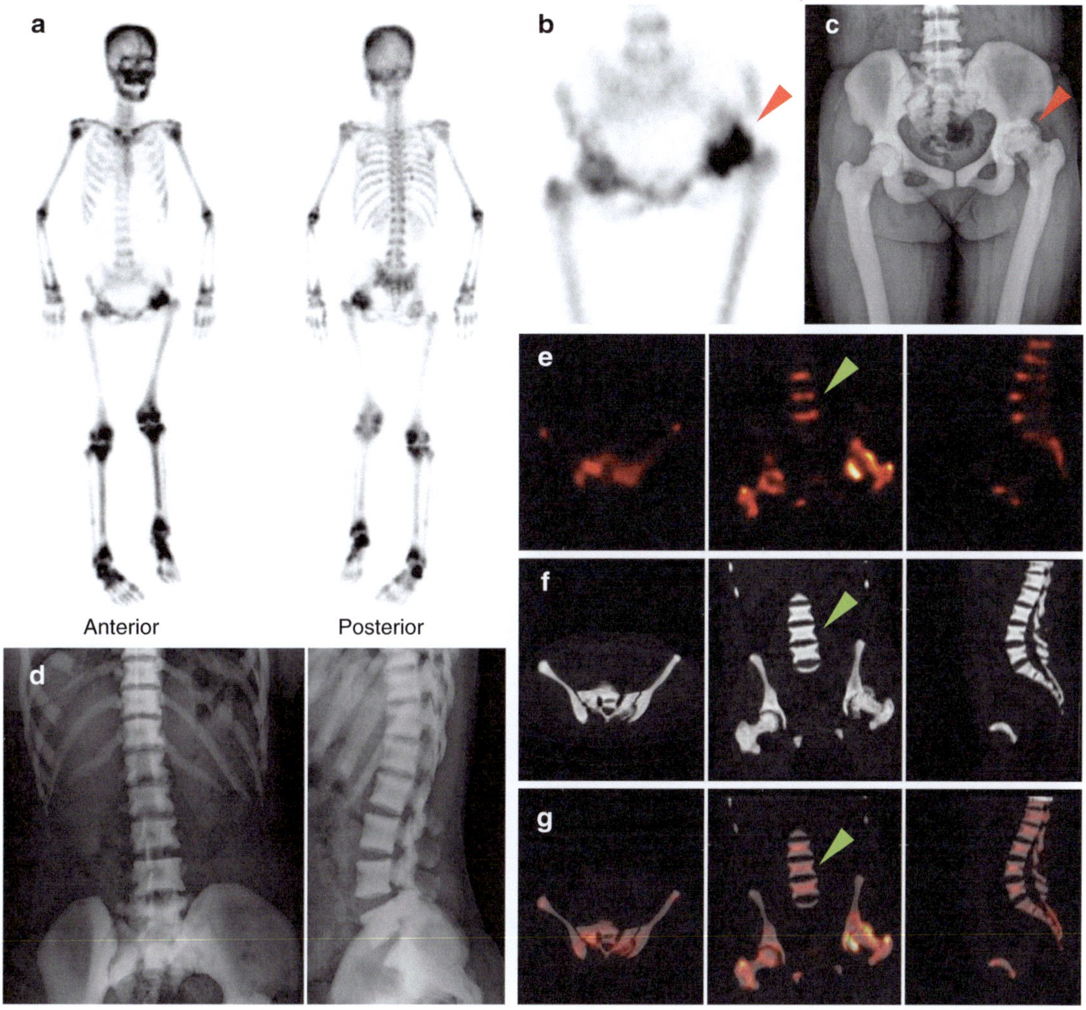

Fig. 14.12 A 39-year-old patient with severe osteopetrosis with hematologic failure. Whole-body bone scan (**a**, **b**) shows diffusely increased uptakes in the whole skeleton, especially in the skull and long bones. Multifocal increased uptakes at the right posterior arc of the eighth and ninth ribs, radial, and fibular shafts suggest earlier fractures. A deformity at the left hip joint reveals intensely increased periarticular bone uptakes (red arrowhead). On the pelvic radiograph (**c**), the entire bones are abnormally dense. Additional abnormalities at the left hip joint, including joint space narrowing, subchondral cystic changes, and subluxation of the left femoral head, are observed, indicating secondary osteoarthritis. Radiographs of the lumbar spine (**d**) show a "sandwich vertebrae" appearance, and bone SPECT/CT images (**e**–**g**) of the L-spine and pelvis demonstrate decreased uptakes in the thick dense upper and lower endplates of the vertebrae and increased uptake in the relatively lucent central zone with narrow marrow spaces (green arrowhead)

[12]. The common symptoms include extremity pain, muscle weakness, cranial nerve impairment, and waddling gait. Patients may also present with hepatosplenomegaly. A small proportion of the patients are asymptomatic.

14.5.2 Imaging

The radiographic hallmark of Camurati–Engelmann disease is cortical thickening of the diaphysis of the long bones. The epiphyses are

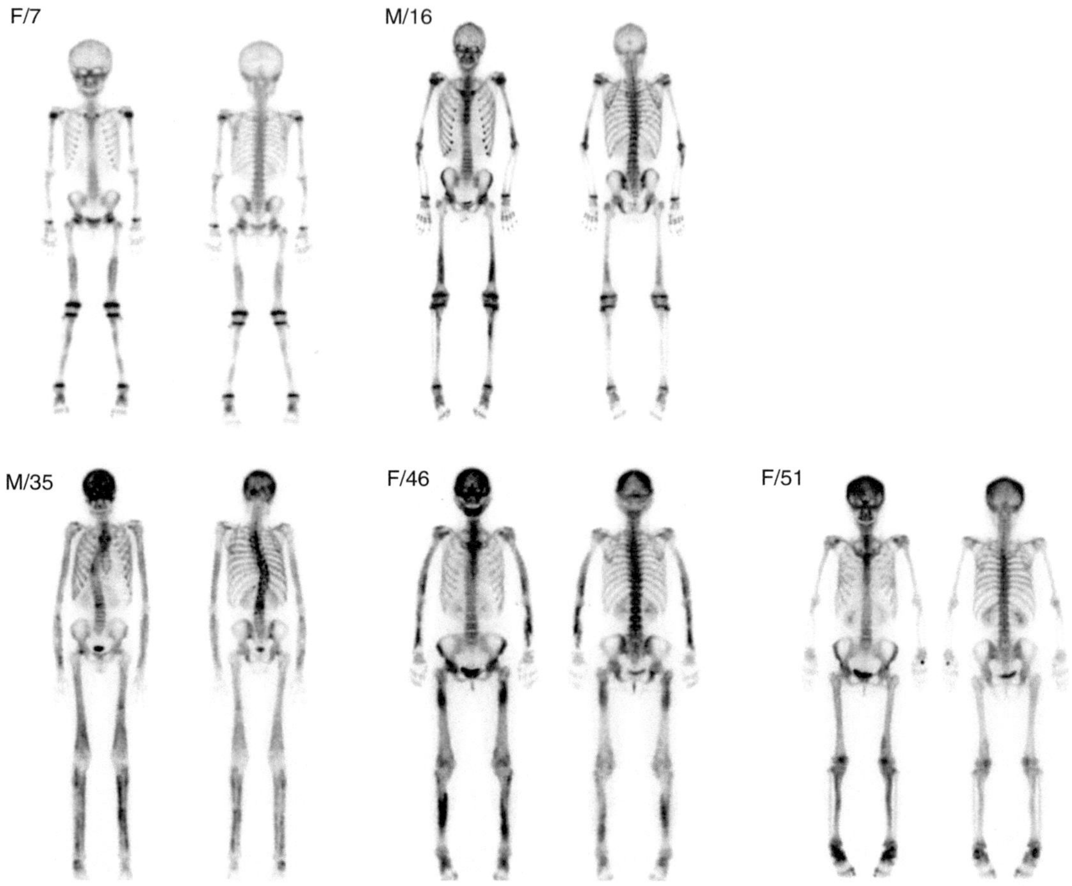

Fig. 14.13 Scintigraphic pattern of Camurati–Engelmann disease (progressive diaphyseal dysplasia) in various stages on bone scan

spared, and narrowing or obliteration of the medullary canal is observed in a bilateral symmetric pattern. In severe cases, osteosclerosis is widespread, and the skull and axial skeleton are also involved [13]. On bone scan, the affected regions show high tracer uptake representing osteoblastic activity, even before it is radiologically visible. Clinical, radiographic, and scintigraphic findings are generally concordant. However, markedly increased uptake with minimal radiographic findings can reflect early and active disease (Fig. 14.13). Therefore, bone scan is a valuable tool for diagnosing early-stage disease.

Case 14.11

An 11-year-old boy with Camurati–Engelmann type I disease visited the medical genetics clinic for further management. At the age of 5 years, he was diagnosed with this disease after a workup for his waddling gait. Molecular analysis revealed the presence of a TGF β1 gene mutation. He complained of discomfort in the right ankle. Skeletal survey and bone scan revealed a typical pattern of bilateral, symmetric hyperostosis at the diaphysis of the long bones (Fig. 14.14). The patient was followed up periodically in the clinic with steroid treatment.

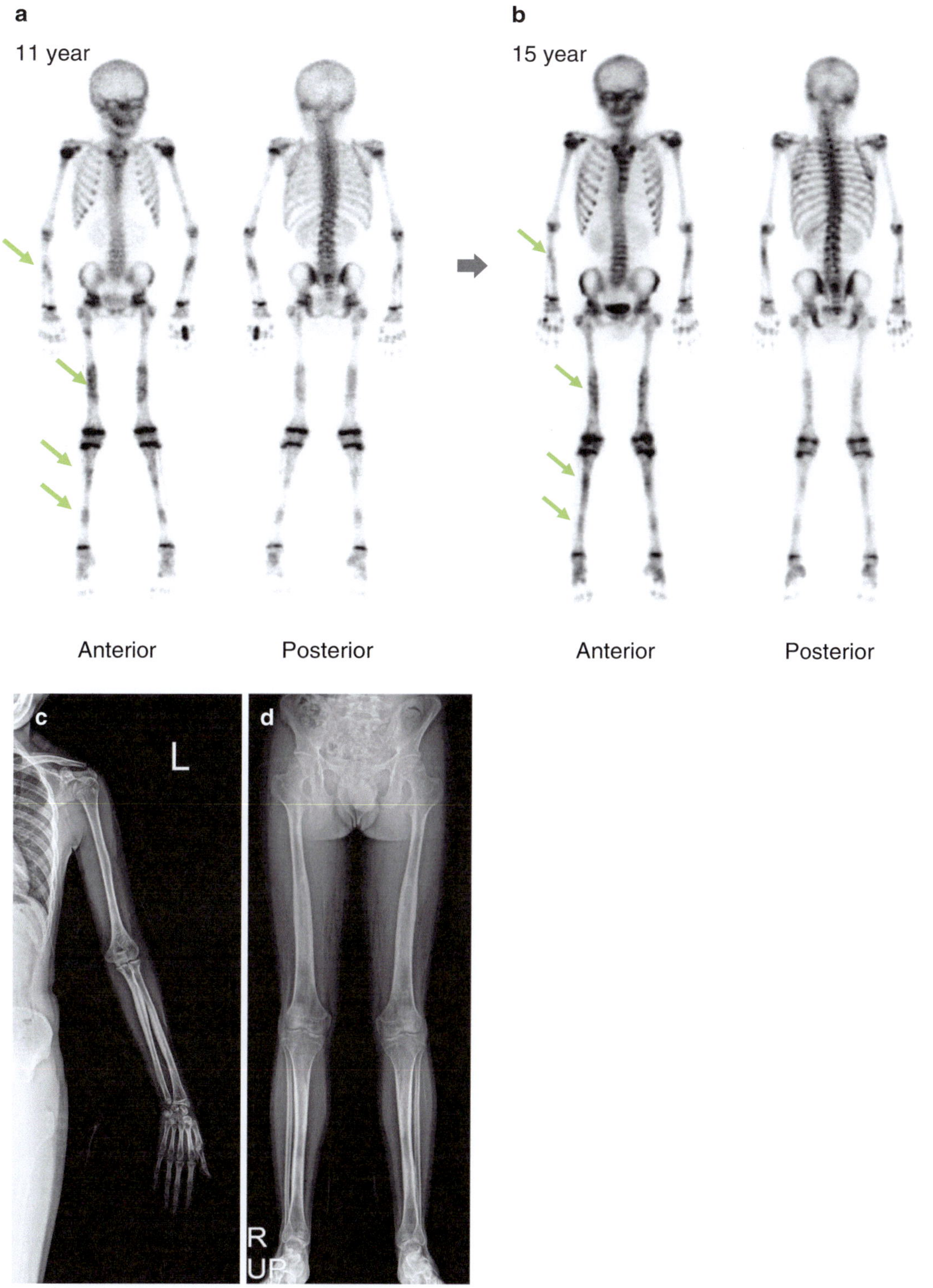

Fig. 14.14 An 11-year-old boy with Camurati–Engelmann type I disease. Initial bone scan (**a**) shows symmetric increased tracer uptakes in the diaphysis of the long bones in the bilateral ulnae, radii, femurs, and tibiae (arrows). On follow-up bone scan 4 years later (**b**) after steroid treatment, similar patterns of increased uptakes in the long bones are persistent in the diaphysis of long bones (arrows). Plain radiographs show cortical thickening of the diaphysis of the long bones in the same location shown on the bone scan (**c**, **d**)

Teaching Points

- Knowledge of the various scintigraphic patterns of each MBD on bone scan assists in obtaining the highest diagnostic assessment.
- The correlative interpretation of various imaging modalities with an understanding of their diverse findings allows for an early and specific diagnosis of MBD.
- The most important practical applications of bone scans in MBD are the detection of focal conditions or focal complications such as insufficiency fractures or pseudofractures of generalized disease. This includes an evaluation of the disease's activity on diagnosis and after treatment.
- An extensive investigation is required to investigate the causes of generalized bone pain in patients with hypophosphatemia. Somatostatin receptor PET/CT imaging with ^{68}Ga-DOTA-peptide is a useful tool for the detection of culprit tumors inducing osteomalacia.
- The scintigraphic appearance of renal osteodystrophy differs with the varying degrees of secondary hyperparathyroidism according to the three major types—high-turnover disease (most common), low-turnover disease, and mixed disease.

References

1. Elgazzar AH. Diagnosis of metabolic, endocrine, and congenital bone disease. In: Orthopedic nuclear medicine. Cham: Springer; 2017. p. 101–45.
2. Chang CY, Rosenthal DI, Mitchell DM, Handa A, Kattapuram SV, Huang AJ. Imaging findings of metabolic bone disease. Radiographics. 2016;36(6):1871–87.
3. Hussein MAM, Cafarelli FP, Paparella MT, Rennie WJ, Guglielmi G. Phosphaturic mesenchymal tumors: radiological aspects and suggested imaging pathway. Radiol Med. 2021;126(12):1609–18.
4. Lee DY, Lee SH, Kim BJ, Kim W, Yoon PW, Lee SJ, et al. Usefulness of ^{68}Ga-DOTATOC PET/CT to localize the culprit tumor inducing osteomalacia. Sci Rep. 2021;11(1):1819.
5. Kim DH, Sung DH, Min YK. Hypophosphatemic osteomalacia induced by low-dose adefovir therapy: focus on manifestations in the skeletal system and literature review. J Bone Miner Metab. 2013;31(2):240–6.
6. Pimentel A, Bover J, Elder G, Cohen-Solal M, Ureña-Torres PA. The Use of imaging techniques in chronic kidney disease-mineral and bone disorders (CKD-MBD)-a systematic review. Diagnostics (Basel). 2021;11(5):772.
7. Elgazzar AH. Synopsis of pathophysiology in nuclear medicine. Cham: Springer; 2014. p. 85.
8. Theodorou DJ, Theodorou SJ, Kakitsubata Y. Imaging of Paget disease of bone and its musculoskeletal complications. Am J Roentgenol. 2011;196(6_supplement):S64–75.
9. Abdelrazek S, Szumowski P, Rogowski F, Kociura-Sawicka A, Mojsak M, Szorc M. Bone scan in metabolic bone diseases. Review. Nucl Med Rev Cent East Eur. 2012;15(2):124–31.
10. Ralston SH, Corral-Gudino L, Cooper C, Francis RM, Fraser WD, Gennari L, et al. Diagnosis and management of Paget's disease of bone in adults: a clinic. Guideline J Bone Miner Res. 2019;34(4):579–604.
11. Sit C, Agrawal K, Fogelman I, Gnanasegaran G. Osteopetrosis: radiological & radionuclide imaging. Indian J Nucl Med. 2015;30(1):55–8.
12. Janssens K, Vanhoenacker F, Bonduelle M, Verbruggen L, Van Maldergem L, Ralston S, et al. Camurati-Engelmann disease: review of the clinical, radiological, and molecular data of 24 families and implications for diagnosis and treatment. J Med Genet. 2006;43(1):1–11.
13. Bartuseviciene A, Samuilis A, Skucas J. Camurati–Engelmann disease: imaging, clinical features and differential diagnosis. Skelet Radiol. 2009;38(11):1037–43.

15 Osteoporosis

Seoung-Oh Yang, Jung Mi Park, Hye Joo Son, Jang Gyu Cha, Jee Won Chai, and So Won Oh

Abstract

Osteoporosis is the most common metabolic bone disorder which is characterized by reduction in the bone density. Osteoporosis is called as "the silent killer" and often diagnosed after the development of fracture because it itself has no overt clinical symptoms. However, osteoporosis must not be neglected since osteoporotic fractures have enormous impacts on patients as well as the whole society. Osteoporotic fracture is the most serious clinical outcome of osteoporosis, and it is more common in women than in men, due to decreased bone mineral density (BMD) after menopause. Thus, active prevention including early diagnosis and proper treatment is crucial in the management of patients with osteoporosis. This chapter includes clinically relevant cases performed by nuclear imaging (bone scan, SPECT/CT, and PET/CT) and other correlative radiologic images for the diagnosis of the vertebral compression fracture, sacral insufficiency fracture, atypical femoral fracture, and medication-related osteonecrosis of the jaw (MRONJ) in patients with osteoporosis.

Keywords

Osteoporosis · Vertebral fracture
Insufficiency fracture · Atypical femoral fracture · Medication-related osteonecrosis of the jaw (MRONJ)

Osteoporosis is the most common musculoskeletal disease in the world. The World Health Organization (WHO) and National Osteoporosis Foundation define osteoporosis as a metabolic bone disease that is characterized by reduction of bone mass and microstructural deterioration of bone tis-

S.-O. Yang (✉)
Department of Nuclear Medicine, Dongnam Institute of Radiological and Medical Sciences, Busan, Republic of Korea
e-mail: soyang@dirams.re.kr

J. M. Park
Department of Nuclear Medicine, Soonchunhyang University Hospital, Bucheon, Republic of Korea
e-mail: jmipark@schmc.ac.kr

H. J. Son
Department of Nuclear Medicine, Dankook University College of Medicine, Cheonan, Republic of Korea
e-mail: hyejooson@dkuh.co.kr

J. G. Cha
Department of Radiology, Soonchunhyang University Hospital, Bucheon, Republic of Korea
e-mail: mj4907@schmc.ac.kr

J. W. Chai
Department of Radiology, Seoul National University Boramae Medical Center, Seoul, Republic of Korea
e-mail: chaijw@snu.ac.kr

S. W. Oh
Department of Nuclear Medicine, Seoul National University Boramae Medical Center, Seoul, Republic of Korea
e-mail: mdosw@snu.ac.kr

S.-O. Yang et al. (eds.), *Atlas of Nuclear Medicine in Musculoskeletal System*,
https://doi.org/10.1007/978-981-19-2677-8_15

sue. Enhanced bone fragility and decreased bone strength are attributed to an increased risk of fracture (osteoporotic fracture). Osteoporotic fracture can be induced by non-traumatic cause, which refers to a fracture resulting from a minor fall from a standing height or less. Osteoporotic fracture commonly occurs in the vertebra, hip, and distal radius.

15.1 Etiology and Pathophysiology

One of the main factors affecting osteoporosis is aging. In general, the bone mass reaches the maximum at the age of 30, and then the process of bone formation and bone resorption that maintains the minerals of the bone tissue slows down. The reduction in skeletal mass results from an imbalance between bone resorption and bone formation; increased bone resorption or decreased bone formation may result in osteoporosis.

Various factors including age, gender, family history, and ethnicity can affect the development of osteoporosis. The balance between bone formation and resorption plays a key role in determining the bone mineral density (BMD). BMD gradually decreases with age after reaching its maximum at the age of 30, and the bone becomes brittle with age after the age of 50. Osteoporosis is more likely to occur in women than men, particularly after menopause. Estrogen regulates bone resorption, and its deficiency leads to a rapid decrease in BMD and deterioration of bone quality. Besides, malnutrition, smoking, lack of weight-bearing exercise, small body shape, and drugs or diseases affecting the BMD are associated with the development of osteoporosis.

Osteoporosis can be classified according to the underlying causes: primary and secondary. Primary osteoporosis occurs in relation to age, which includes postmenopausal (type 1) and senile (type 2). Secondary osteoporosis is caused by certain medical conditions and medications such as prolonged immobilization, steroid therapy, and diabetes mellitus. Senile osteoporosis is the most common type of osteoporosis and followed by postmenopausal osteoporosis.

Osteoporosis and osteoporotic fracture can impose significant economic and healthcare burdens not only on the individual level but also on the public level. For example, osteoporotic hip fracture pays a considerable amount of social costs. Hip fracture requires a long period of hospitalization, and furthermore, it is associated with serious medical complications such as pressure sores, pneumonia, urinary tract infection, and venous thrombosis (pulmonary embolism) that are followed by the immobilization. In addition, loss of labor during the hospitalization and subsequent rehabilitation causes enormous socioeconomical loss. The incidence of hip fractures is anticipated to increase from 1.1 million in 2018 to 2.6 million in 2050, by the Asian Federation of Osteoporosis Societies [1]. Recently, osteoporotic fracture is rapidly increasing in South Korea, as South Korea already became an aged society and is about to enter a super-aged society by 2026. It deserves to be called as "Osteoporosis Tsunami."

15.2 Diagnosis of Osteoporosis

Osteoporosis is diagnosed by the measurement of BMD using dual energy X-ray absorptiometry (DXA). DXA measures BMD as the ratio of bone mineral content (BMC) to the area of region of interest (ROI). Other than single-photon absorptiometry (SPA) and dual-photon absorptiometry (DPA), radioisotopic modality is not used to measure BMD. Quantitative imaging techniques like DXA and quantitative computed tomography (QCT) measure the BMD from the segmented bone regions of the acquired images. However, the measurement of BMD alone cannot accurately predict the risk of fracture.

Bone scan can help in detecting early fractures and determining the stage of vertebral fractures as a supplementary tool to radiographic imaging. Bone scan is advantageous to screen the whole skeleton identifying osteoporotic fractures [2]. Bone scan is also helpful in the case of avascular necrosis that occurs as a complication of osteoporotic fracture and in detecting osteomyelitis or clinically unpredicted lesions that may be accompanied by the fractures. However, a sensitivity of bone scan decreases in elderly patients with osteoporotic fractures and in patients with steroid medication. In addition, a specificity of bone scan is low because increased uptakes are also seen at the sites of fractures, infection, metabolic bone disease, and metastases.

Other imaging modalities can be used for the assessment of osteoporosis. Magnetic resonance imaging (MRI) is the most sensitive exam for diagnosing vertebral fractures, due to visualization of the bone marrow swelling. Unfortunately, the clinical accessibility of MRI is often limited because of high cost and/or various medical conditions of patients, e.g., metallic devices. Computed tomography (CT) is also useful since it provides three-dimensional reconstructed images. However, the application of PET/CT is still limited. Schmitz et al. evaluated fluorodeoxyglucose (FDG) PET in patients with osteoporosis or preclinical osteoporosis to differentiate pathological fractures from benign fractures, and they suggested that a high FDG uptake is characteristic for malignant and inflammatory processes [3].

15.3 Osteoporotic Vertebral Compression Fracture

Vertebral compression fractures are the most common type of insufficiency fractures because the axial skeletons are primarily composed of cancellous bone that is more metabolically active than cortical bone. It is difficult to diagnose osteoporotic vertebral fractures with simple radiography, when only minimal compressions occurred at an initial stage of the fracture. Besides, secondary vertebral fractures were reported to develop in nearly 20% of the patients within 1 year. Multiple vertebral fractures may lead to kyphosis, scoliosis, chronic back pain, loss of height, decreased pulmonary function, decreased movement and fatigue, and imbalance. In this regard, detection of the early stage of vertebral fracture is necessary to prevent the serial development of multiple vertebral fractures.

Densitometric vertebral facture assessment (VFA) combined with BMD increased clinical diagnosis of osteoporosis by detecting previously unknown vertebral fractures and suggested VFA with BMD for the first BMD assessment in postmenopausal women [4]. Bone scan is also useful to detect microtrauma in patients with low back pain without definite radiographic abnormalities, as it demonstrates multiple or single linear areas of increased uptake with reduction of the vertebral height and loss of normal vertebral contour. Three-phase bone scan may help to determine the stages of vertebral fractures. The intensity of radiotracer uptake of the vertebral fracture gradually diminishes until 12–24 months. On the other hand, spine MRI shows low signal intensity on T1-weighted image and band-like pattern in 46.7% of patients with acute osteoporotic compression fracture. However, it can be difficult to differentiate malignant fractures from benign fractures in cases that acute stage of compression fracture was accompanied by severe bone marrow edema on MRI [5, 6]. Acute vertebral fractures originating from osteoporosis or preclinical osteoporosis tend to have not pathologically increased FDG uptake [7]. Because high FDG uptake is characteristic of malignant and inflammatory processes, FDG-PET may be potentially useful for differentiating osteoporotic vertebral fractures and pathologic fractures. In certain clinical fracture cases where CT and MRI images are inconclusive in differentiating benign from malignant etiologies, PET/CT can be acquired, which can also discover additional skeletal or extra-skeletal metastases. The standardized uptake value (SUV), a dimensionless parameter, is commonly used as a relative measure of FDG tissue uptake with correction for the amount of injected FDG and the patient's weight [8].

Case 15.1

An 80-year-old male presented to the emergency room for the chest pain after fall-down injury. Bone scan showed intense bone uptake in recent compression fracture site of T10, L1, and L2 and mildly increased uptake in T11–12 suggesting old compression fracture sequela. Furthermore, there were focal increased uptakes in the known fracture sites of right third and left third to sixth anterior arc and right tenth and 11th and left tenth rib posterior arc (a). In addition to multiple compression fractures in thoraco-lumbar (T-L) spine, degenerative spondylosis in L5-S1 with probable lumbosacral transitional vertebra in L5-S1 was noted in the radiograph (b). In the patient's BMD of the lumbar spines, mean T-score of L3–4 was −3.0 indicating osteoporosis (c). The International Society for Clinical Densitometry (ISCD) recommends that BMD of more than two lumbar vertebrae should be used when interpreting BMD of the lumbar spine (Fig. 15.1).

Case 15.2

A 70-year-old woman came to the emergency room for back pain by slip down on the floor. Bone scan showed rib fractures in the left hemithorax and increased radioactivity in L2 vertebral body (a). Simple radiography and CT of lumbar spine showed anterior ossifications at the level of disc spaces indicating diffuse idiopathic skeletal hyperostosis (DISH), diffuse osteoporosis, and

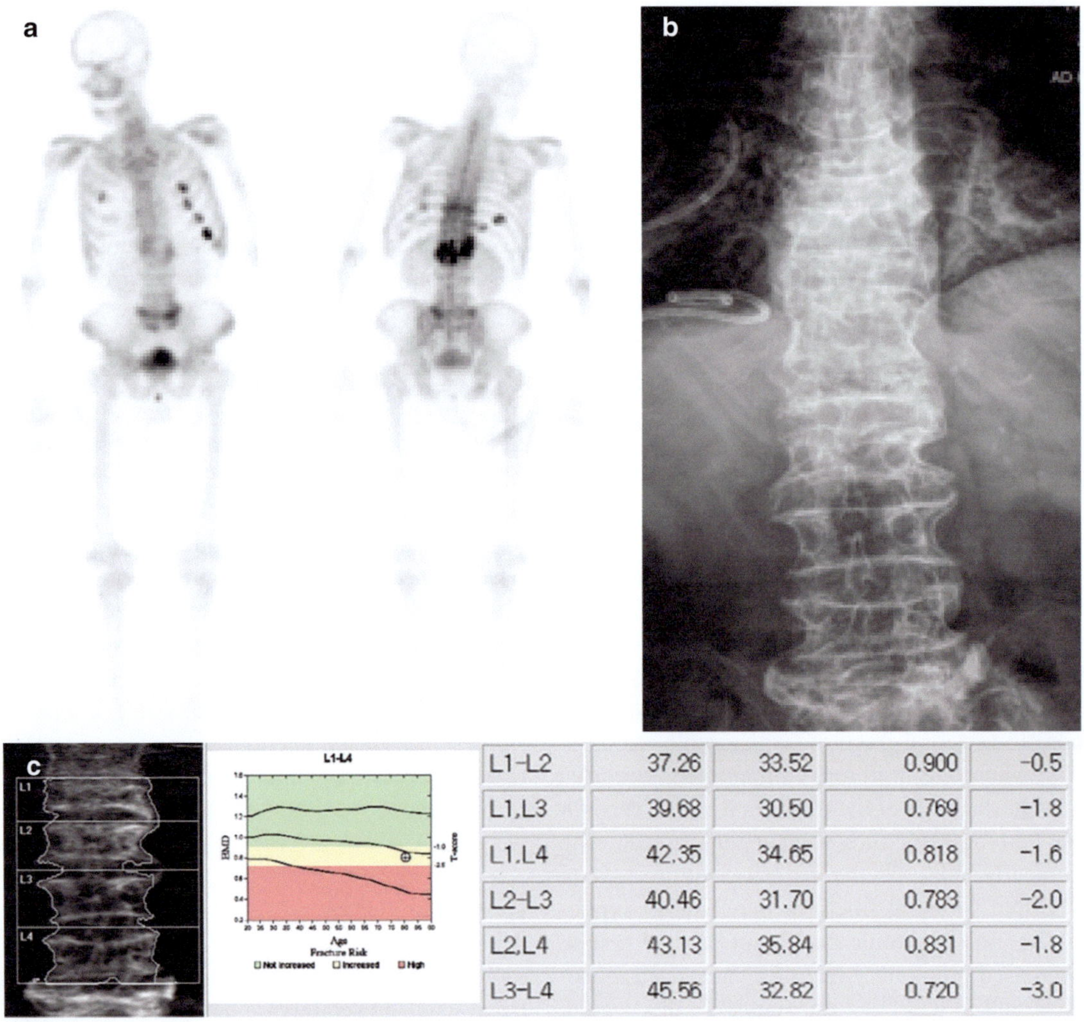

L1-L2	37.26	33.52	0.900	-0.5
L1,L3	39.68	30.50	0.769	-1.8
L1,L4	42.35	34.65	0.818	-1.6
L2-L3	40.46	31.70	0.783	-2.0
L2,L4	43.13	35.84	0.831	-1.8
L3-L4	45.56	32.82	0.720	-3.0

Fig. 15.1 Bone scan shows intense bone uptake in T10, L1, and L2 and mildly increased uptake in T11–12. There are focal increased uptakes in the osteoporotic fracture sites of anterior arcs of right third and left third–sixth ribs and posterior arcs of right 10–11th and left 10th ribs (**a**). Multiple compression fractures in T-L spines and degenerative spondylosis in L5-S1 with probable lumbosacral transitional vertebra in L5-S1 are noted in the radiograph (**b**). Mean T-score of L3–4 is −3.0 indicating osteoporosis (**c**)

trabecular loss of L2 with preserved vertebral height (b, c). Bone SPECT/CT showed increased uptake in the endplate area of L2 with more decreased uptake in the left anterior column (d). In the patient's initial BMD of the lumbar spines, mean T-score was −2.1 indicating osteopenia. She received pain management and treatment with teriparatide (recombinant human parathyroid hormone) injection for 3 months. Follow-up L-spine CT showed interval increased bone density and wedge-shaped vertebral collapse of L2 body, which suggested osteonecrosis 5 months after the acute trauma (e).

Delayed thoraco-lumbar fractures appear often in osteoporosis or old age. Its main mechanism is hyperflexion injury. The posterior two-thirds of vertebral bodies receive collateral blood from four arteries derived from two intervertebral levels, whereas the anterior one-third of the vertebral body is defined as the watershed zone associated with a higher risk of ischemic AVN [9] (Fig. 15.2).

Case 15.3
A 62-year-old woman with known lung cancer suffered back pain for several years. PET/CT for initial staging of lung cancer showed compression fractures in T11 and L4 vertebral bodies with low FDG uptakes (a). After 17 months from initial PET/CT, bone scan showed increased horizontal radioactivity in the L2, L3, and L4 vertebral bodies which suggest recent compression fracture (b). BMD at the total femur showed a T-score of −3.3, and lateral radiograph of the L-spine showed multiple compression fractures in T11, L2, L3, L4, and L5 after 1 week from bone scan (c, d). In this case, we can assume the dating of the compression fracture that T11 and L4 lesions were old ones and L2, L3, and L5 lesions were relatively acute lesions by uptake patterns on bone scan (Fig. 15.3).

15.4 Insufficiency Fractures of Pelvis and Sacrum

Insufficiency (fragility) fractures of the pelvis are common in patients with over 65 years of age after a low energy fall. In severe osteoporotic bones, insufficiency fractures can occur without trauma. These fractures can be important because they lead to immobility and are associated with high mortality. The 1-year mortality rate is 16.3%, and the 5-year mortality rate is 58.1% [10]. In most cases, pubic rami fractures and sacral injuries are ipsilateral. CT can detect fracture sites in 25% of all the sacral fractures and 30% of the femoral neck fractures [11]. MRI and bone scan are more sensitive to detect the fractures than CT.

Insufficiency fractures of the sacrum are also common and usually occur in osteoporotic bone with minimal or unremembered trauma. Sacral insufficiency fractures are also common and are often difficult to diagnose radiographically or by CT. Owing to its relationship with osteoporosis, the majority occur in elderly females and are frequently bilateral, often presenting as low back pain.

Plain radiographs are generally normal, and both clinician and radiologist need to consider the possibility of sacral insufficiency fracture to allow prompt accurate diagnosis and proper treatment. Lumbar spine MRI is among the first investigations performed and can enable the correct diagnosis to be made. Occasionally the MR appearances can mimic tumor or osteomyelitis. The most common pattern is the "H" or butterfly pattern, with a horizontal band of increased uptake across the body of the sacrum and two vertical limbs of activity in the sacrum. Several pattern variations may be seen, including asymmetry of the alar activity. Less severe fractures may show only horizontal linear uptake. The "H" sign on bone scan is considered diagnostic finding in the appropriate clinical setting, but this sign is often absent. CT is useful to confirm the diagnosis and exclude tumor or infection.

Case 15.4
A 76-year-old woman with osteoporosis presented with fall-down injury at stairs. She took medication for 10 years for rheumatoid arthritis with neck and shoulder pain. Pelvic CT showed multiple fractures at left sacral ala and superior and inferior pubic rami with swelling of left obturator and pectineus muscle by contusion (a).

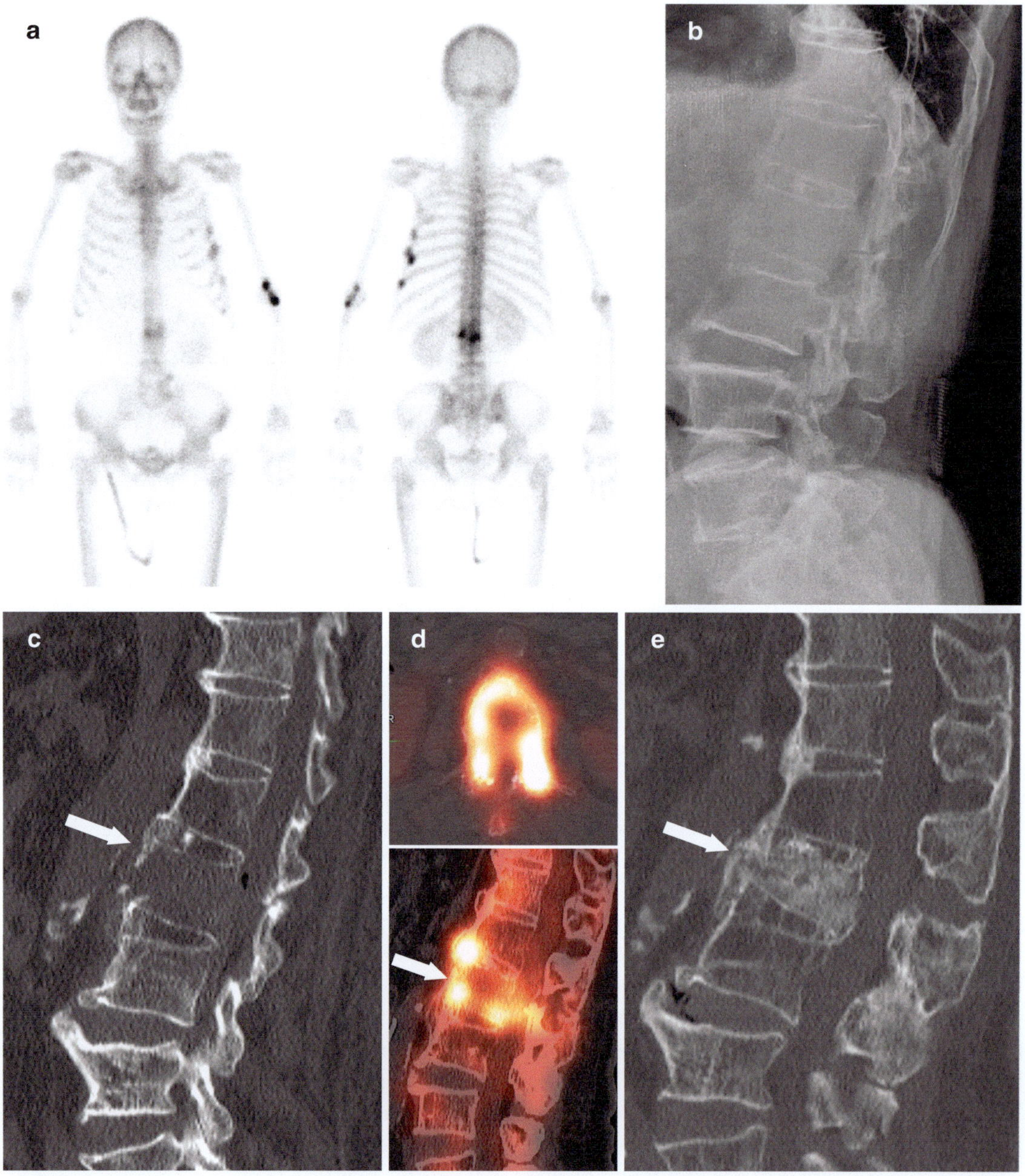

Fig. 15.2 Multiple rib fractures in the left hemithorax and increased radioactivity in L2 vertebral body are seen on bone scan (**a**). Simple radiography and CT of lumbar spine show anterior ossifications at the level of disc spaces indicating DISH, diffuse osteoporosis, and trabecular loss of L2 (arrow) with preserved vertebral height (**b**, **c**). Bone SPECT/CT shows increased uptake in L2 (arrow) with more decreased uptake in the left anterior column (**d**). Follow-up L-spine CT shows increased bone density and wedge-shaped vertebral collapse of L2 body (arrow) suggesting osteonecrosis, 5 months after the acute trauma (**e**)

Bone scan showed increased bone uptakes in the left sacral ala, left pubic ramus, and left acetabulum, sternal fracture, and multiple compression fractures of T spines (b). In her BMD of the lumbar spines and femur neck, T-scores were −2.8 and −2.1, respectively (Fig. 15.4).

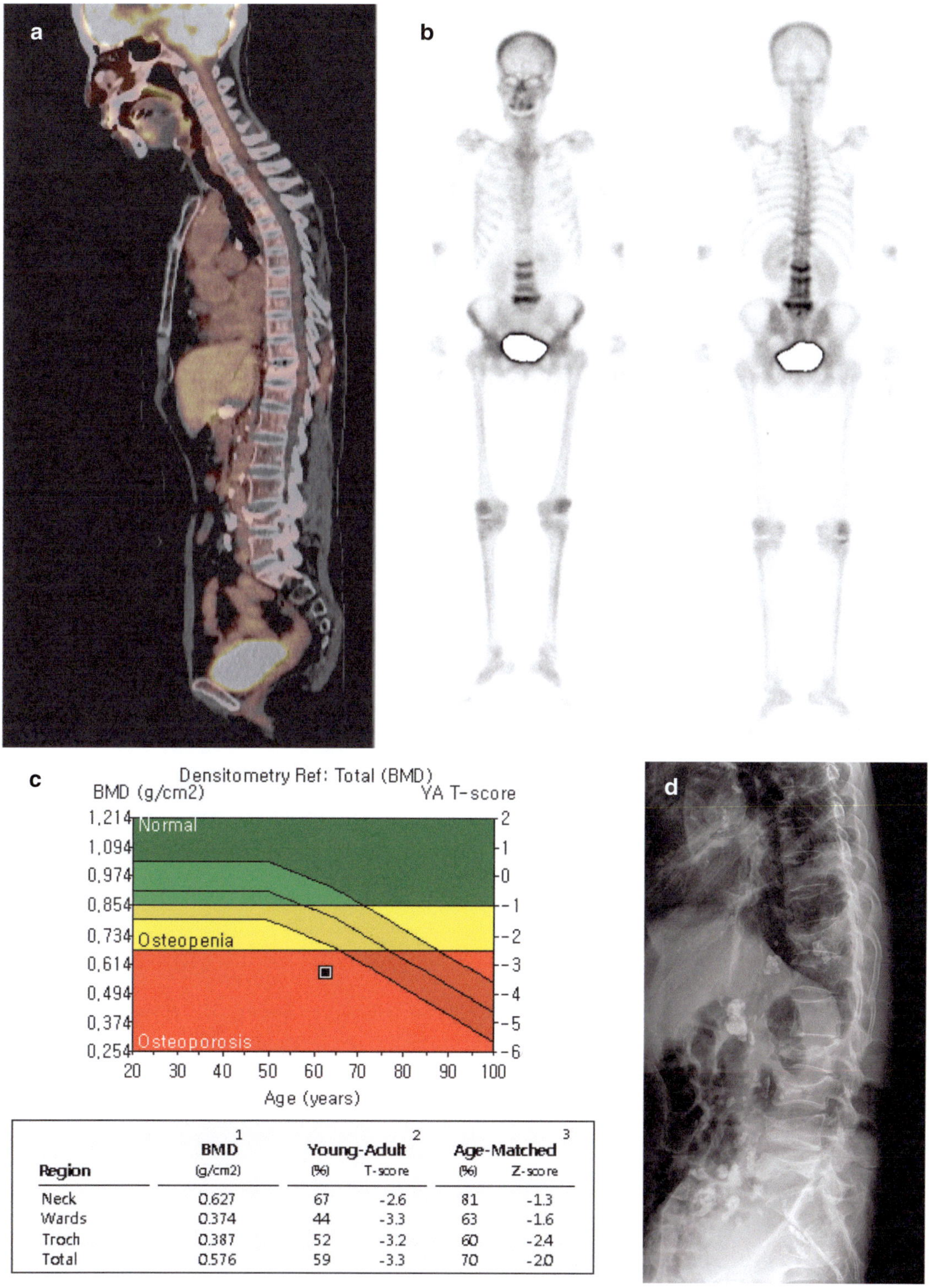

Region	BMD[1] (g/cm2)	Young-Adult[2] (%)	T-score	Age-Matched[3] (%)	Z-score
Neck	0.627	67	-2.6	81	-1.3
Wards	0.374	44	-3.3	63	-1.6
Troch	0.387	52	-3.2	60	-2.4
Total	0.576	59	-3.3	70	-2.0

Fig. 15.3 PET/CT shows compression fractures in T11 and L4 vertebral bodies with low FDG uptakes (**a**). Bone scan 17 months later from PET/CT shows increased horizontal radioactivities in the L2-4 vertebral bodies which suggest recent compression fracture (**b**). BMD at the total femur shows a T-score of −3.3 (**c**). Lateral radiograph of the L-spine shows multiple compression fractures in T11 and L2-5 vertebrae (**d**)

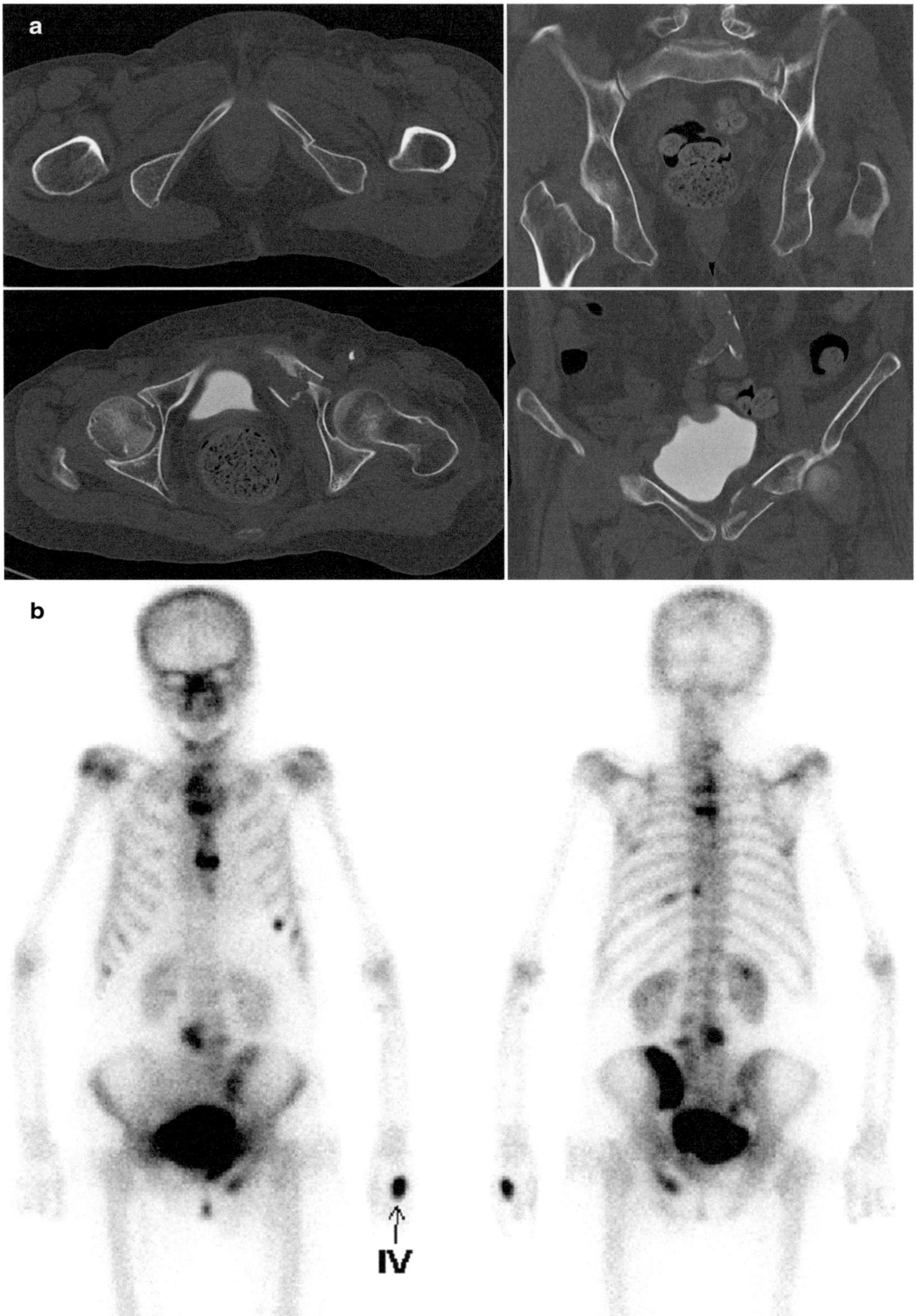

Fig. 15.4 Pelvic CT shows fractures at left sacral ala and superior and inferior pubic rami with swelling of left obturator and pectineus muscle (**a**). Increased uptakes in the left sacral ala, left pubic ramus, and left acetabulum are seen including sternal fracture and multiple compression fractures of T spines on bone scan (**b**)

Case 15.5

A 68-year-old woman with back pain for 2 months was given MRI order in the outpatient clinic. MRI showed irregular permeative low T1 signal intensity with heterogeneously gadolinium enhancing lesion in the upper sacrum. Differential diagnoses of MRI included metastasis, infiltrative bone marrow lesion (lymphoma, leukemia), and recent bone contusion (a). To evaluate the possibility of metastasis or other malignancy, PET/CT was performed. On maximum intensity projection (MIP) image, moderate degree of FDG uptakes (maxSUV; 2.7) in the sacral body was noted without evidence of primary malignancy outside of the sacrum (b). In three-orthogonal CT images, sclerotic change in the sacrum was also seen (c). PET/CT diagnosis was suggestive of insufficiency fracture of the sacrum, so bone scan was done as a next imaging study. Bone scan showed relatively characteristic flat H-shaped increased radioactivity of insufficiency fracture in the sacral body with two vertebral compression fractures (d) (Fig. 15.5).

Case 15.6

In a 75-year-old female patient who underwent surgery 6 months ago for rectal cancer, ^{18}F-FDG PET/CT was performed for further evaluation of metastasis. She complained pain in the back and left hip joint at that time. In the patient's PET/CT, increased FDG uptakes were observed on the sacrum mainly in the right side (maxSUV; 7.3) and left acetabular roof (maxSUV; 3.1), suggesting possible metastasis (a). The patient also underwent bone scan which showed intense hot uptakes in the right upper sacrum and left acetabular roof which were consistent with the PET/CT lesions (b). Due to horizontal radioactivity crossing the sacral body (arrow in b), sacral insufficiency fracture was suggested. MRI was performed the next day to exclude the possibility of metastasis. MRI showed suspicious low signal intensity line in the right sacral ala and low signal intensity lesion in the left acetabular roof on T1 WI (c, d). Final imaging diagnosis was stress fracture more likely rather than metastasis. After 8 years until now, she is well alive without evidence of skeletal metastasis (Fig. 15.6).

15.5 Atypical Femoral Fracture (AFF)

Bisphosphonate, which has been used for the longest time for treatment of osteoporosis, has been proven to have an excellent effect of reducing the incidence of osteoporotic fractures by about 50% through several randomized clinical trials. Bisphosphonates are antiresorptive agents that inactivate osteoclastic bone resorption, decreasing bone turnover and bone loss. However, since 2005, it has been reported that there is a risk of deterioration of bone quality due to the suppression of the normal bone remodeling process. Furthermore, unusual types of femur fractures have been reported even with minor trauma in patients with long-term bisphosphonate treatment [12]. It occurs frequently in the femur and mandible, which requires the most bone remodeling process in the human body. As a clinical feature, it does not heal properly during the remodeling process, so the fracture line spreads and continues to cause unstable fractures.

The characteristics of AFF are non-comminuted, transverse fractures originating at the lateral cortex of the subtrochanteric femur with localized periosteal or endosteal thickening that occurs with minimal trauma. The shape of AFF plane has distinct feature that the fracture line is horizontal on the outside but the fracture progressing obliquely toward the inside is characteristic. Adults with long-term bisphosphonate use are at increased risk of AFF, estimated 100 per 100,000 person-years [13].

Case 15.7

A 65-year-old woman with pain on the left thigh visited orthopedic surgery clinic. She had a renal transplant 21 years ago. There is no history of trauma. Preoperative radiograph showed bilateral cortical abnormalities in the lateral side of femoral shafts (a). Bone scan showed focal increased radioactivity more prominent in the left femur (b). Surgery (intramedullary nailing) was performed to prevent overt fracture (c). After 18 months, she slipped down at home and got overt fracture in her right femur (d) (Fig. 15.7).

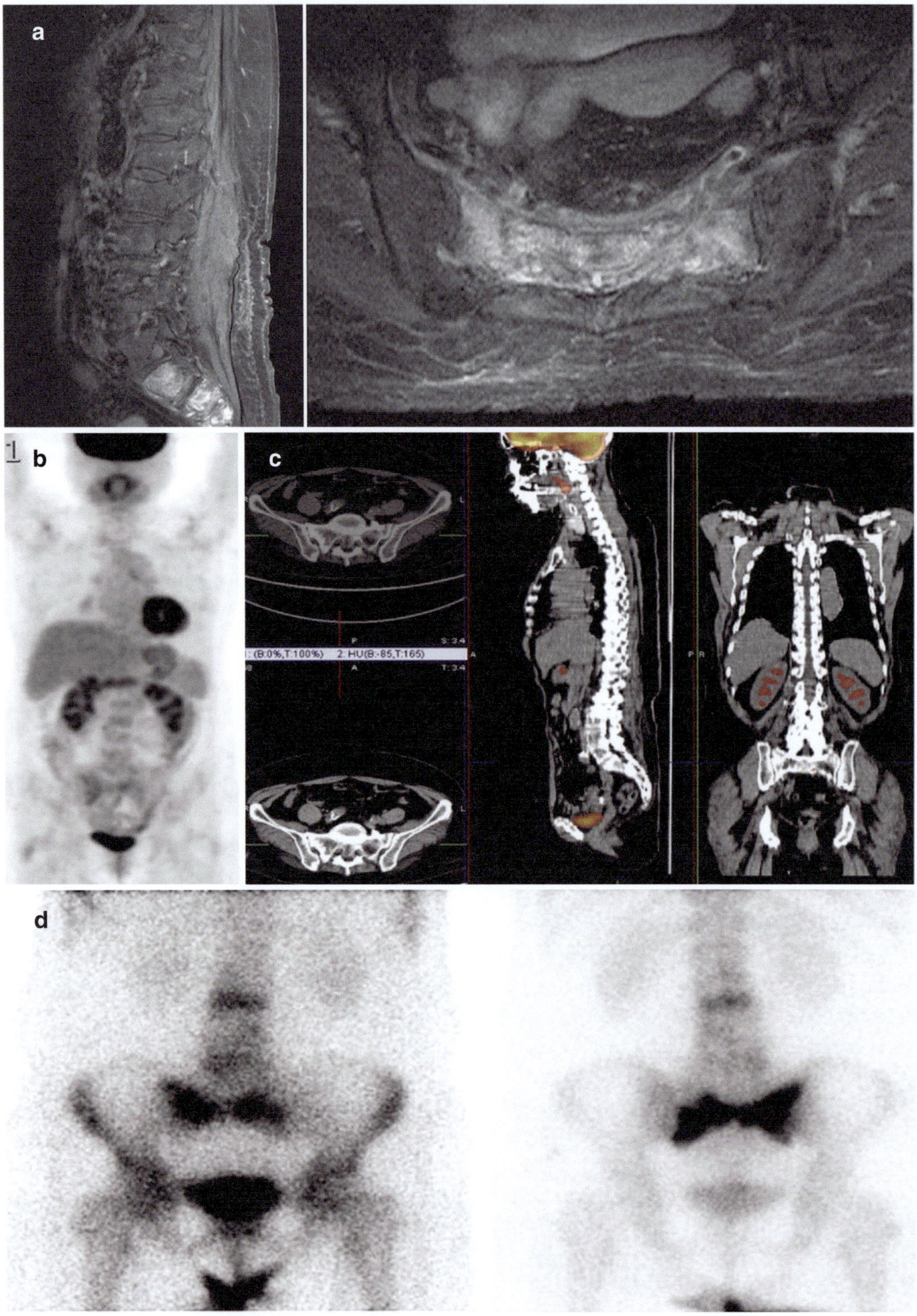

Fig. 15.5 MRI shows irregular permeative low T1 signal intensity with heterogeneously gadolinium-enhancing lesion in the upper sacrum (**a**). On maximum intensity projection (MIP) image of PET/CT, moderate degree of FDG uptakes in the sacral body is noted without evidence of primary malignancy outside of the sacrum (**b**). In three-orthogonal CT images, sclerotic change in the sacrum is also seen (**c**). Bone scans (anterior and posterior spot view) show relatively characteristic flat H-shaped pattern with a horizontal band of increased uptake across the body of the sacrum and vertebral compression fractures in L3 and L5 (**d**)

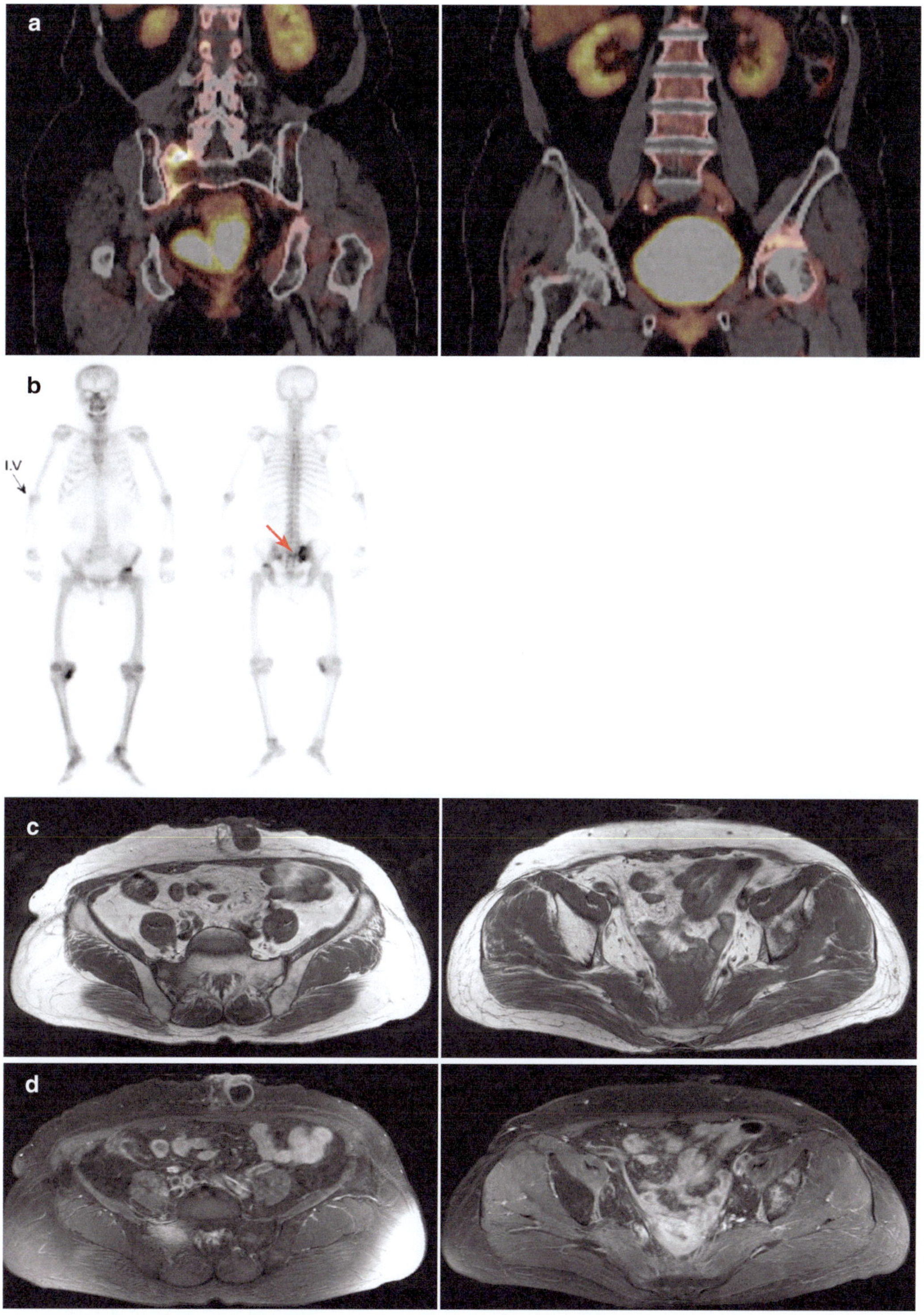

Fig. 15.6 PET/CT shows increased FDG uptakes on the sacrum mainly in the right side and left acetabular roof (**a**). Bone scan shows intense hot uptakes in the right upper sacrum and left acetabular roof with a horizontal radioactivity crossing the sacral body (arrow) (**b**). MRI shows suspicious low signal intensity line in the right sacral ala and low signal intensity lesion in the left acetabular roof on T1 WI with mild gadolinium enhancement (**c**, **d**)

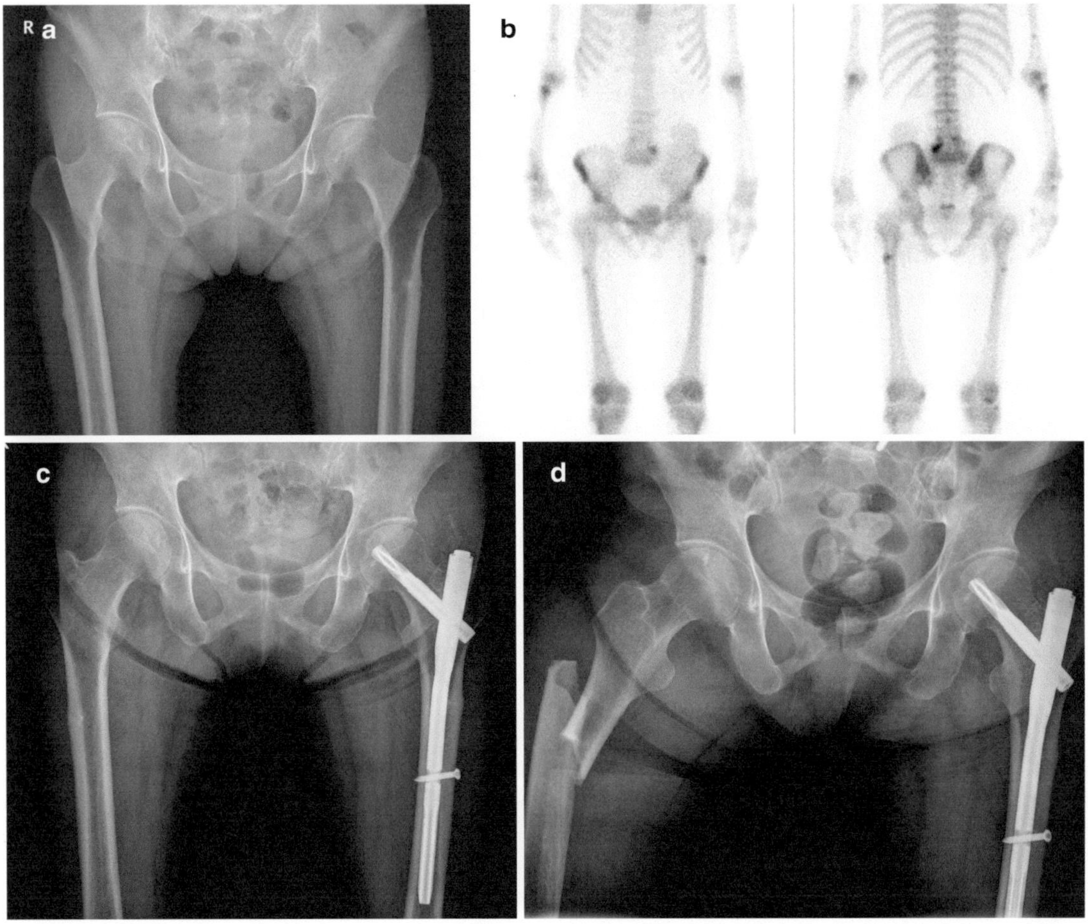

Fig. 15.7 Preoperative radiograph shows bilateral cortical abnormalities in the lateral side of femoral shafts (**a**). Bone scan shows focal increased radioactivities more prominent in the left femur (**b**). Surgery (intramedullary nailing) was performed to prevent overt fracture (**c**) After 18 months, she slipped down at home and got overt fracture in her right femur (**d**). [Courtesy of Kwang-kyoun Kim, MD, Konyang University Hospital]

Case 15.8

A 77-year-old woman with pain on both thighs visited orthopedic surgery clinic. She was on bisphosphonate treatment for 6 years for osteoporosis. Initial radiograph of the femur showed focal cortical thickening in the lateral sides of femoral shaft predominantly in the right femur (a). Bone scan showed focal intense horizontal radioactivity in the right femoral shaft (b). One week later after taking bone scan, she had fall-down injury resulting in fracture of the right femur (c) (Fig. 15.8).

15.6 Medication-Related Osteonecrosis of the Jaw (MRONJ)

MRONJ is a rare complication of certain medication, occurring in about 1 in 10,000–100,000 patients. Bone resorption inhibitors such as bisphosphonates are widely used for the treatment and symptom relief of various bone diseases such as osteoporosis and bone metastasis of malignant tumors. Nevertheless, MRONJ is a serious complication that has been reported, and related stud-

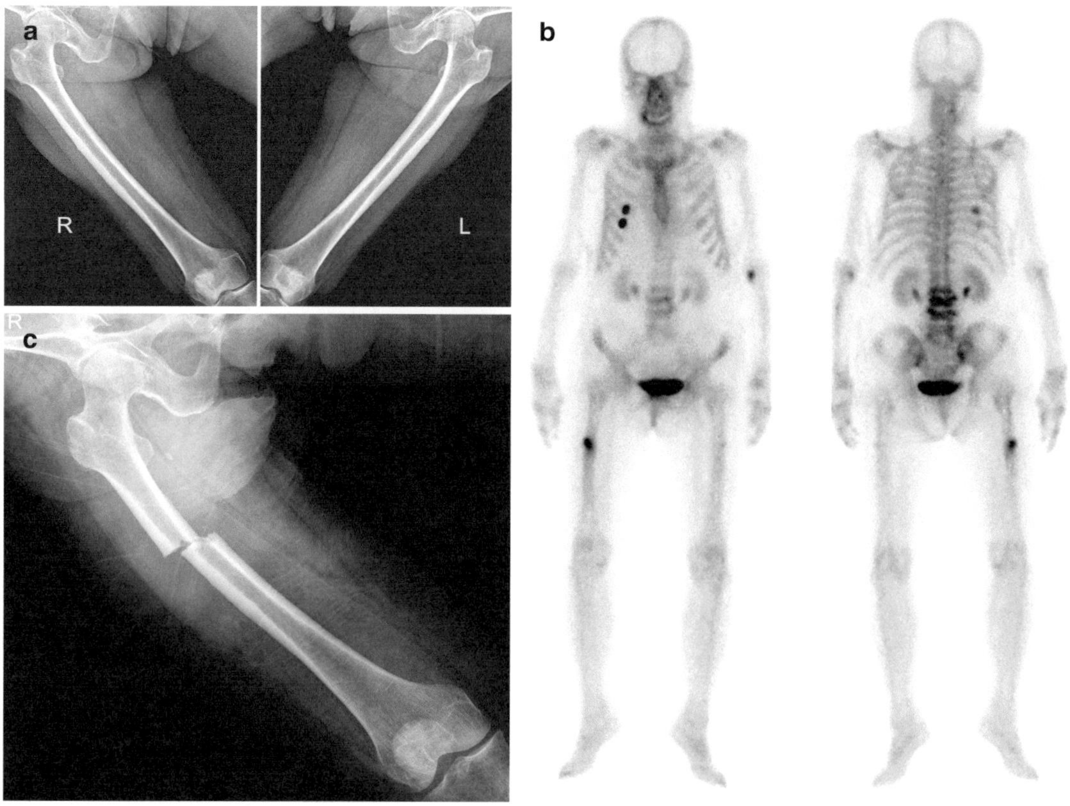

Fig. 15.8 Initial radiograph of the femur shows focal cortical thickening in the lateral sides of femoral shaft predominantly in the right femur (**a**). Bone scan shows focal intense horizontal radioactivity in the right femoral shaft (**b**). After 1 week from bone scanning date, she had fall-down injury resulting in fracture of the right femur (**c**). [Courtesy of Kwang-kyoun Kim, MD, Konyang University Hospital]

ies have been conducted, but a clear mechanism of development and treatment has not been established so far. Although the etiology and pathogenesis of MRONJ remain obscure, it has been proposed that the jaw bones are highly susceptible to osteonecrosis due to certain anatomical and physiological factors [14]. MRONJ is characterized by pain, exposed bone, infection, and pathological fracture. Incidence of osteonecrosis of the jaw is expected to continue to increase. Definition of MRONJ includes the following characteristics to be defined as (1) current or previous administration of bone resorption inhibitors or angiogenesis inhibitors, (2) bone exposure in the maxillofacial region or bone probed through internal or external fistula of oral cavity lasting for more than 8 weeks, and (3) no history of radiotherapy or definite metastatic bone tumors in the maxilla.

MRONJ is a bone disease that frequently affects the soft tissues, so it requires targeted imaging methods for diagnostic definition. Although radiographic findings are often nonspecific, an increasing volume of evidence recognizes some radiological characteristics are associated with MRONJ [15]. In dental panoramic radiographs and apical radiographs, osteolytic radiographic lesions with uneven borders and radiopaque osteosclerosis can be observed. In CT, osteophytes or osteonecrosis is clearly observed. Bone scan with three-phase imaging is important for the diagnosis of osteonecrosis and is considered useful for the detection of early changes, but it is difficult to detect minor inflammation and necrosis due to its low resolution. Thus, SPECT/CT improves both sensitivity and specificity, providing cross-sectional images combined with anatomical CT information. In MRI, the T1 signal of osteonecrosis is often decreased, and the low signal of STIR, T2, and vascular components is often attenuated.

Medications Associated with MRONJ

The following is the list of drugs which are known to cause MRONJ.

1. Antiresorptives.
   (a) Bisphosphonates: pamidronate, alendronate, risedronate, ibandronate, zolendronate.
   (b) Human monoclonal antibody of RANKL (receptor activator of nuclear factor kappa-B ligand): denosumab.
2. Sclerostin-binding monoclonal antibody: romosozumab.
3. Drugs that are not used for osteoporosis but known to cause drug-related osteonecrosis (antiangiogenic or targets of the vascular endothelial growth factor (VEGF) pathway).
   (a) Tyrosine kinase inhibitor: sunitinib, sorafenib.
   (b) Humanized monoclonal antibody: bevacizumab.
   (c) Mammalian target of rapamycin pathway: sirolimus.

Case 15.9

A 74-year-old woman was referred to the Department of Endocrinology and Metabolism for evaluation of pain and persistent abnormal exposure of jaw after teeth extraction. She had a history of taking alendronate (70 mg weekly) for 5 years for the treatment of osteoporosis. She had no clinical history of cranial or oral radiation therapy.

The left mandibular first and second molars were extracted; however, the wound did not heal and persisted. Short-term (three treatment periods comprising of 4 days administration each) antibiotic (amoxicillin) treatment was given, but there was no improvement. Curettage and debridement were performed repeatedly until the patient was referred to the Endocrinology Clinic. Panoramic radiograph showed bilateral bony destruction in both mandibular bodies with more involvement in the left side (a). She had open wound in her left mandibular bone (arrow in b). Three-phase bone scan showed diffusely increased uptake in both mandibular bodies (c–e) predominantly in the left side (Fig. 15.9).

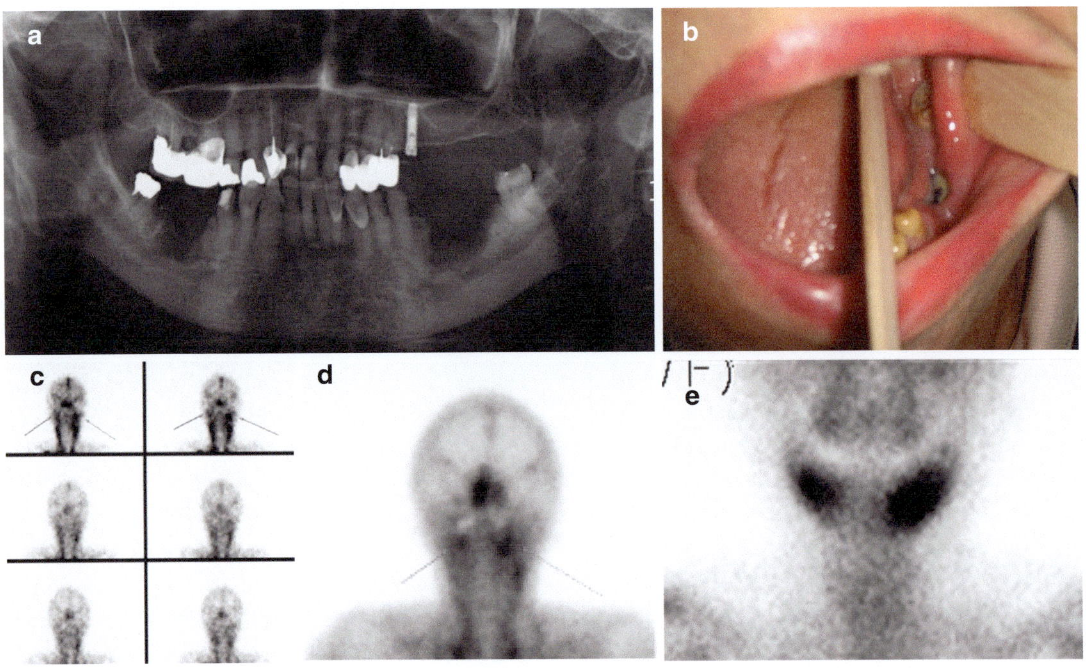

Fig. 15.9 Bilateral bony destruction in both mandibular bodies is seen on panoramic radiography (**a**). Open wound in her left mandibular bone was noted (arrow in **b**). Three-phase bone scan (blood flow, blood pool, delayed image from left) show diffusely increased radioactivities in both mandibular bodies (**c**–**e**). [Courtesy of Yoon-Sok Chung, MD, Ajou University Hospital]

In conclusion, BMD measures the bone quantity and not the bone structure; it is insufficient to predict the risk of insufficiency fracture. The role of nuclear imaging in diagnosing osteoporotic fractures is often complementary and very sensitive.

Teaching Points

- Early diagnosis, treatment, and patient education about osteoporosis are important to reduce future additional fractures.
- Compression fractures of the spine are common and may show abnormal uptake in bone scan before radiographic changes.
- The insufficiency osteoporotic fractures may show persistent uptake for months or years on bone scan, so it can be difficult to determine if the fracture is acute.
- Combination of bone scan and MRI is often complementary in the diagnosis of vertebral fracture and sacral insufficiency fracture.
- The characteristics of AFF are non-comminuted, transverse fractures originating at the lateral cortex of the subtrochanteric femur which can be frequently observed in the long term of bisphosphonate treatment by radiographs and bone scan.
- In the diagnosis of MRONJ, three-phase bone scan is important for the diagnosis of osteonecrosis and is considered useful for the detection of early changes.
- Correctly diagnosing osteoporotic fractures with all available imaging modalities is one of the major responsibilities we have as nuclear physicians and radiologists.

References

1. Cheung C-L, Ang SB, Chadha M, Chow ES-L, Chung Y-S, Hew FL, et al. An updated hip fracture projection in Asia: the Asian Federation of Osteoporosis. Osteoporos Sarcopenia. 2018;4(1):16–21.
2. Elgazzar AH. Diagnosis of metabolic, endocrine and congenital bone disease. In: Elgazzar AH, editor. Orthopedic nuclear medicine. Springer; 2017. p. 111.
3. Schmitz A, Risse JH, Textor J. FDG-PET findings of vertebral compression fractures in osteoporosis: preliminary results. Osteoporos Int. 2002;13(9):755–61.
4. Cai S, Yu H, Li Y, He X, Yan L, Huang X, et al. Bone mineral density measurement combined with vertebral fracture assessment increases diagnosis of osteoporosis in postmenopausal women. Skelet Radiol. 2020;49(2):273–80.
5. Ahn SE, Ryu KN, Park JS, et al. Early bone marrow edema pattern of the osteoporotic vertebral compression fracture can be predictor of vertebral deformity types and prognosis? J Korean Neurosurg Soc. 2016;59:137–42.
6. Yang SO, Kim S, Juhng SK. Imaging diagnosis of osteoporotic fracture. J Korean Med Assoc. 2010;53:67–75.
7. Bredella MA, Essary B, Torriani M, Ouellette HA, Palmer WE. Use of FDG-PET in differentiating benign from malignant compression fractures. Skelet Radiol. 2008;37:405–13.
8. Shin DS, Shon OJ, Byun SJ, Choi JH, Chun KA, Cho IH. Differentiation between malignant and benign pathologic fractures with F-18-fluoro-2-deoxy-D-glucose positron emission tomography/computed tomography. Skelet Radiol. 2008;37:415–21.
9. Maheshwari PR, Nagar AM, Prasad SS, Shah JR, Patkar DP. Avascular necrosis of spine: a rare appearance. Spine. 2004;29(6):E119–22.
10. Hamilton CB, Harnett JD, Stone NC, et al. Morbidity and mortality following pelvis ramus fractures in an older Atlantic Canadian cohort. Can J Surg. 2019;62:270–4.
11. Cabarrus MC, Ambekar A, Lu Y, et al. MRI and CT of insufficiency fractures of the pelvis and the proximal femur. AJR. 2008;191:995–1001.
12. Yoon RS, Hwang JS, Beebe KS. Long-term bisphosphonate usage and subtrochanteric insufficiency fractures? A cause for concern? J Bone Joint Surg Br. 2011;93(10):1289–95.
13. Shane E, Burr D, Abrahamsen B, Adler RA, Brown TD, Cheung AM, et al. Atypical subtrochanteric and diaphyseal femoral fractures: second report of a task force of the American Society for Bone and Mineral Research. J Bone Miner Res. 2014;29(1):1–23.
14. Varun B, Sivakumar T, Nair BJ, Joseph AP. Bisphosphonate induced osteonecrosis of jaw in breast cancer patients: a systematic review. J Oral Maxillofac Pathol. 2012;16:210–4.
15. Mallya SM, Tetradis S. Imaging of radiation- and medication-related osteonecrosis. Radiol Clin N Am. 2018;56(1):77–89.

Fibrous Dysplasia

16

Yong-il Kim and Jin-Sook Ryu

Abstract

Fibrous dysplasia is a disease in which fibrous tissues replace the normal bone medullary space. Monostotic fibrous dysplasia accounts for 70–85% of cases of fibrous dysplasia and develops in areas such as the rib and femur. Polyostotic fibrous dysplasia accounts for 15–30% of cases and develops in areas such as the femur and tibia. Bone scan is a valuable imaging technique for differentiating between monostotic and polyostotic fibrous dysplasia and mostly shows the area of intensely increased uptake. Bone scan can be useful for assessing the activity of fibrous dysplasia because the uptake decreases in the quiescent state. Fibrous dysplasia requires a differential diagnosis with other diseases because small lesions can show false-negative results. Bone SPECT/CT can be used to accurately determine the extent of disease invasion. ^{18}F-FDG PET/CT shows variable uptake for fibrous dysplasia.

Keywords

Fibrous dysplasia of bone · Fibrous dysplasia, monostotic · Fibrous dysplasia, polyostotic · Radionuclide imaging · Single-photon emission computed tomography/computed tomography · Positron emission tomography/computed tomography

16.1 Clinical Features and Pathophysiology

Fibrous dysplasia is a benign, non-genetic bone developmental disease in which the fibrous connective tissues of the bone grow abnormally and form immature bone fragments. Fibrous dysplasia accounts for 5–7% of benign bone tumors and is most commonly detected in children and adolescents [1].

Monostotic fibrous dysplasia and polyostotic fibrous dysplasia comprise 70–85% and 15–30% of cases of fibrous dysplasia, respectively [2]. Monostotic fibrous dysplasia develops in the rib, femur, tibia, skull, and facial bones (in order of frequency) and rarely invades the spine. Polyostotic fibrous dysplasia occurs in the femur, tibia, pelvis, metatarsal bone, metacarpal bone, sternum, skull, humerus, and facial bones. Polyostotic fibrous dysplasia often invades the spine and can be accompanied by systemic conditions. In cases with precocious puberty and café au lait spots, the disease is referred to as McCune-Albright syndrome [3], and in cases with myxoma, the disease is referred to as Mazabraud syndrome [4].

The cause of this disease is known to be the ongoing activation of adenylyl cyclase (G protein

Y.-i. Kim (✉) · J.-S. Ryu
Department of Nuclear Medicine, Asan Medical Center, University of Ulsan College of Medicine, Seoul, Republic of Korea
e-mail: kyi821209@amc.seoul.kr; jsryu2@amc.seoul.kr

S.-O. Yang et al. (eds.), *Atlas of Nuclear Medicine in Musculoskeletal System*,
https://doi.org/10.1007/978-981-19-2677-8_16

effector) through the mutation of stimulatory G (Gs) protein genes (guanine nucleotide-binding protein, alpha-stimulating activity polypeptide 1: GNAS1), which subsequently induces cell proliferation in response to cyclic adenosine monophosphate (cAMP) [5] (Fig. 16.1).

Most cases of fibrous dysplasia have no clinical symptoms, and non-specific symptoms can occur depending on the site of fibrous dysplasia, which is often detected by chance on X-ray images [6]. When the disease is followed up, most cases do not show any disease progression. However, some symptoms can occur due to painless swelling with nasal obstruction, nasal bleeding, facial asymmetry, exophthalmos, diplopia, headache, and anosmia [7]. Surgical interventions are necessary if the disease leads to either functional or cosmetic problems, causes severe pain, or is likely to be malignant [1].

16.2 Radiologic Findings and Nuclear Medicine Imaging

On X-ray images, radiolucency changes are observed according to the amount of fibrous and bone tissues in the bone marrow space, the extent of loss of normal trabecular patterns, and ground-glass opacities. If the bone endosteum shows endosteal scalloping with the replacement of normal tissues in the bone marrow space with fibrous collagen tissues, the bone is expanded, and the boundaries of the bone cortex disappear. Radiolucent lesions are sometimes observed as cystic lesions with sclerotic bone rims or show multilocular or bubble shapes. Computed tomography (CT) is used to assess the extent of lesion invasion, especially in the skull and facial bones [8].

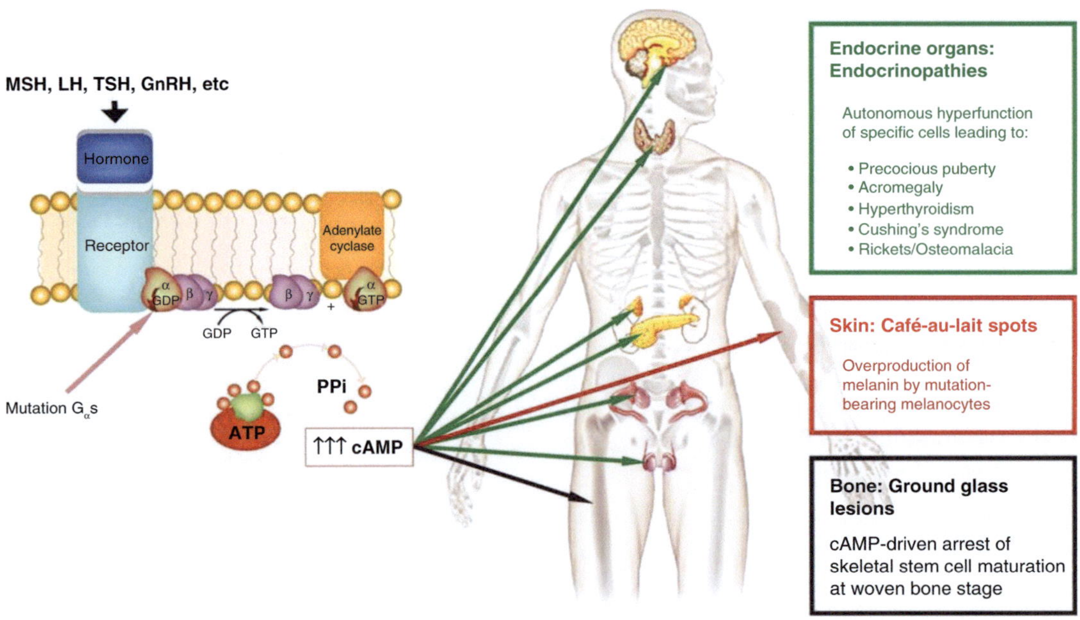

Fig. 16.1 Pathophysiology of fibrous dysplasia. Mutations of stimulatory G (Gs) protein genes (GNAS1) can lead to the inappropriate production of cAMP. The increased concentration of cAMP causes the incomplete differentiation of bone marrow stromal cells into abnormal osteoblasts, which results in the abnormal maturation of the bony matrix. Adapted from [5] with permission

Bone scan is a sensitive nuclear medicine imaging method that can detect early-stage lesions for fibrous dysplasia and can screen for polyostotic fibrous dysplasia as it examines the entire body. Blood flow and metabolism are increased due to active osteoblasts; thus, the area of significantly increased uptake usually appears on bone scan. In addition, bone single-photon emission computed tomography (SPECT)/CT can be used to accurately assess the extent of lesion invasion [9]. When lesions enter the quiescent state during disease progression, an area of increased uptake might not appear on bone scan even if the lesions are evident on X-ray images. Therefore, bone scan is more advantageous when assessing the disease's activity. However, small lesions can show false-negative results in some cases. Hence, if an osteolytic lesion shows no uptake on bone scan, a differential diagnosis is required, which may include hemangioma, giant cell tumor, and aneurysmal bone cyst. ^{18}F-FDG positron emission tomography (PET)/CT shows variable uptake for fibrous dysplasia based on active fibroblasts, which may cause problems in differentiating between fibrous dysplasia and bone metastasis [10] (Fig. 16.2).

Teaching Points

- Bone scan of fibrous dysplasia usually shows increased radiotracer uptake and can be useful to assess the disease activity.
- Bone SPECT/CT is known to be helpful in determining the extent of fibrous dysplasia.
- ^{18}F-FDG PET/CT of fibrous dysplasia demonstrates variable radiotracer uptake.

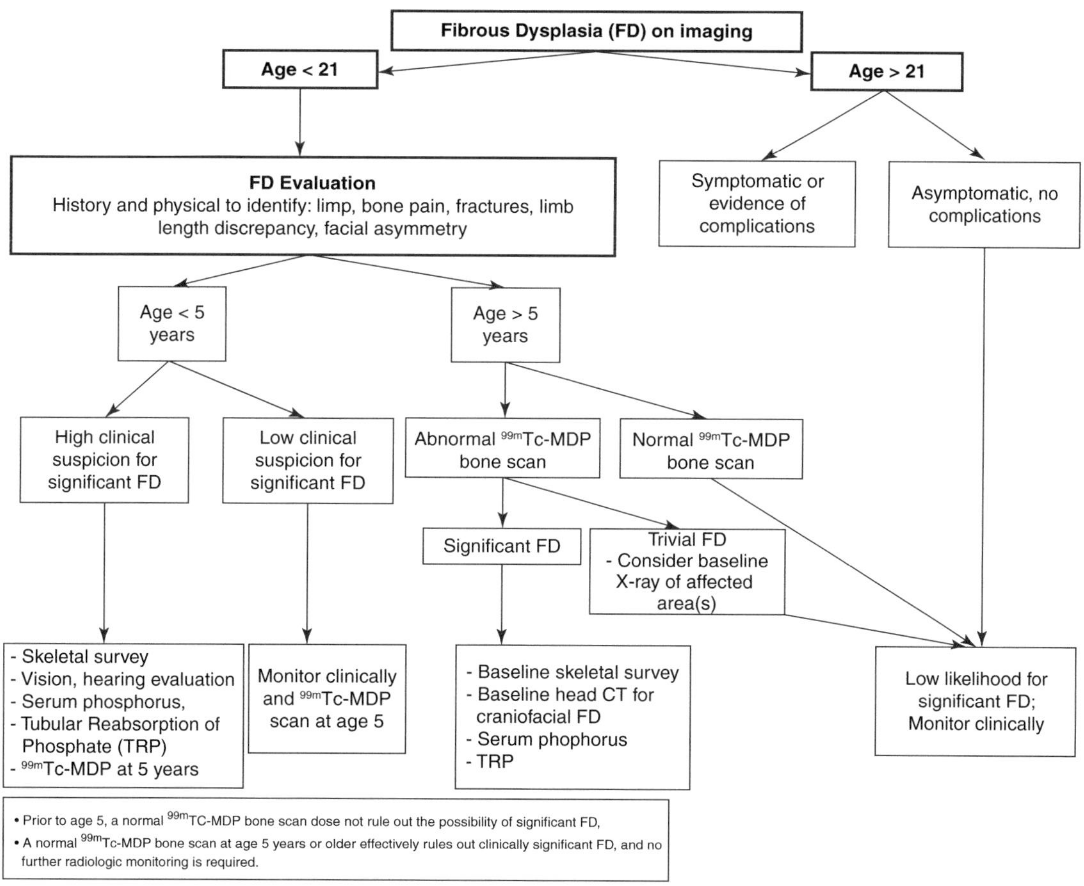

Fig. 16.2 Fibrous dysplasia management algorithm. Adapted from [5] with permission

Case 16.1
A 46-year-old woman underwent bone scan and chest computed tomography (CT) to evaluate her right upper chest wall area protrusion. The right second rib lesion was diagnosed as fibrous dysplasia by excisional biopsy (Fig. 16.3).

Case 16.2
A 10-year-old boy underwent bone scan and lower extremity CT to assess his left calf area pain. The left femur lesion was diagnosed as fibrous dysplasia by excisional biopsy. In addition, typical café au lait spots on the patient's back/lower extremities and precocious puberty were found. The patient was finally diagnosed as McCune-Albright syndrome (Fig. 16.4).

Case 16.3
A 40-year-old woman underwent bone scan and bone SPECT/CT to evaluate an incidentally found spine and rib mass. The left third rib lesion was diagnosed as fibrous dysplasia by a needle biopsy (Fig. 16.5).

Case 16.4
A 41-year-old woman underwent bone scan and ^{18}F-FDG PET/CT to assess her rib and spinal mass by chance. The right fifth rib lesion was diagnosed as fibrous dysplasia by excisional biopsy (Fig. 16.6).

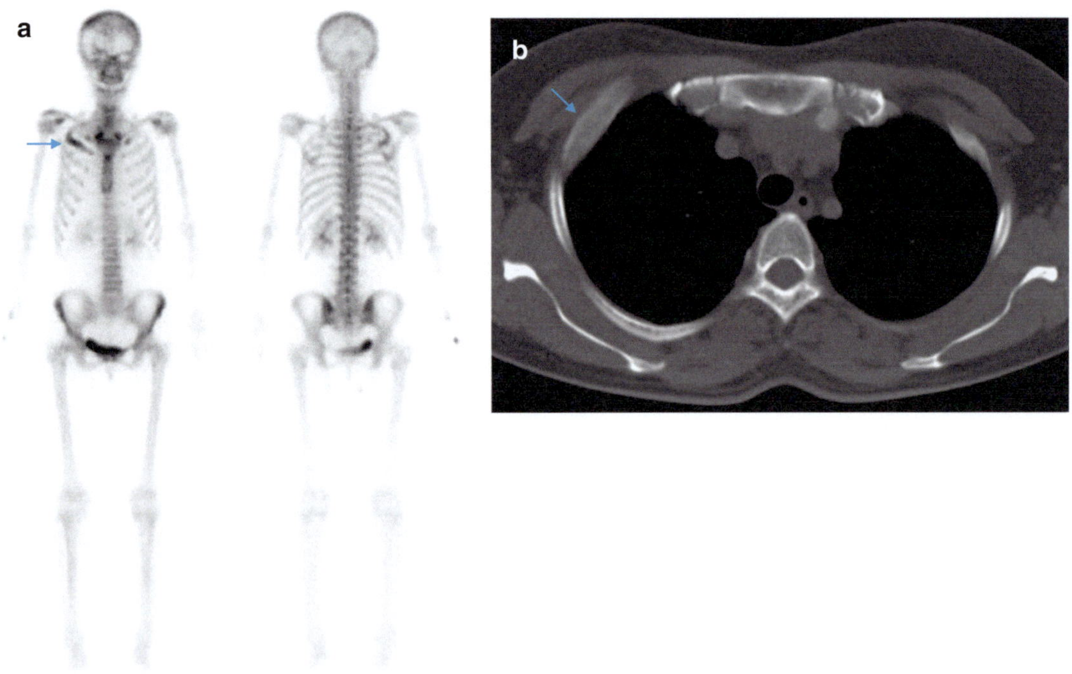

Fig. 16.3 A case of monostotic fibrous dysplasia in a 46-year-old woman. On the bone scan (**a**), diffusely increased uptake is observed in the right second rib (blue arrow). On the chest CT (**b**), diffuse swelling is noted in the right second rib (blue arrow)

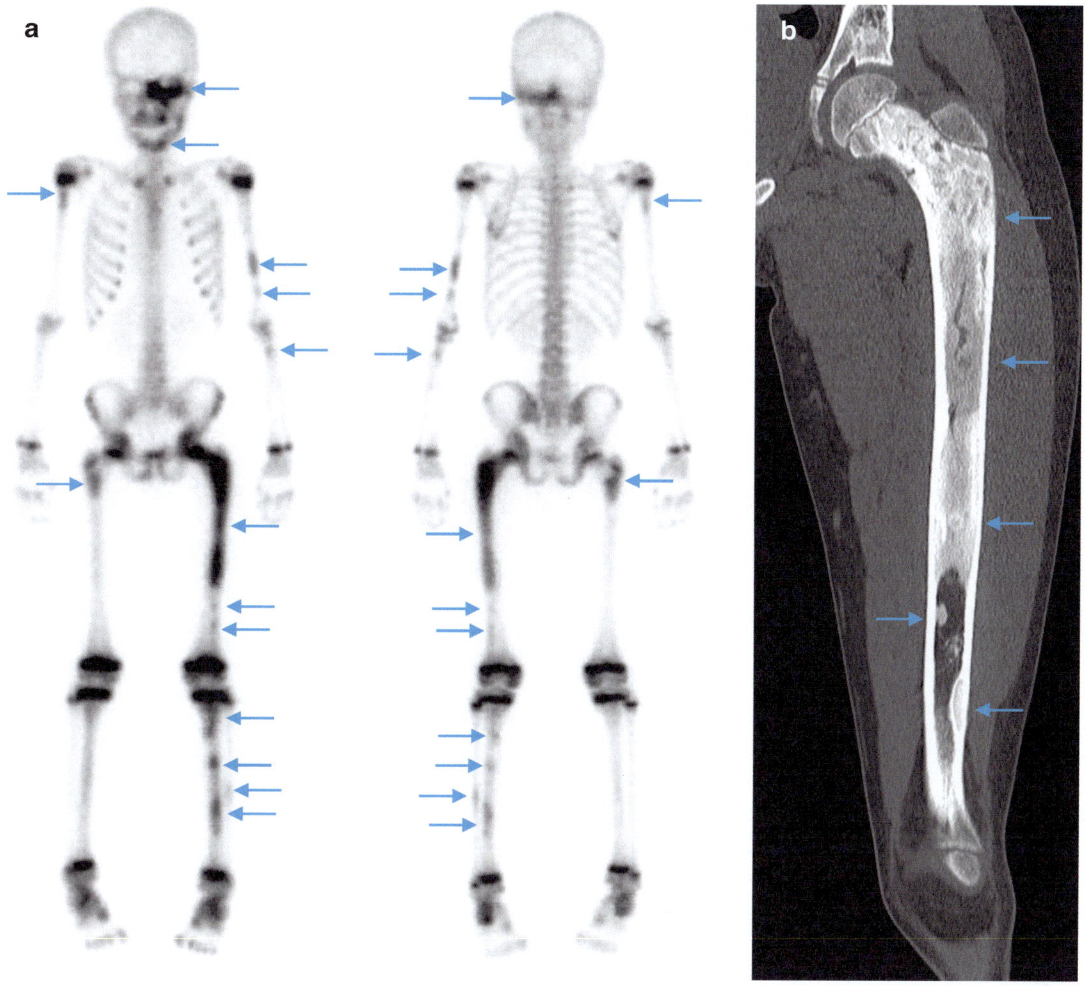

Fig. 16.4 A 10-year-old boy with McCune-Albright syndrome. On the bone scan (**a**), multiple increased uptakes are found in the left side skull base, mandible, both humeri, left proximal radius, both femurs, and left tibia (blue arrows). On the lower extremity CT (**b**), an extensive ground glass attenuated mass and other small multifocal lesions are found in the left femur (blue arrows)

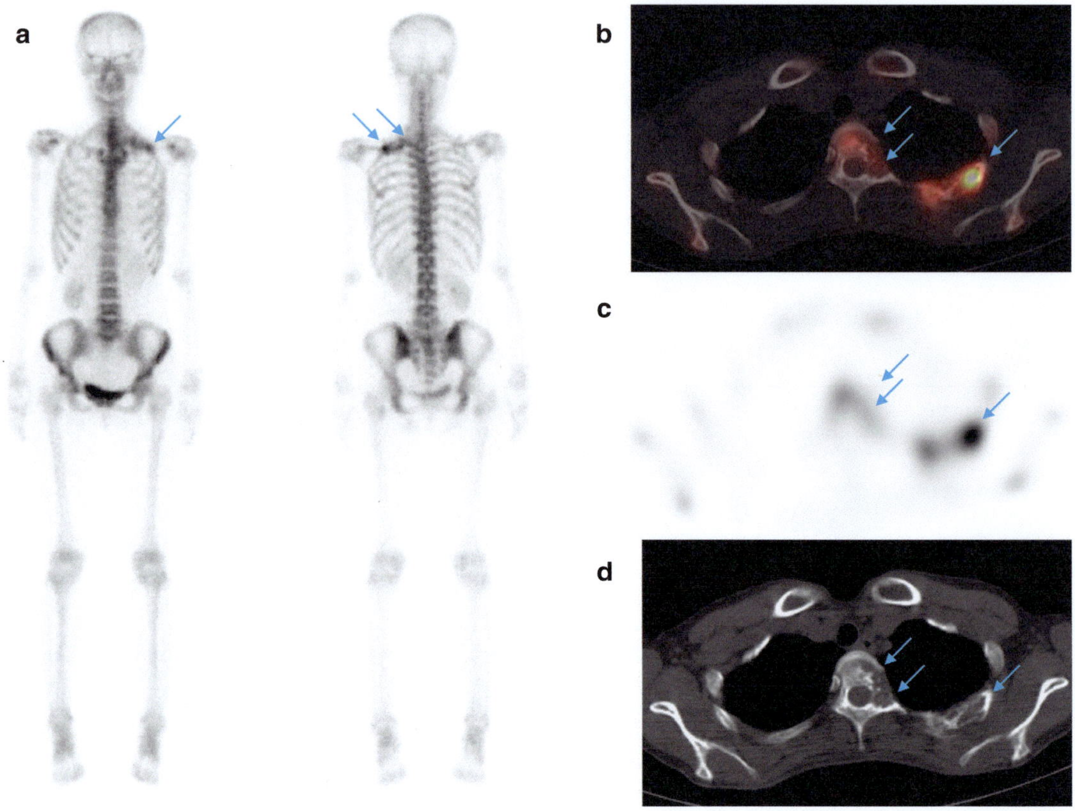

Fig. 16.5 A case demonstrating the usefulness of bone SPECT/CT in fibrous dysplasia. On the bone scan (**a**), irregularly increased uptakes are shown in the left third rib (blue arrows). On the bone SPECT/CT images (**b–d**), the osteolytic and sclerotic lesions with uneven increased uptake are found in the body, left pedicle, left transverse process of T3 vertebra in addition to left third rib posterior arc (blue arrows)

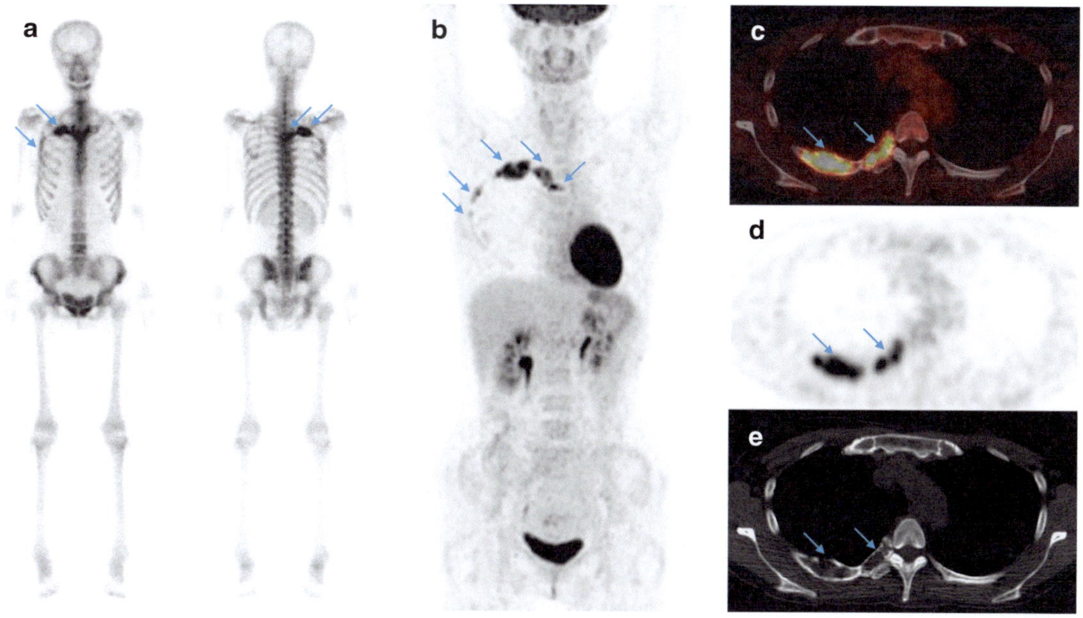

Fig. 16.6 A case of fibrous dysplasia with hypermetabolic activity on ^{18}F-FDG PET/CT. On the bone scan (**a**), intensely increased uptakes are found in the right fifth rib and T5 vertebra (blue arrows). On the ^{18}F-FDG PET/CT images (**b**–**e**), the right fifth rib and T5 lesions are demonstrated as hypermetabolic osteolytic lesions [maximum standardized uptake value (SUV) of the right fifth rib; 8.1] (blue arrows)

References

1. Ramsey HE, Strong EW, Frazell EL. Fibrous dysplasia of the craniofacial bones. Am J Surg. 1968;116:542–7. https://doi.org/10.1016/0002-9610(68)90390-5.
2. Funk FJ Jr, Wells RE. Hip problems in fibrous dysplasia. Clin Orthop Relat Res. 1973;90:77–82.
3. Dumitrescu CE, Collins MT. McCune-Albright syndrome. Orphanet J Rare Dis. 2008;3:12. https://doi.org/10.1186/1750-1172-3-12.
4. Piciu D, Barbus E, Piciu A, Fetica B. Mazabraud's syndrome and thyroid cancer, a very rare and confusing association: a case report. BMC Endocr Disord. 2015;15:39. https://doi.org/10.1186/s12902-015-0036-z.
5. Kushchayeva YS, Kushchayev SV, Glushko TY, Tella SH, Teytelboym OM, Collins MT, et al. Fibrous dysplasia for radiologists: beyond ground glass bone matrix. Insights Imaging. 2018;9:1035–56. https://doi.org/10.1007/s13244-018-0666-6.
6. DiCaprio MR, Enneking WF. Fibrous dysplasia. Pathophysiology, evaluation, and treatment. J Bone Joint Surg Am. 2005;87:1848–64. https://doi.org/10.2106/jbjs.D.02942.
7. Ozcan KM, Akdogan O, Gedikli Y, Ozcan I, Dere H, Unal T. Fibrous dysplasia of inferior turbinate, middle turbinate, and frontal sinus. B-ENT. 2007;3:35–8.
8. Lisle DA, Monsour PA, Maskiell CD. Imaging of craniofacial fibrous dysplasia. J Med Imaging Radiat Oncol. 2008;52:325–32. https://doi.org/10.1111/j.1440-1673.2008.01963.x.
9. Zhang L, He Q, Li W, Zhang R. The value of (99m) Tc-methylene diphosphonate single photon emission computed tomography/computed tomography in diagnosis of fibrous dysplasia. BMC Med Imaging. 2017;17:46. https://doi.org/10.1186/s12880-017-0218-4.
10. Kim M, Kim HS, Kim JH, Jang JH, Chung KJ, Shin MK, et al. F-18 FDG PET-positive fibrous dysplasia in a patient with intestinal non-Hodgkin's lymphoma. Cancer Res Treat. 2009;41:171–4. https://doi.org/10.4143/crt.2009.41.3.171.

Part V

Musculoskeletal Neoplastic Disorders

Primary Bone and Soft Tissue Tumors

17

Jin Chul Paeng and Seoung-Oh Yang

Abstract

Primary bone and soft tissue tumors comprise many diverse pathologic types that may be benign or malignant. Radiological imaging including plain radiograph, CT, MRI, and ultrasonography is the primary imaging method for diagnosing such tumors. Bone scan is usually performed to determine extent of bone invasion or distant bone metastasis. FDG PET is effective for initial staging, monitoring treatment response, and detecting recurrence. Although there are quite a large variation in image findings of primary bone and soft tissue tumors and overlap between benign and malignant tumors, bone scan and FDG PET have effective roles. Particularly, it has been consistently reported that FDG PET has a significant correlation with pathologic grade and patients' prognosis, in certain pathologic types. Some representative pathologic types and cases of primary bone and soft tissue tumors are presented in this chapter.

J. C. Paeng (✉)
Department of Nuclear Medicine, Seoul National University College of Medicine, Seoul, Republic of Korea
e-mail: paengjc@snu.ac.kr

S.-O. Yang
Department of Nuclear Medicine, Dongnam Institute of Radiological and Medical Sciences, Busan, Republic of Korea
e-mail: soyang@dirams.re.kr

Keywords

Bone scan · FDG PET · Primary bone tumor · Primary soft tissue tumor · Sarcoma

17.1 Pathologic Classification

Bone and soft tissue are composed of diverse cells of several origins, and each of them can be transformed to malignancy. According to the 2020 WHO classification of soft tissue and bone tumors, the classification of primary bone and soft tissue tumors is categorized based on the cell origins (Table 17.1) [1].

Table 17.1 WHO classification of primary bone and soft tissue tumors

Primary bone tumors	Primary soft tissue tumors
Chondrogenic tumors	Adipocytic tumors
Osteogenic tumors	Fibroblastic and myofibroblastic tumors
Fibrogenic tumors	Fibrohistiocytic tumors
Vascular tumors of bone	Vascular tumors
Osteoclastic giant cell-rich tumors	Pericytic tumors
Notochordal tumors	Smooth muscle tumors
Other mesenchymal tumors of bone	Skeletal muscle tumors
Hematopoietic neoplasm of bone	Gastrointestinal stromal tumors
	Chondro-osseous tumors
	Peripheral nerve sheath tumors
	Undifferentiated small round cell tumor

S.-O. Yang et al. (eds.), *Atlas of Nuclear Medicine in Musculoskeletal System*,
https://doi.org/10.1007/978-981-19-2677-8_17

17.2 Diagnosis

Plain radiograph is usually used for the initial evaluation of primary bone and soft tissue tumors, and it may provide basic information on tumor characteristics such as location, extent, calcification, and related bone changes. Ultrasonography and computed tomography (CT) are effective in some specific conditions such as superficially located tumors or tumors in head and neck or mediastinum. However, general diagnostic efficacy of ultrasonography and CT in bone and soft tissue tumor is not optimal. Currently, magnetic resonance imaging (MRI) is used as the essential imaging modality for bone and soft tissue tumors. MRI can visualize the exact tumor extent, invasion to adjacent tissues, and metastatic lesions in the covered field of view. MRI can also provide much information on the pathologic characteristics.

17.3 Nuclear Imaging

Bone scan is usually used as one of basic image studies in bone and soft tissue tumors. The purpose of bone scan is to determine extent of bone invasion or distant bone metastasis. It also shows tumor characteristics regarding osteoblastic activity. Thus, baseline bone scan is necessary for future follow-up and surveillance of a patient. Most of primary malignant bone tumors show high uptake on bone scan. However, benign bone tumors may show variable uptake, and the degree of uptake cannot be used for differentiation of malignant from benign tumors or high-grade from low-grade tumors. Bone positron emission tomography (PET) using ^{18}F-NaF may also be used for the same purpose. However, ^{18}F-NaF PET is not so widely used due to high cost despite higher image quality than bone scan.

^{18}F-fluorodeoxyglucose (FDG) PET is effective in the initial staging and diagnosis of recurrence. FDG PET is a sensitive imaging to detect tumors and effective in detecting metastasis. Because FDG PET covers the whole body on a single scan, unexpected distant metastasis may be detected in initial staging or surveillance. FDG PET can also be used for determining biopsy site when the biopsy of primary site is risky or initial biopsy result is insufficient due to large necrotic portion. FDG uptake is related to the degree of malignancy, and high uptake is usually observed in high-grade or poorly differentiated tumors. Thus, FDG PET finding is associated with a patient's prognosis, although specific pathologic types are cannot be differentiated on PET images

FDG PET is also effective for treatment response evaluation. Currently, chemotherapy and/or radiotherapy is often used for some bone and soft tissue sarcomas as neoadjuvant therapy or palliative therapy (Fig. 17.1). FDG PET shows metabolic change of a tumor and is a sensitive imaging to show response to treatment. During follow-up and surveillance after initial treatment, local recurrence is the most common treatment failure. Although MRI is the most effective imaging in diagnosing recurrence, FDG PET is effective when there are metallic prostheses that cause severe metallic artifact and/or post-radiation changes (Fig. 17.2).

In contrast to usual cancers, bone and soft tissue sarcomas often metastasize to atypical sites including peripheral bone and soft tissues. Thus, it is recommended to obtain total body images in the case of these sarcomas, rather than usual torso images.

17.4 Image Findings of Common Primary Bone and Soft Tissue Tumors

17.4.1 Osteosarcoma

Although various ossification patterns are observed on plain radiographs, osteoblastic activity is enhanced in most of osteosarcoma. Thus, osteosarcoma shows high uptake on bone scan. Additionally, high uptake is also observed in extraskeletal metastatic sites such as the lungs. FDG PET also shows high uptake in osteosarcoma [2]. FDG PET is effective for response monitoring and recurrence detection.

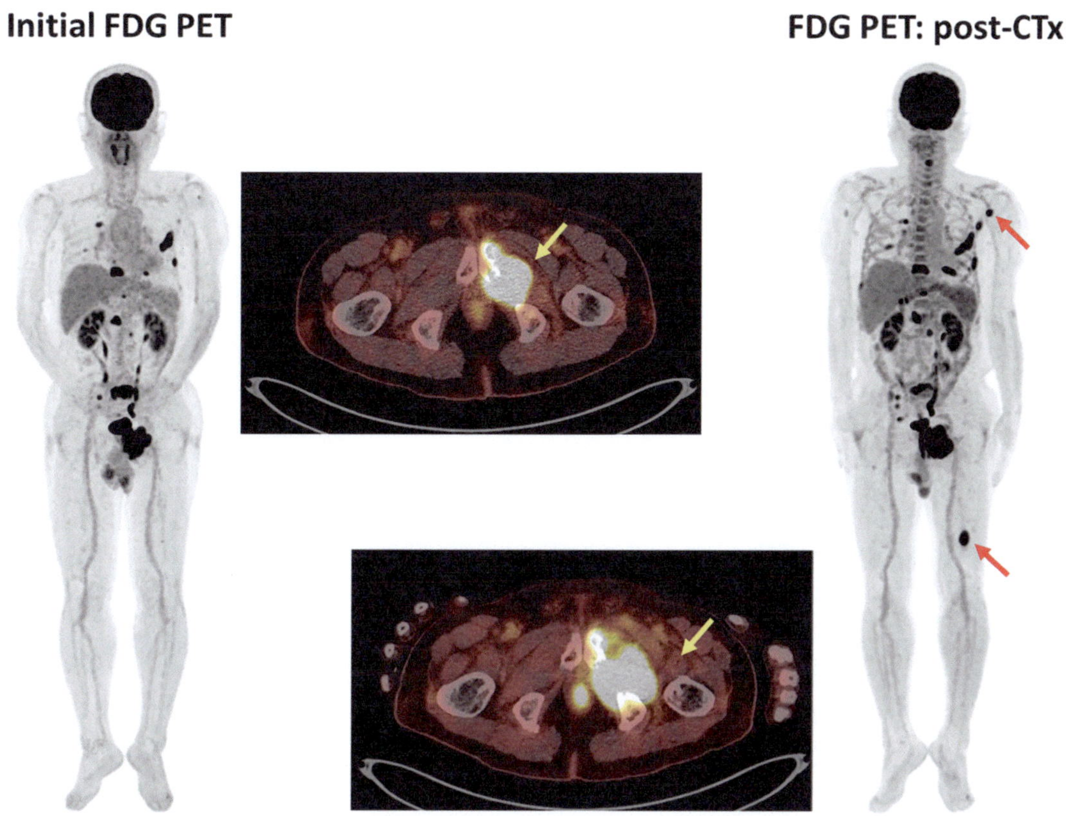

Fig. 17.1 Intense uptake was observed in multiple lesions on FDG PET (maximum SUV 18.5). Despite chemotherapy of second-line regimen, the tumor of the primary site progressed (yellow arrows, maximum SUV 34.4), and multiple new lesions appeared (red arrows)

17.4.2 Chondrosarcoma

Chondrosarcoma usually shows intense uptake on bone scan, whereas benign enchondroma shows mild to moderate uptake [3]. Thus, bone scan can be used for monitoring malignant transformation of benign chondrogenic tumors. On FDG PET, although chondrosarcoma usually shows moderate uptake, the uptake is higher in high-grade chondrosarcoma [4].

17.4.3 Liposarcoma

Liposarcoma is a relatively common bone and soft tissue tumor. Bone scan is helpful in bone metastasis of liposarcoma like other sarcoma. The uptake of FDG by liposarcoma is usually lower than that of other sarcoma, in line with relatively favorable prognosis. Thus, discrimination between benign and malignant lipomatous tumors based on FDG uptake is often difficult [5]. However, FDG uptake is well correlated with grade of liposarcoma, and high-grade liposarcoma may show intense uptake. FDG uptake is also associated with patients' prognosis [6].

17.4.4 Giant Cell Tumor

As giant cell tumor is caused by hyperproliferation of osteoclasts, it is usually shown as a radiolucent mass without surrounding sclerosis or calcification on CT and a T1-low tumor with high

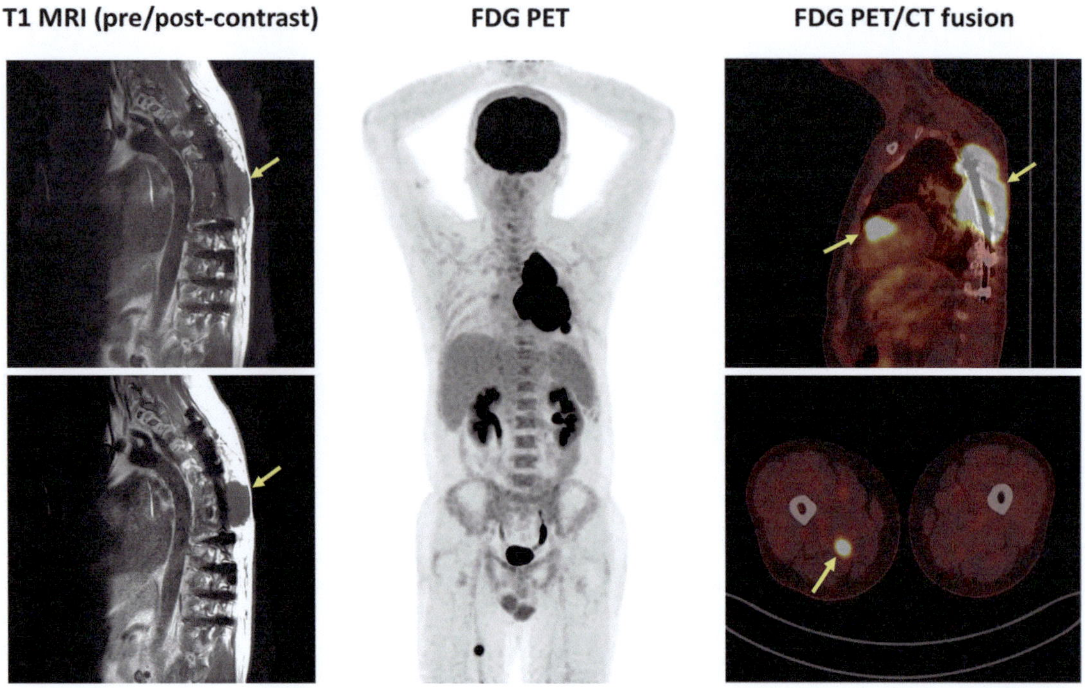

Fig. 17.2 On MRI, irregular enhancement pattern was observed in the back mass (arrows on MRI), which can be interpreted as a benign postoperative change. On FDG PET, the mass showed intense uptake, suggesting malignancy (maximum SUV 22.6). Atypical metastases were observed in the lung, myocardium, and thigh muscle (arrows on PET)

enhancement on MRI. On bone scan, most giant cell tumor shows high uptake. The uptake is often combined with a central defect, which is called "doughnut sign." Although giant cell tumor is classified as a malignancy, it usually shows high uptake on FDG PET with a large variability [7].

17.4.5 Ewing Sarcoma

Ewing sarcoma is classified as undifferentiated small round cell sarcoma of bone and soft tissue. Ewing sarcoma usually shows intense FDG uptake [2], with sensitivity and specificity of FDG PET >95% [8]. Ewing sarcoma may show variable uptake on bone scan, although a typical lesion usually shows moderate uptake.

17.4.6 Fibrogenic and Fibroblastic Tumors

Fibrous dysplasia is a benign bone lesion of intramedullary fibrous proliferation, often combined with altered osteogenesis. It may be monostotic or polyostotic forms. Fibrous dysplasia usually shows intense uptake on bone scan and variable FDG uptake on PET [9]. Malignant transformation may occur in fibrous dysplasia, although it is rare. Other fibrogenic, fibroblastic, and fibrohistocytic tumors also show variable FDG uptake, and the uptake is usually associated with grade of tumors. Because a large mass may show heterogeneous uptake pattern due to necrosis and/or internal heterogeneous tissue components, FDG PET is helpful to determine biopsy target.

17.4.7 Langerhans Cell Histiocytosis

Langerhans cell histiocytosis is a disorder of abnormal proliferation of a certain immune cell type. The bone is the most common site of involvement and usually presented in children or young adults. The skull is the most common site and it can involve any site of the skeleton. On plain radiographs, osteolytic lesion without rim is the typical finding. On bone scan, increased uptake with internal defect is a typical finding, and the uptake is normalized after treatment. FDG PET is usually not necessary for diagnosis of follow-up of Langerhans cell histiocytosis. However, FDG PET may be used in initial diagnosis when diagnosis is uncertain. On FDG PET, high uptake is often observed, although it may be variable.

17.4.8 Other Tumors

There are many other types of bone and soft tissue tumors, with variable pathology. The tumors may show variable findings on bone scan or FDG PET. In most tumors, FDG uptake is related to tumor grade, degree of malignancy, and patients' prognosis. Thus, FDG PET is recommended to be considered in initial staging, selection of biopsy site, evaluation of treatment response, and recurrence detection. However, it should be noted that many benign bone tumors also show high uptake on bone scan or FDG PET.

Teaching Points

- Most of primary malignant bone tumors and bone involvement of malignant soft tissue tumors show high uptake on bone scan, whereas benign bone tumors may show variable uptake.
- Although some tumors such as osteosarcoma, giant cell tumor, fibrous dysplasia, and Langerhans cell histiocytosis present relatively typical findings on bone scan, it is difficult to diagnose pathologic types on bone scan.
- On FDG PET scan, there are considerable variations of uptake even in the same pathologic types, and thus, it is inappropriate to discriminate malignant from benign tumors or to determine pathologic types on FDG PET.
- FDG uptake in the same pathology is usually associated with pathologic grades and patients' prognosis.
- In primary bone and soft tissue tumors, FDG PET can be used for determining biopsy sites, initial staging, prognosis prediction, treatment response monitoring, and detection of recurrence.

Case 1

A 68-year-old male patient was diagnosed with osteosarcoma and showed multiple metastases to the bones and lungs. The patient received palliate chemotherapy, and new nodules were detected on chest CT. Second-line chemotherapy was started, and FDG PET was performed after two cycles of chemotherapy. On the PET images, disease progression was determined (Fig. 17.1), and radiotherapy with changed chemotherapy regimen was started.

Case 2

A 30-year-old male patient presented with a growing mass in the upper back. He had undergone resection of a giant cell tumor in T-spines 5 years ago, and the new mass recurred in the operation site. On MRI, a new mass was observed in the soft tissue with prominent metallic artifact. He underwent FDG PET, and the mass showed intense hypermetabolism, suggesting recurrence of tumor. Additionally, atypical metastases were observed in multiple organs including myocardium (Fig. 17.2).

Case 3

A 14-year-old male patient presented with a mass in the right humerus. From bone biopsy, the mass was confirmed as osteosarcoma. Bone scan and FDG PET were performed for initial staging of the tumor. On both images, increased uptake was observed in the primary tumor, and no other lesion was detected. After neoadjuvant chemotherapy and limb-salvage surgery, the patient was followed up using bone scan for surveillance of recurrence. Three months after surgery, a new uptake on bone scan was observed in the right humerus. On other images, it was confirmed as a benign screw fracture (Fig. 17.3).

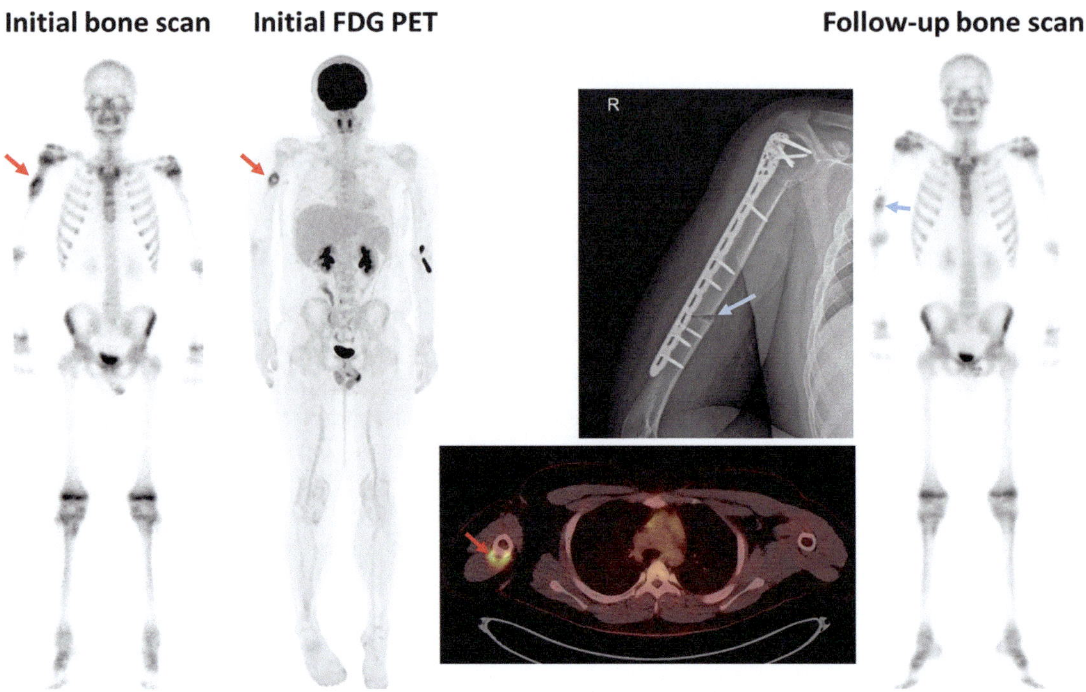

Fig. 17.3 On initial bone scan and FDG PET, the primary tumor in the right humerus shows uptake (red arrows, maximum SUV 6.9). Three months after surgery, bone scan uptake in the primary site had disappeared, whereas a new uptake was observed in the screw fracture site (blue arrows)

Case 4

A 40-year-old male patient who had been confirmed as hereditary multiple osteochondroma complained of expansile upper back mass during follow-up. On bone scan, multiple osteochondroma lesions showed moderately increased uptake. Particularly, intense uptake was observed in a mass of the upper T-spine. On MRI, the mass showed was suspected as a malignant tumor rather than a benign osteochondroma. On FDG PET, only mild uptake was shown (Fig. 17.4). The mass was excised and confirmed as grade 1 chondrosarcoma.

Case 5

A 45-year-old female patient presented with a left pelvic mass. The mass had slowly grown over 5 years and fat component was observed on CT. On FDG PET, the mass showed mild uptake. The mass was excised and confirmed as dedifferentiated liposarcoma (Fig. 17.5a).

Case 6

A 65-year-old female patient presented with aggravating cough. Multiple lung nodules were detected on chest radiograph, and FDG PET was performed to determine probable primary site and metastatic lesions. On FDG PET, large and intense hypermetabolic mass was detected in the right psoas muscle. From the muscle biopsy, the mass was confirmed as a high-grade dedifferentiated liposarcoma (Fig. 17.5b).

Case 7

A 19-year-old male patient presented with multiple tumors. From bone biopsy, the tumors were diagnosed with synchronous giant cell tumors. After tumor removal of right femur head and total hip replacement surgery, he still had several giant cell tumors (Fig. 17.6).

Case 8

A 44-year-old male patient presented with a tumor in the left gluteal muscle. From the muscle

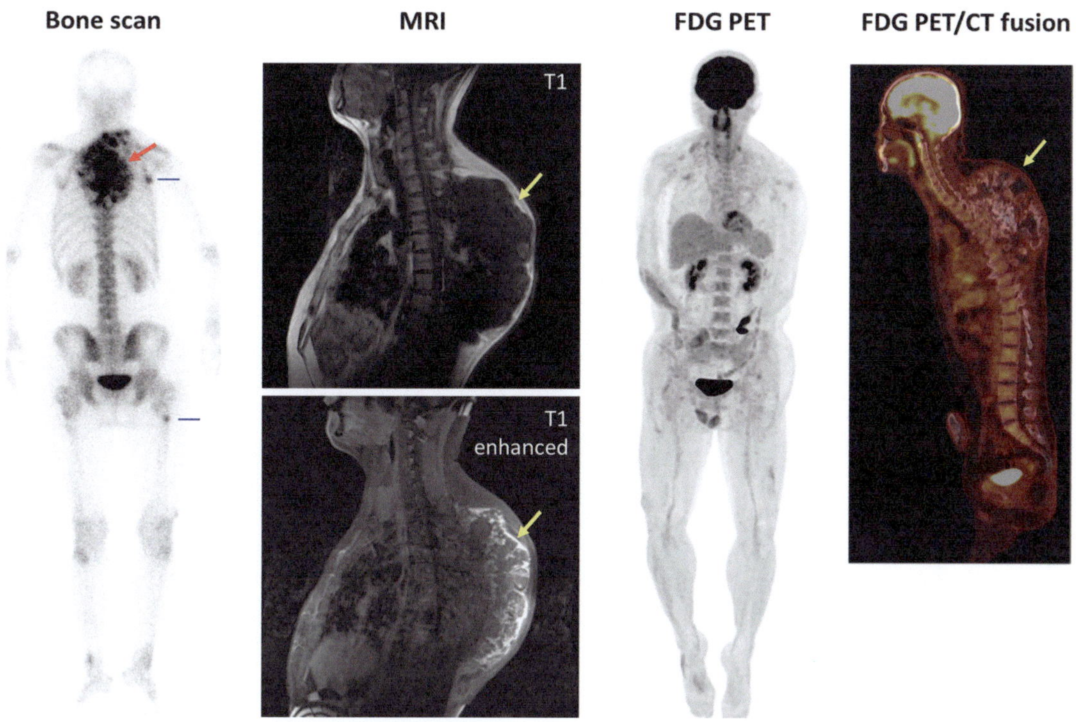

Fig. 17.4 On bone scan, multiple osteochondroma lesions show high uptake (blue lines), and intense uptake was observed in upper T-spine mass (red arrow). On MRI, the mass shows peripheral and septal enhancement (yellow arrows). On FDG PET, the mass showed mild uptake (maximum SUV 2.7), although the mass was confirmed as grade 1 chondrosarcoma

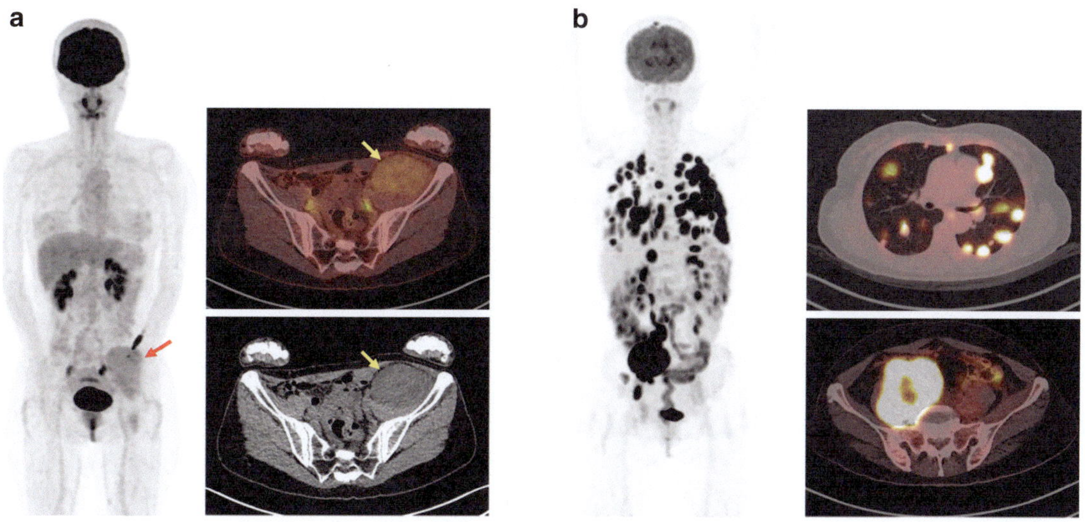

Fig. 17.5 (**a**) A left pelvic mass with fat component showed mild uptake on FDG PET (maximum SUV 2.5). The mass was confirmed as dedifferentiated liposarcoma. (**b**) Multiple metastatic lung nodules show intense uptake on FDG PET. A large and intense hypermetabolic mass was detected in the right psoas muscle (maximum SUV 43.1), which was confirmed as high-grade dedifferentiated liposarcoma

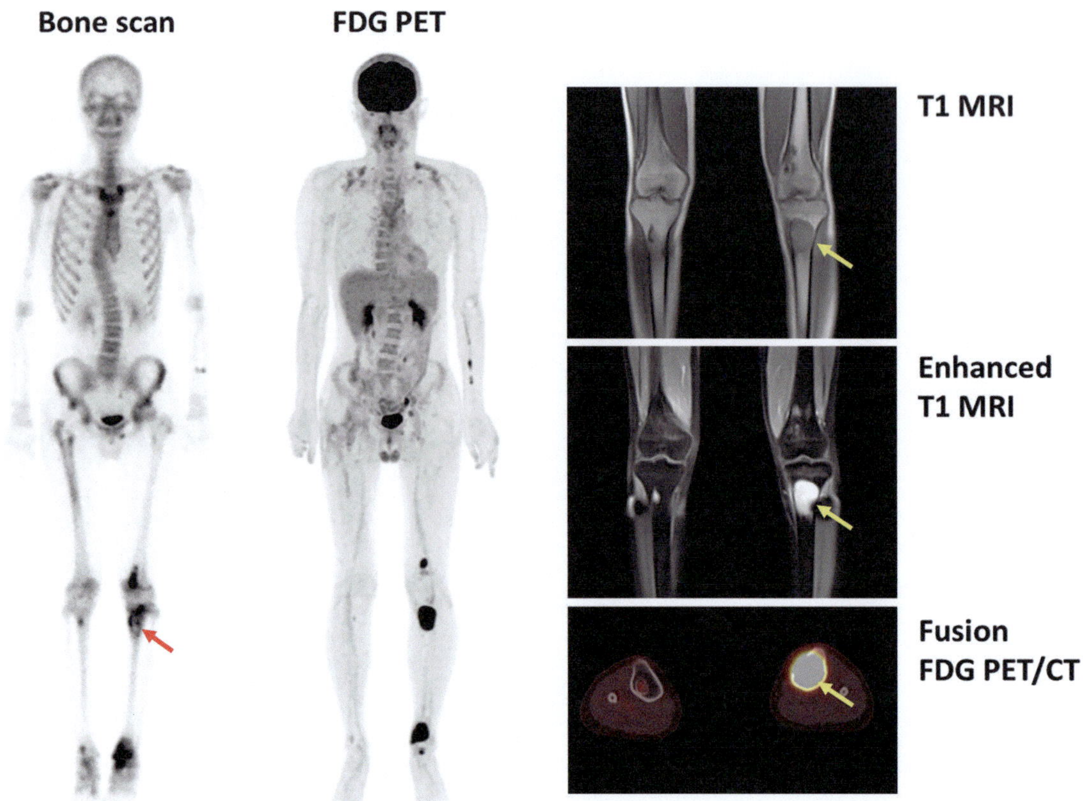

Fig. 17.6 In a patient with multiple synchronous giant cell tumors, several giant cell tumors are shown. A tumor in the left proximal tibia shows central defect on bone scan (red arrow), which is called "doughnut cell." MRI showed typical finding of giant cell tumor, low T1 signal, and high enhancement. FDG PET shows multiple foci of high uptake (maximum SUV 14.7)

biopsy, the tumor was confirmed as Ewing sarcoma. FDG PET showed intense uptake of the primary tumor and multiple metastatic lesions including lymph nodes and bones. On bone scan, the metastatic site of bone showed moderate uptake (Fig. 17.7).

Case 9
A 35-year-old man presented with fibrous dysplasia. He showed multiple bone lesions, which showed intense uptake on bone scan. During follow-up, a mass in the left ilium enlarged and biopsy was performed. It was confirmed to be a chondrosarcoma (red arrows), which was deemed a transformed malignancy from the fibrous dysplasia. Interestingly, whereas fibrous dysplasia lesions showed variable FDG, malignant chondrosarcoma showed relatively mild uptake (Fig. 17.8a).

Case 10
A 81-year-old man presented with a large tumor in the left medial thigh. The mass was diagnosed with myxoid fibrosarcoma on biopsy. On FDG PET, despite intense uptake in some part (maximum SUV 19.6), a considerable heterogeneity was observed. When the tumor was surgically resected, similar heterogeneity was observed on the gross tumor and microscopic findings (Fig. 17.8b).

Case 11
A 2-year-old boy presented with left femoral pain. On plain radiograph an osteolytic lesion was observed in the left proximal femur. On bone scan, high uptake was observed in the margin area with internal defect. FDG PET was performed to rule out malignancy and showed high uptake in the lesion. Bone biopsy showed that it

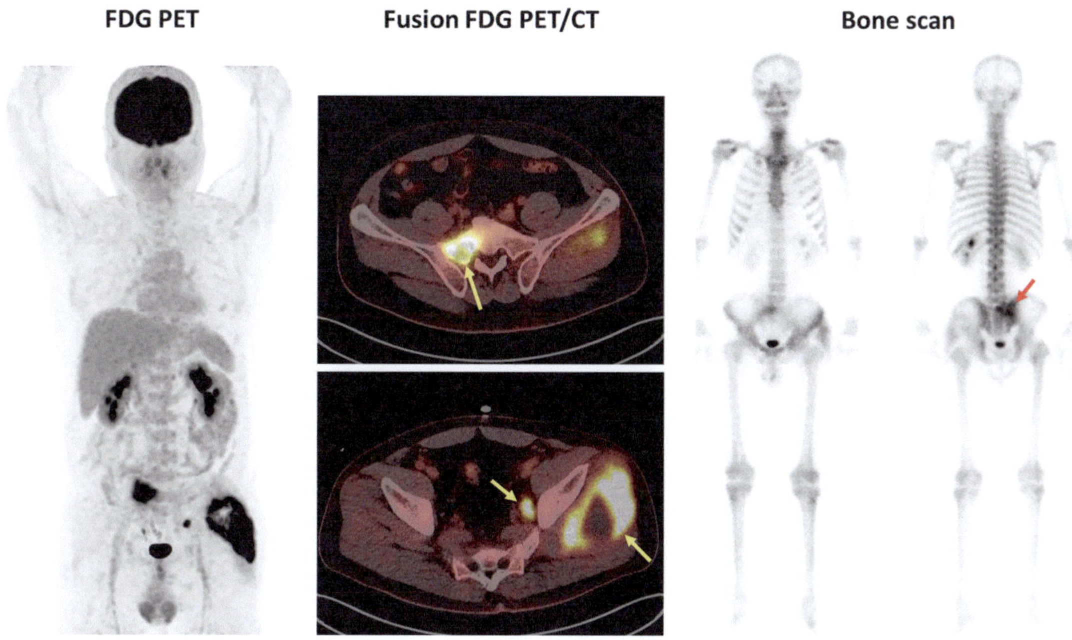

Fig. 17.7 Ewing sarcoma in the left gluteal muscle shows intense FDG uptake on PET (maximum SUV 18.8). Metastatic lesions are also shown in the left obturator lymph node and right side of sacrum (yellow arrows). On bone scan, the sacral metastasis shows moderate uptake (red arrow)

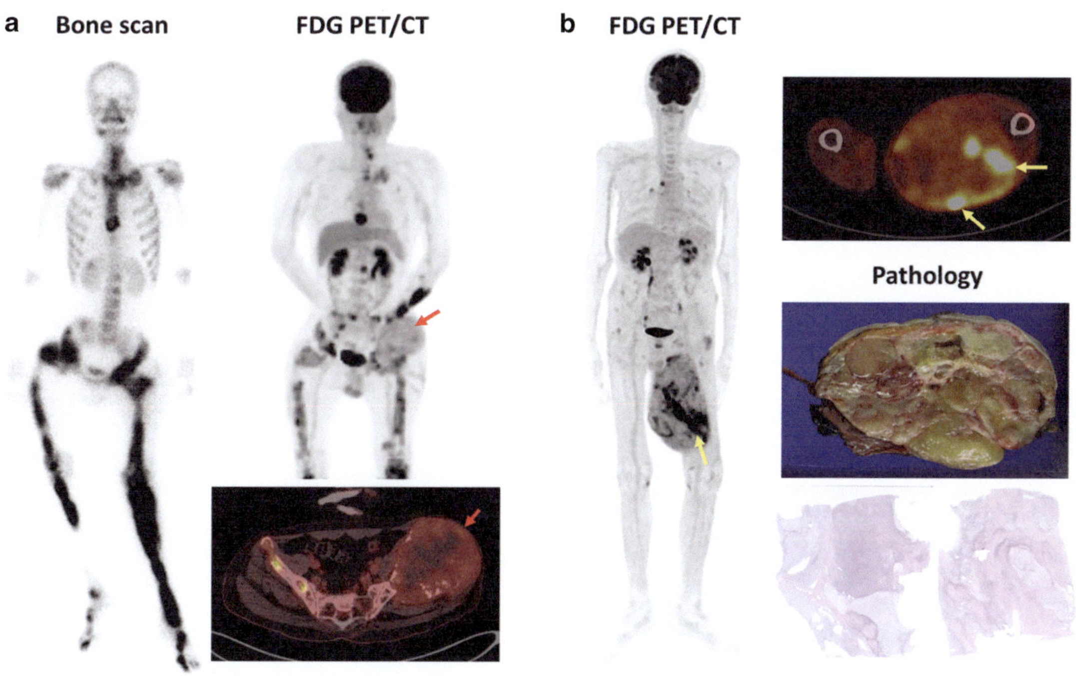

Fig. 17.8 (**a**) Polyostotic fibrous dysplasia in multiple bones shows intense uptake on bone scan. A chondrosarcoma transformed from the fibrous dysplasia (red arrows) shows mild uptake (maximum SUV 3.5), whereas fibrous dysplasia lesions show variable FDG uptake (maximum SUV up to 13.7. (**b**) A myxoid fibrosarcoma shows intense uptake in some part on FDG PET (yellow arrows, maximum SUV 19.6), which is matched with a considerable heterogeneity in gross/microscopic pathology

was Langerhans cell histiocytosis. After indomethacin treatment, the lesion on bone scan normalized, and pain disappeared (Fig. 17.9).

Case 12

A 42-year-old male patient presented with a palpable mass in the left knee and discomfort on walking. MRI revealed a soft tissue mass in the anterior knee area, which showed intense FDG uptake. He underwent tumor resection, and the pathologic diagnosis was clear cell sarcoma. After 1-year follow-up, a new nodule was detected in the right subscapularis muscle, which was confirmed as recurred clear cell sarcoma from muscle biopsy. FDG PET also showed another metastatic lesion (Fig. 17.10).

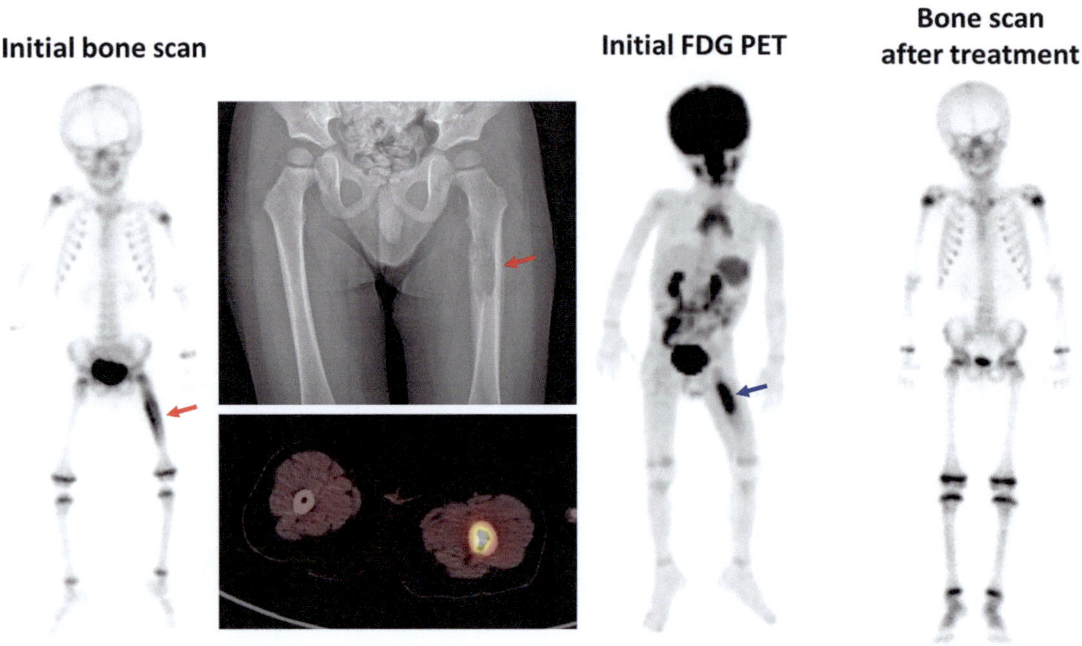

Fig. 17.9 On plain radiograph, an osteolytic lesion is observed in the left proximal femur (red arrow). On bone scan, high uptake is observed in the margin area with internal defect. FDG PET shows also high uptake in the lesion (blue arrow)

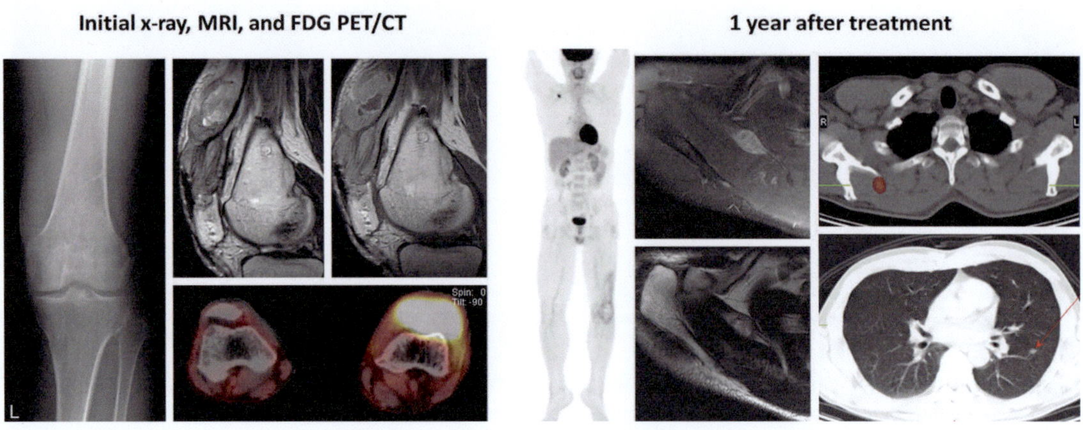

Fig. 17.10 On MRI, a soft tissue mass is observed in the anterior knee area, which showed intense FDG uptake (maximum SUV 11.6). In 1-year follow-up FDG PET, a new nodule with high FDG uptake was detected in the right subscapularis muscle (maximum SUV 6.4), which was confirmed as metastasis. Another small metastatic lesion in the left lung was not detected on PET, probably due to partial volume effect and motion artifact

References

1. The WHO. Classification of tumours editorial board. WHO Classification of Tumours Soft Tissue and Bone Tumours. 5th ed. Lyon: IARC Press; 2020.
2. Charest M, Hickeson M, Lisbona R, Novales-Diaz JA, Derbekyan V, Turcotte RE. Eur J Nucl Med Mol Imaging. 2009;36:1944–51. https://doi.org/10.1007/s00259-009-1203-0.
3. Murphey MD, Flemming DJ, Boyea SR, Bojescul JA, Sweet DE, Temple HT. Radiographics. 1998;18:1213–37; quiz 44-5. https://doi.org/10.1148/radiographics.18.5.9747616.
4. Brenner W, Conrad EU, Eary JF. Eur J Nucl Med Mol Imaging. 2004;31:189–95. https://doi.org/10.1007/s00259-003-1353-4.
5. Baffour FI, Wenger DE, Broski SM. Am J Nucl Med Mol Imaging. 2020;10:74–82.
6. Brenner W, Eary JF, Hwang W, Vernon C, Conrad EU. Eur J Nucl Med Mol Imaging. 2006;33:1290–5. https://doi.org/10.1007/s00259-006-0170-y.
7. Muheremu A, Ma Y, Huang Z, Shan H, Li Y, Niu X. Oncol Lett. 2017;14:1985–8. https://doi.org/10.3892/ol.2017.6379.
8. Treglia G, Salsano M, Stefanelli A, Mattoli MV, Giordano A, Bonomo L. Skelet Radiol. 2012;41:249–56. https://doi.org/10.1007/s00256-011-1298-9.
9. Choi YY, Kim JY, Yang SO. Semin Musculoskelet Radiol. 2014;18:133–48. https://doi.org/10.1055/s-0034-1371016.

18 Metastatic Musculoskeletal Tumors

Young-Sil An and Seoung-Oh Yang

Abstract

Bone metastasis from solid tumors may appear at various sites, mainly cancer from the breast and prostate. Bone metastases are mainly distributed in the axial skeleton, which contains red bone marrow. The role of imaging studies in bone metastasis is to establish a treatment plan for the patient and predict prognosis. For nuclear medicine imaging, bone scan and ^{18}F-FDG PET are the most commonly used clinically, and bone PET using ^{18}F-NaF can also be used to evaluate bone metastasis. Here, we introduce a variety of nuclear medicine imaging cases showing metastatic bone lesions, and we would like to inform you about what points to keep in mind when evaluating bone metastases with nuclear medicine imaging.

Keywords

Bone metastasis · Bone scan · ^{18}F-NaF PET
^{18}F-FDG PET · Flare phenomenon
Osteolytic · Osteosclerotic

Y.-S. An (✉)
Department of Nuclear Medicine and Molecular Imaging, Ajou University School of Medicine, Suwon, Republic of Korea
e-mail: aysays@aumc.ac.kr

S.-O. Yang
Department of Nuclear Medicine, Dongnam Institute of Radiological and Medical Sciences, Busan, Republic of Korea
e-mail: soyang@dirams.re.kr

18.1 Etiology and Pathophysiology

Bone metastasis indicates that cancer cells escape from the primary cancer site and colonize the bone, which is seen in various primary cancers, such as the breast, prostate, lungs, and kidneys [1]. The process by which a solid tumor can metastasize to bone includes pre-metastatic niche formation [2], circulation-mediated dissemination of tumor cells, and complex interaction between circulating tumor cells and the bone microenvironment, known as the "seed and soil" hypothesis [3, 4].

Cancer cells settle in the bone and cause bone destruction mediated by osteoclast-mediated osteolysis, and these bone changes cause bone pain and fracture, which lowers the patient's quality of life and may increase morbidity [5]. Systemic chemotherapy, radiation therapy, and orthopedic surgery can be performed to treat bone metastases; however, there is no ideal treatment that can offer a complete cure. Clinical treatment and supportive care in patients with bone metastasis mainly focus on reducing metastatic bone pain, improving the patient's quality of life, and increasing life expectancy.

S.-O. Yang et al. (eds.), *Atlas of Nuclear Medicine in Musculoskeletal System*,
https://doi.org/10.1007/978-981-19-2677-8_18

18.2 Diagnosis

Assessing bone metastasis in cancer patients using imaging tools is an essential element in establishing a patient's treatment plan and predicting prognosis. In the field of nuclear medicine, bone scans using bone-seeking radiopharmaceuticals (^{99m}Tc-MDP, ^{99m}Tc-DPD, and ^{99m}Tc-HDP) and ^{18}F-FDG PET reflecting glucose metabolism of metastatic sites are currently widely used in clinics to evaluate metastatic bone lesions.

Bone scan is the most commonly used clinical nuclear medicine imaging method for evaluating bone metastasis in patients with various cancers (including breast, stomach, lung, and prostate cancer). This imaging tool focuses on the fact that osteoblastic (bone-forming) activity occurs actively at the site of bone metastasis, which can show hot uptake of bone-seeking radiopharmaceuticals. Bone metastasis is known to predominantly occur in the axial skeleton (spine, pelvis, skull, and ribs) where red bone marrow is widely distributed [6]; therefore, this area should be carefully examined when reading a bone scan. In the case of extensive bone metastasis, it may involve the appendicular skeleton and may appear as a superscan. In addition, some metastases could be found as a single lesion in an unexpected area (e.g., single metastasis of the sternum in breast cancer); therefore, caution is required when evaluating bone scans. In detecting bone metastases, bone scans are generally known to have high sensitivity but relatively low specificity [6, 7]. Therefore, if metastasis is suspected on a bone scan, it may be necessary to obtain further images such as computed tomography (CT), magnetic resonance imaging (MRI), or ^{18}F-fluorodeoxyglucose (^{18}F-FDG) positron emission tomography (PET) to evaluate metastasis. In addition, a bone scan has a limitation in that lesions may be missed in cases of predominantly osteolytic (bone destructive) metastatic bone lesions that do not have increased osteoblastic activity.

Bone PET using ^{18}F-NaF, a bone-seeking radiopharmaceutical that emits positrons, can also be used to evaluate bone metastasis. ^{18}F-NaF bone PET can obtain high-resolution images compared to bone scans and, in particular, has the advantage of acquiring 3D images; therefore, it can be superior to bone scan in evaluating bone metastasis [8]. Currently, it is not widely used because of its weakness compared to bone scans in terms of cost. However, bone PET is expected to be more widely used clinically because it is more convenient for patients than bone scan because the waiting time from radiopharmaceutical injection to image acquisition in bone PET is shorter than bone scan (1 h versus 3–4 h).

^{18}F-FDG PET is widely used clinically to evaluate distant metastasis to various organs, including the bone in cancer patients. It is generally known that ^{18}F-FDG PET shows better diagnostic performance than bone scans in evaluating bone metastasis [9]. However, in the case of osteosclerotic metastasis, the degree of ^{18}F-FDG uptake may be low, and in this case, it might be necessary to evaluate the lesion complementarily by performing a bone scan [10]. In particular, when evaluating the response to chemotherapy, it is thought that evaluating the viability of the lesion on ^{18}F-FDG PET rather than the activity of the metastatic lesion remaining on the bone scan is better for predicting the patient's prognosis [11].

When evaluating bone metastases using nuclear medicine imaging, it is essential to consider the patient's current treatment status. If a patient underwent imaging studies during chemotherapy and/or hormone therapy, a flare phenomenon that may appear as if the bone metastasis has temporarily worsened may be observed. If the patient's current clinical information is not properly understood, it may be mistakenly judged that metastasis had progressed. The flare phenomenon is known to occur in both bone scan [12] and ^{18}F-FDG PET [13], and this is a factor that can predict a good prognosis for patients. When reading nuclear medicine images, we must fully understand the patient's clinical information.

In this chapter, we would like to introduce cases in which physicians should carefully consider when reading nuclear medicine images to evaluate bone metastases.

Teaching Points

- Superscan is a finding suggestive of extensive metastasis.
- The possibility of metastasis should be considered for hot uptake lesions with a linear pattern of the rib.
- In the case of bone scans in breast cancer patients, metastasis should be suspected even with a single lesion of the sternum.
- ^{18}F-sodium fluoride (^{18}F-NaF) PET/CT can detect bone metastases more sensitively than bone scan.
- When reading a bone scan or ^{18}F-FDG PET/CT in a patient with bone metastasis, be aware of the patient's current treatment status, and be mindful of the possibility of a flare phenomenon.
- Non-^{18}F-FDG-avid osteosclerotic bone metastasis lesions may consistently appear as hot uptake lesions on bone scan after treatment, but this may suggest a good prognosis.

Case 18.1

A 78-year-old woman diagnosed with advanced gastric cancer visited our department to evaluate bone metastasis and underwent a bone scan. A diffuse pattern of hot uptake lesions was observed in the thoracic and lumbar spines, both ribs, pelvic bones, and femur on the patient's bone scan, whereas the bilateral kidneys and soft tissue activity were almost nonexistent (Fig. 18.1). This finding is reasonable for superscans, suggesting extensive metastasis.

Case 18.2

A 59-year-old woman diagnosed with left breast cancer underwent periodic bone scans to evaluate bone metastasis. During her bone scan follow-up every 6 months after surgery and chemotherapy, a linear pattern of hot uptake lesion on the left posterior third rib and a faintly hot uptake lesion on the right humeral shaft area were newly noted (Fig. 18.2b). The focal pattern of hot uptakes in the right posterior ninth rib observed on a previous bone scan was more likely to be a benign posttraumatic change than metastasis (Fig. 18.2a). The patient underwent a repeat bone scan after 3 months, and as a result, multiple hot uptake lesions were newly observed in the skull, L2 spine, and both ilium, all of which were likely metastases (Fig. 18.2c). The linear pattern of hot uptake in the left posterior third rib was still observed, indicating a metastatic pattern, but focal hot uptakes in the right anterior seventh and posterior ninth ribs were most likely due to a benign posttraumatic change. Another notable lesion was the right humeral shaft lesion, which showed an increased uptake activity pattern during the follow-up scan. Eventually, this lesion caused a pathologic fracture during chemotherapy and was pathologically confirmed as metastasis by operation. In this case, the linear hot pattern of rib lesions should be suspected as metastasis, and further evaluation should be strongly considered in cancer patients.

Case 18.3

A single hot uptake in the sternum was found in a 39-year-old woman diagnosed with left breast cancer during a periodic follow-up of bone scans to evaluate bone metastasis (Fig. 18.3a). The patient did not have any previous history of trauma; hence, ^{18}F-FDG PET/CT was additionally performed, and hot uptake of ^{18}F-FDG in the sternum (Fig. 18.3b, d and e) was accompanied by an osteolytic lesion on CT image (Fig. 18.3c). Additional metastatic lesions were found in the left supraclavicular lymph node and liver on ^{18}F-FDG PET/CT (Fig. 18.3b). It is known that a hot uptake of the sternum in the bone scan can be a non-specific finding, but in the case of breast cancer, a single metastasis of the sternum should be considered and must be carefully evaluated.

Case 18.4

A 50-year-old woman who was diagnosed with right breast cancer 4 years prior and was undergoing follow-up after mastectomy and chemotherapy was suspected to have bone metastases.

The patient underwent a bone scan, and the bone scan showed focal hot uptakes on the right ischium, upper cervical spine, and C7 spine,

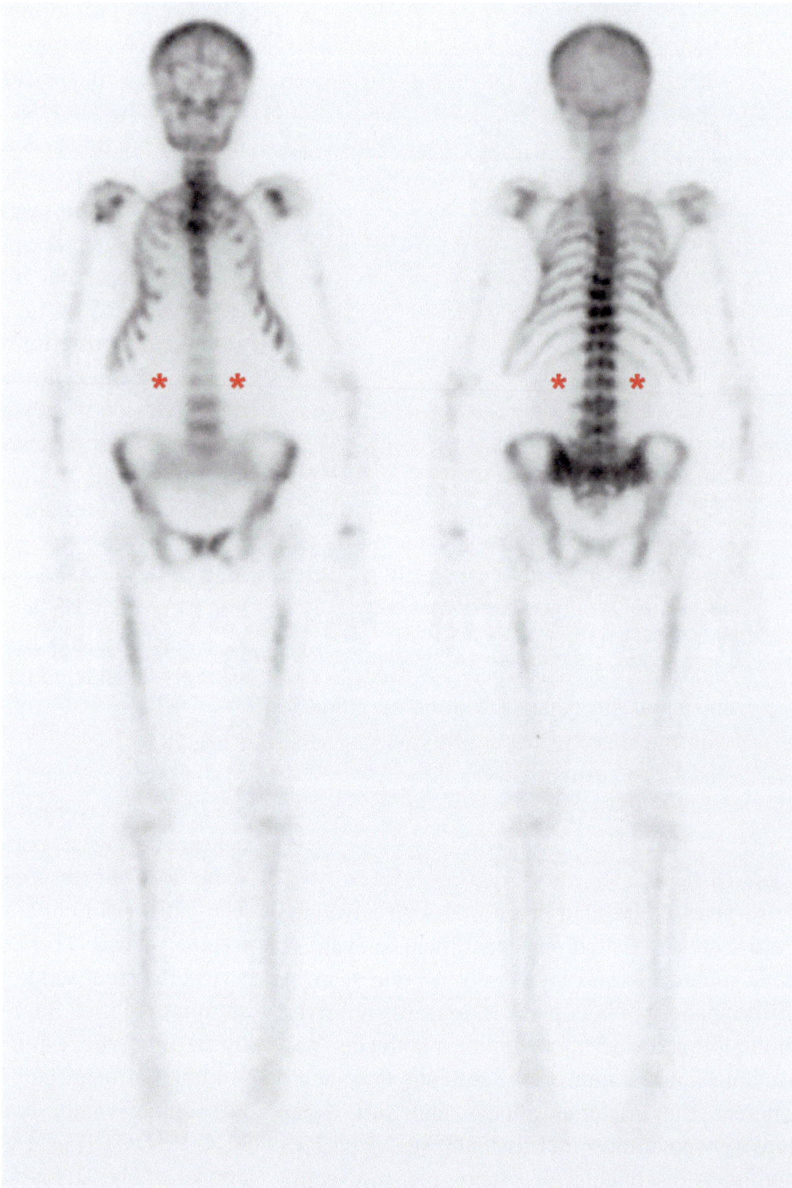

Fig. 18.1 Extensive diffuse hot uptakes were observed in the axial skeleton and femur on bone scan, but neither both kidneys (asterisks) nor soft tissue activity was observed

suggesting a possible metastasis (Fig. 18.4a). For a more detailed evaluation, ^{18}F-NaF PET/CT performed 2 weeks later showed multiple hot uptakes in the left parietal bone; C2, C7, and L1 spine; left acetabulum; and right ischium, all of which were highly suggestive of metastases (Fig. 18.4b). In the body region of the L1 spine, a sclerotic change lesion was also found on CT, and hot uptake was also observed on PET in the same region (Fig. 18.4c–e) which suggested metastasis. In this case, we were able to identify more metastatic lesions on ^{18}F-NaF PET/CT than on a bone scan.

Case 18.5

A 46-year-old woman diagnosed with right breast cancer with bone metastases underwent a bone scan to evaluate bone metastases. At the time of diagnosis of bone metastasis, the patient showed a hot uptake in the lower cervical spine; T7, T9,

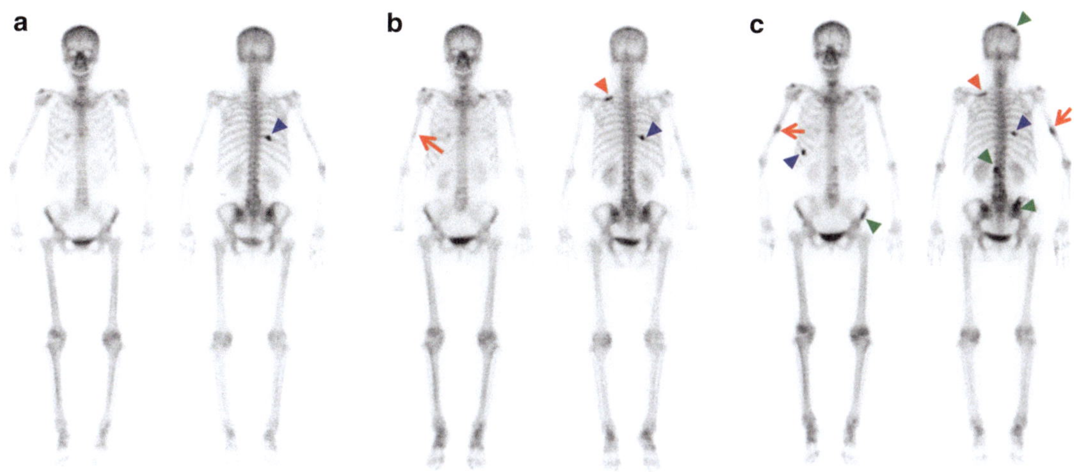

Fig. 18.2 (**a**) The focal hot uptake lesion was observed in the right posterior ninth rib, suggesting posttraumatic change (blue arrowhead). (**b**) On a bone scan performed 6 months later, the hot lesion of the right posterior ninth rib was still seen without significant change (blue arrowhead), and hot uptake lesions were newly appeared on the left posterior third rib (red arrowhead) and the right humeral shaft (arrow). (**c**) New hot uptakes were observed in the skull, L2 spine, and both ilium on a bone scan performed 3 months later (green arrowheads). The linear pattern of hot uptake in the left posterior third rib was still observed (red arrowhead), and focal hot uptakes in the right anterior seventh and posterior ninth ribs (blue arrowheads) were noted. The right humeral shaft lesion showed an increased uptake activity during follow-up (arrows)

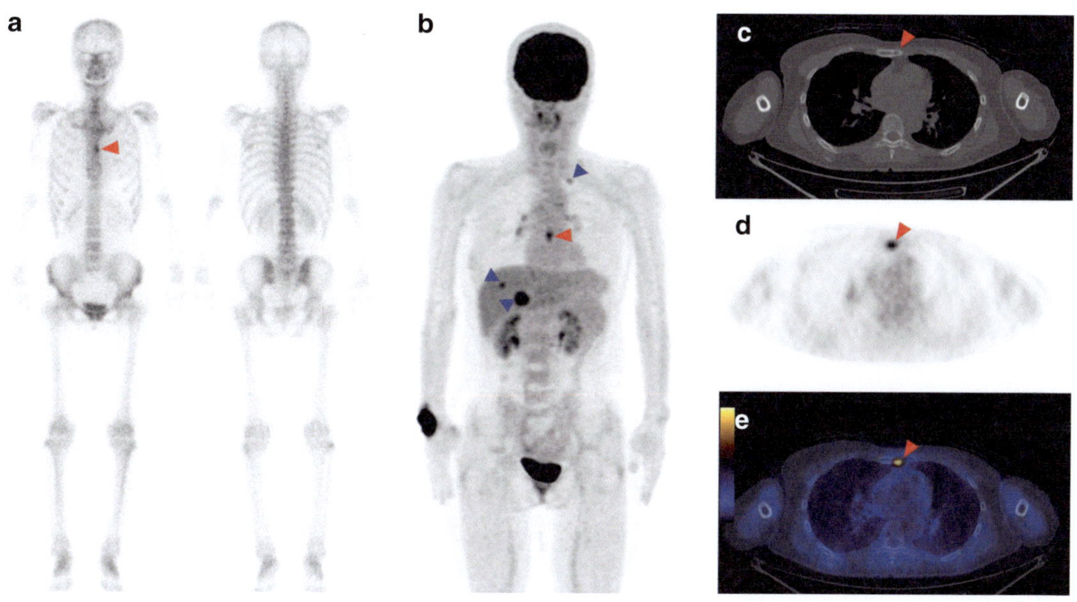

Fig. 18.3 (**a**) A hot uptake lesion is observed in the sternum on the bone scan (red arrowhead). (**b–e**) On ^{18}F-FDG PET/CT, hot uptake with osteolytic lesion was observed in the sternum (red arrowhead in **b** [MIP image], **c** [CT image], **d** [PET image], and **e** [PET fusion with CT]). Also, abnormal hypermetabolic lesions in the left supraclavicular lymph node and liver were noted (blue arrowhead in **b**)

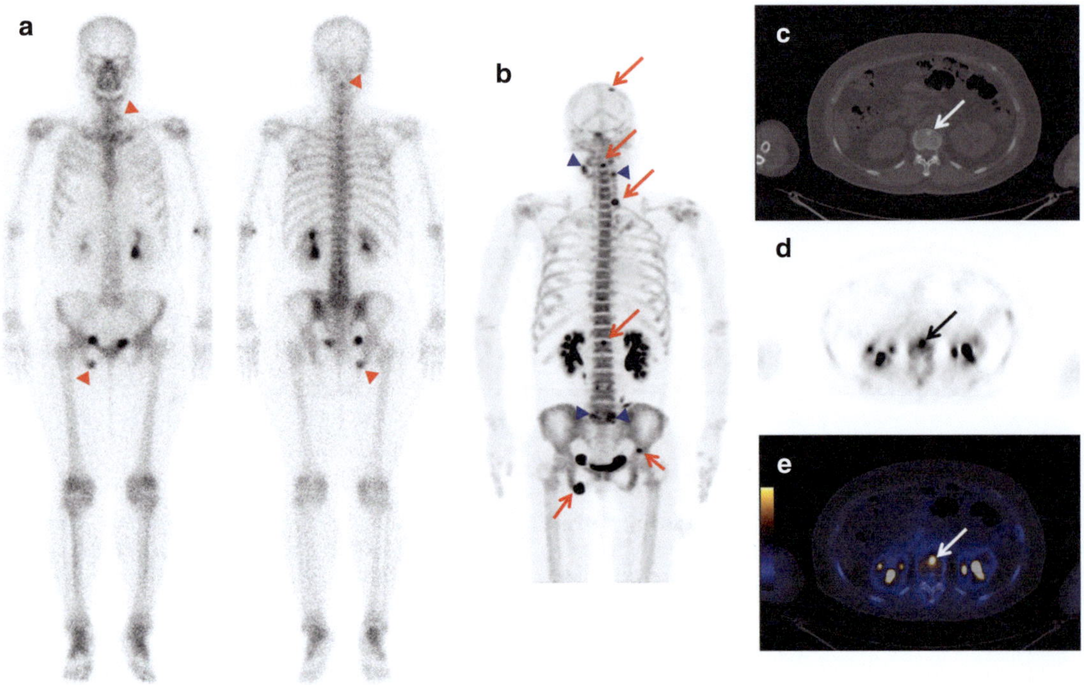

Fig. 18.4 (**a**) Focal hot uptakes were seen on the right ischium, upper cervical spine, and C7 spine in bone scan (red arrowheads). (**b–e**) Multiple hot uptakes were observed in the left parietal bone; C2, C7, and L1 spine; left acetabulum; and right ischium on ^{18}F-NaF PET/CT (arrows in b [maximum intensity projection (MIP) image]). The body of L1 spine lesion showed hot uptake with sclerotic change on the transaxial images (arrows in **c** [CT], **d** [PET], and **f** [PET/CT fusion image]). The hot uptakes observed in the L4 and L5 spine and mandibles were attributed to benign degenerative change and dental problems, respectively (blue arrowheads in **b**)

T10, and T12 spine; left posterior tenth rib; and both ischium on a bone scan (Fig. 18.5a), all of which were metastatic lesions. A follow-up bone scan was performed 3 months after the start of chemotherapy. In most of the lesions seen in the previous image, activity and extent were overall increased, and there were newly appeared hot uptake lesions in the sternum, L5 spine, both ilium, right scapula, and right femoral head (Fig. 18.5b). The patient underwent a bone scan 6 months after the completion of chemotherapy. As a result, hot uptakes of T-spines, left posterior tenth rib, and both ischia still remained, but overall activity and extent decreased compared to before, and other previously seen lesions almost disappeared (Fig. 18.5c). In this patient, a temporary worsening of bone scans performed during chemotherapy is referred to as the flare phenomenon. Since this is a phenomenon that occurs temporarily when bone metastasis lesions respond to chemotherapy, it is necessary to evaluate whether a patient is undergoing treatment when reading a bone scan.

Case 18.6

A 63-year-old woman who underwent mastectomy for left breast cancer visited our department for evaluation of bone metastasis and underwent ^{18}F-FDG PET/CT. On initial ^{18}F-FDG PET/CT in this patient, hot uptake was observed in T5, L2 spine, and right ilium, showing metastasis (Fig. 18.6a). The patient started chemotherapy, and on ^{18}F-FDG PET/CT performed 3 months during chemotherapy, multiple hot uptake lesions were observed in the skull, C-T-L spine, both pelvic bones, ribs, right distal clavicle, and left femur, all of which were metastatic lesions (Fig. 18.6b). Compared with previous images, most of the lesions showed increased activity and extent, and many newly appearing metastatic lesions were also identified. The patient underwent ^{18}F-FDG PET/CT follow-up examination 4 months after the end of chemotherapy, and the ^{18}F-FDG uptake in multiple metastatic bone uptake lesions that had been seen in a previous study was generally reduced, showing improve-

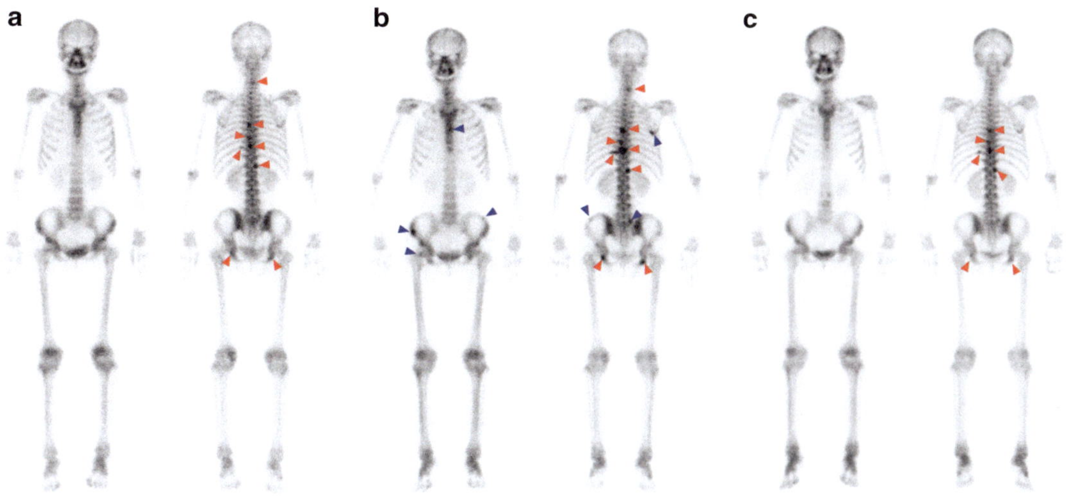

Fig. 18.5 (**a**) Bone scan showed multiple hot uptake lesions in the lower cervical spine; T7, T9, T10, and T12 spine; left posterior tenth rib; and both ischium, suggesting metastasis (red arrowheads). (**b**) A follow-up bone scan during the chemotherapy revealed that activity and extent were overall increased in most of the lesions seen in the previous image (red arrowheads), and metastatic hot uptake lesions in the sternum, L5 spine, both ilium, right scapula, and right femoral head were newly appeared (blue arrowheads). (**c**) Hot uptakes in T-spines, left posterior tenth rib, and both ischia were remained with overall activity and extent decreased than previous image (red arrowheads), and other previously seen lesions disappeared on bone scan after the completion of chemotherapy

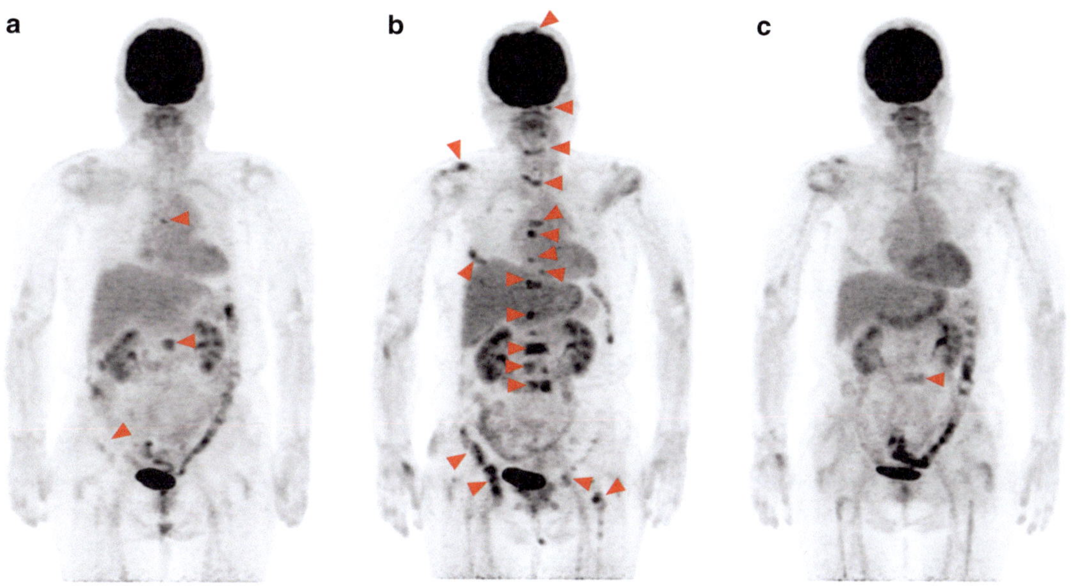

Fig. 18.6 (**a**) Hypermetabolic lesions were noted in T5, L2 spine, and right ilium on initial ^{18}F-FDG PET/CT (arrowheads). (**b**) ^{18}F-FDG PET/CT during chemotherapy revealed multiple hot uptakes in the skull, C-T-L spine, both pelvic bones, ribs, right distal clavicle, and left femur with new lesions, compared to previous image (arrowheads). (**c**) Only mild hypermetabolic lesion in the L2 spine (arrowhead) was remained on ^{18}F-FDG PET/CT after the end of chemotherapy

ment with only remaining mild hypermetabolic lesion in the L2 spine (Fig. 18.6c). This can be interpreted as a flare phenomenon that can appear temporarily aggravated during chemotherapy in patients with bone metastases. The flare phenomenon is mainly observed in bone scans, but as in this case, this phenomenon can also be seen in ^{18}F-FDG PET. It should be noted that there may also be a metabolic flare phenomenon that may appear to be temporarily exacerbated in response to therapy.

Case 18.7

A 70-year-old woman diagnosed with left breast cancer who underwent mastectomy visited our department to evaluate bone metastasis and underwent a bone scan. On a bone scan, hot uptake lesions were observed on the sternum and lower cervical spine (Fig. 18.7a), and MRI was performed for further evaluation. MRI showed signs indicative of metastasis in the sternum and manubrium (Fig. 18.7b), and benign endplate degeneration of cervical spines

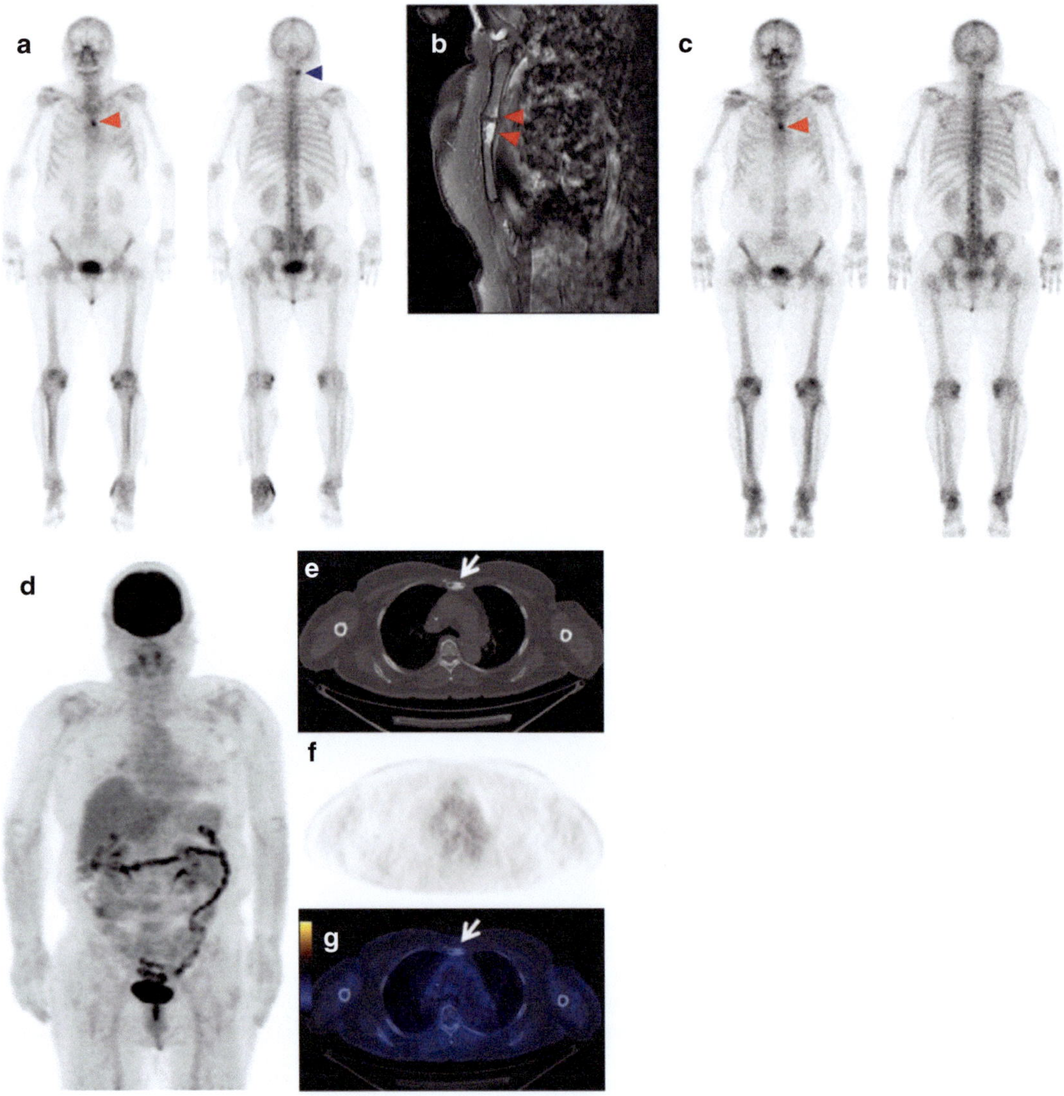

Fig. 18.7 (**a**) Hot uptakes were noted in the sternum (red arrowhead) and lower cervical spine (blue arrowhead) on bone scan. (**b**) MRI showed signs indicative of metastasis in the sternum and manubrium (red arrowheads). (**c**) A hot uptake lesion in the sternum was still observed on bone scan performed after the completion of chemotherapy (red arrowhead). (**d**) ^{18}F-FDG PET/CT showed osteosclerotic lesions in the sternum on CT scan (arrow in **e** and **g**) without significant ^{18}F-FDG activity (**d** and **f**)

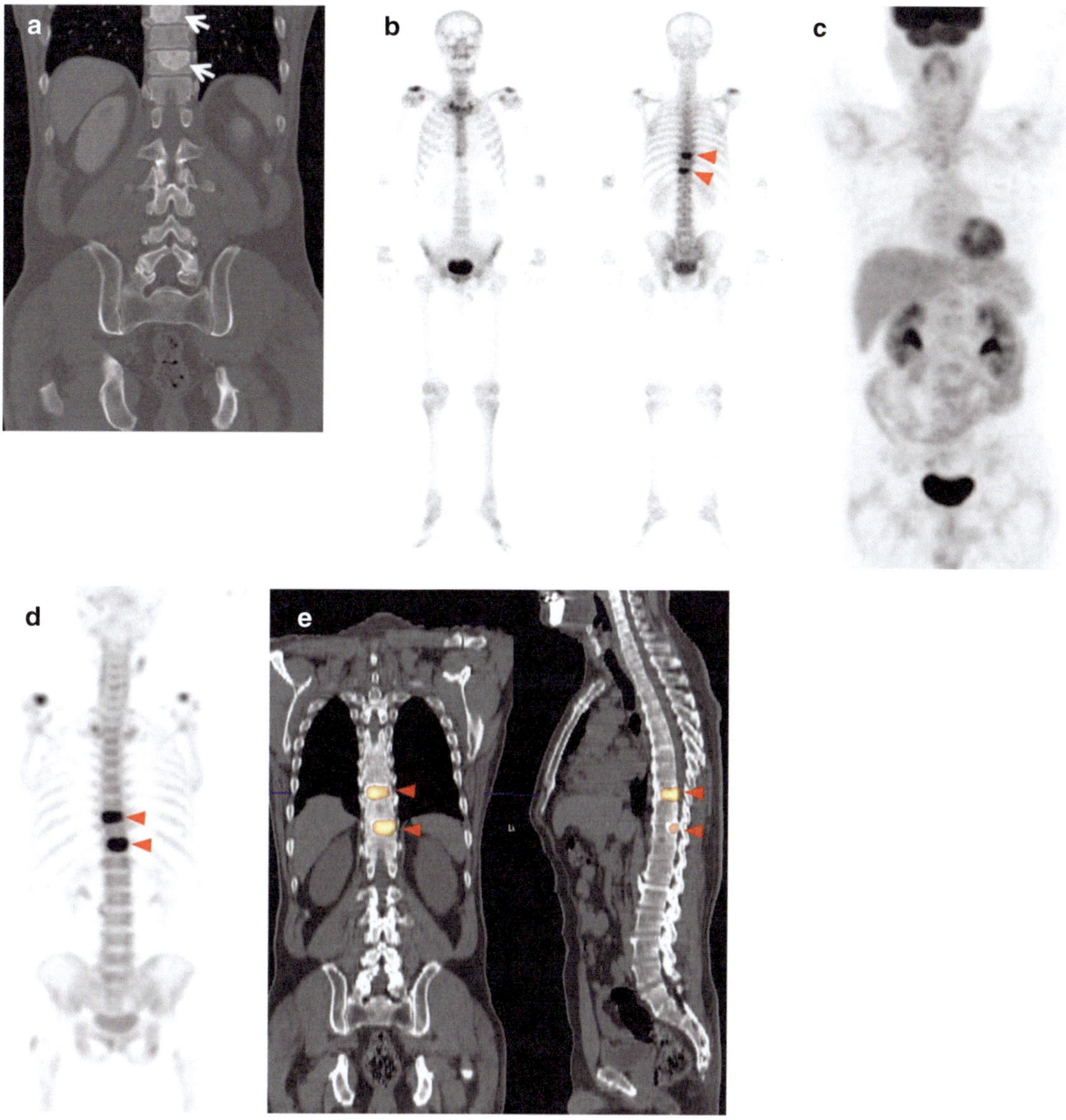

Fig. 18.8 (**a**) There were osteosclerotic lesions in T9 and T11 spines on CT image (arrows). (**b**) Intensely hot uptake lesions were observed in T9 and T11 spines on bone scan (arrowheads). (**c**) There were no abnormal findings on ^{18}F-FDG PET/CT. (**d** and **e**) ^{18}F-NaF PET/CT revealed intense hot uptakes in T9 and T11 spines (arrowheads in **d** [MIP image] and **e** [PET/CT fusion images])

was observed (image not shown). The patient underwent chemotherapy, and a hot uptake lesion of the sternum still remained on the bone scan performed 7 months after the end of the chemotherapy (Fig. 18.7c), but ^{18}F-FDG PET/CT performed concurrently showed osteosclerotic lesions in the sternum on CT scan without significant ^{18}F-FDG activity (Fig. 18.7d–g). As such, in the non-^{18}F-FDG-avid osteosclerotic bone lesions, which showed a hot uptake only in the bone scan, it can be considered that the viability of metastatic lesions is lost in response to chemotherapy, which can suggest a good prognosis.

Case 18.8

Osteosclerotic lesions were found on the T9 and T11 spines on a bone CT (Fig. 18.8a) of a 50-year-old male patient who underwent surgery 3 months ago for sigmoid colon cancer, and nuclear medicine examinations were performed for further evaluation of metastasis.

In the patient's bone scan, intense hot uptakes were observed on the T9 and T11 spines, which are the same sites as the lesions seen on CT, suggesting metastasis (Fig. 18.8b). The patient also underwent ^{18}F-FDG PET/CT, and no abnormal findings were accompanied (Fig. 18.8c). Additional bone PET/CT using ^{18}F-NaF showed intense hot uptakes in the T9 and T11 spines, which was consistent with the bone scan findings (Fig. 18.8d and e). In this case, we showed that osteosclerotic metastasis is indicated by hot uptake on bone scan or ^{18}F-NaF PET, but accumulation of ^{18}F-FDG may be absent.

References

1. Krishnamurthy GT, Tubis M, Hiss J, Blahd WH. Distribution pattern of metastatic bone disease. A need for total body skeletal image. JAMA. 1977;237(23):2504–6.
2. Peinado H, Zhang H, Matei IR, Costa-Silva B, Hoshino A, Rodrigues G, et al. Pre-metastatic niches: organ-specific homes for metastases. Nat Rev Cancer. 2017;17(5):302–17. https://doi.org/10.1038/nrc.2017.6.
3. Fidler IJ. The pathogenesis of cancer metastasis: the 'seed and soil' hypothesis revisited. Nat Rev Cancer. 2003;3(6):453–8. https://doi.org/10.1038/nrc1098.
4. Fornetti J, Welm AL, Stewart SA. Understanding the bone in cancer metastasis. J Bone Miner Res. 2018;33(12):2099–113. https://doi.org/10.1002/jbmr.3618.
5. Coleman RE, Croucher PI, Padhani AR, Clezardin P, Chow E, Fallon M, et al. Bone metastases. Nat Rev Dis Primers. 2020;6(1):83. https://doi.org/10.1038/s41572-020-00216-3.
6. Macedo F, Ladeira K, Pinho F, Saraiva N, Bonito N, Pinto L, et al. Bone metastases: an overview. Oncol Rev. 2017;11(1):321. https://doi.org/10.4081/oncol.2017.321.
7. Min JW, Um SW, Yim JJ, Yoo CG, Han SK, Shim YS, et al. The role of whole-body FDG PET/CT, Tc 99m MDP bone scintigraphy, and serum alkaline phosphatase in detecting bone metastasis in patients with newly diagnosed lung cancer. J Korean Med Sci. 2009;24(2):275–80. https://doi.org/10.3346/jkms.2009.24.2.275.
8. Bastawrous S, Bhargava P, Behnia F, Djang DS, Haseley DR. Newer PET application with an old tracer: role of 18F-NaF skeletal PET/CT in oncologic practice. Radiographics. 2014;34(5):1295–316. https://doi.org/10.1148/rg.345130061.
9. Chang CY, Gill CM, Joseph Simeone F, Taneja AK, Huang AJ, Torriani M, et al. Comparison of the diagnostic accuracy of 99 m-Tc-MDP bone scintigraphy and 18 F-FDG PET/CT for the detection of skeletal metastases. Acta Radiol. 2016;57(1):58–65. https://doi.org/10.1177/0284185114564438.
10. Uchida K, Nakajima H, Miyazaki T, Tsuchida T, Hirai T, Sugita D, et al. (18)F-FDG PET/CT for diagnosis of osteosclerotic and osteolytic vertebral metastatic lesions: comparison with bone scintigraphy. Asian Spine J. 2013;7(2):96–103. https://doi.org/10.4184/asj.2013.7.2.96.
11. Park S, Yoon JK, Jin Lee S, Kang SY, Yim H, An YS. Prognostic utility of FDG PET/CT and bone scintigraphy in breast cancer patients with bone-only metastasis. Medicine (Baltimore). 2017;96(50):e8985. https://doi.org/10.1097/MD.0000000000008985.
12. Cook GJ, Venkitaraman R, Sohaib AS, Lewington VJ, Chua SC, Huddart RA, et al. The diagnostic utility of the flare phenomenon on bone scintigraphy in staging prostate cancer. Eur J Nucl Med Mol Imaging. 2011;38(1):7–13. https://doi.org/10.1007/s00259-010-1576-0.
13. Balasubramanian Harisankar CN, Preethi R, John J. Metabolic flare phenomenon on 18 fluoride-fluorodeoxy glucose positron emission tomography-computed tomography scans in a patient with bilateral breast cancer treated with second-line chemotherapy and bevacizumab. Indian J Nucl Med. 2015;30(2):145–7. https://doi.org/10.4103/0972-3919.152978.

Marrow Replacement Disorders 19

Joo Hyun O and Ie Ryung Yoo

Abstract

Disorders of the plasma cells and lymphoid progenitor cells will involve the bone marrow as well as lymphoid tissues. PET/CT utilizing ^{18}F-fluorodeoxyglucose (FDG) is suitable for detection of both intramedullary and extramedullary diseases due to the capability of the FDG PET/CT to survey the whole body and the high FDG uptake demonstrated by most of the aggressive tumors.

Keywords

Bone marrow · Multiple myeloma
Lymphoma · Leukemia

19.1 Plasma Cell Disorders (Multiple Myeloma)

19.1.1 Clinical Findings

Multiple myeloma (MM) is a proliferative disorder of cytogenetically heterogeneous clonal plasma cells characterized by the autonomous proliferation of monoclonal plasma cells in the bone marrow (BM), leading to the overproduction of the intact immunoglobulin molecule M-protein or immunoglobulin free light chains kappa or lambda [1–3]. MM is the second most common hematological malignancy, rare before the age of 40, but with increasing incidence with age. There is a slight male predominance [3]. In majority of the MM cases, monoclonal gammopathy of undetermined significance (MGUS) or smoldering multiple myeloma (SMM) precedes. MGUS and SMM are not associated with end-organ damage. On the other hand, overt MM manifests as hypercalcemia, renal failure, anemia, or bone lesions known as the CRAB features [4–6]. During the past decade, new biologic drugs were developed, and more effective multidrug combinations were applied, and these remarkable advances have led to improved prognosis for the patients [7].

19.1.2 Image Findings

Bone involvement has very important clinical significance in MM, since bone damage is the critical cause of impaired quality of life, morbidity, and mortality [8]. For such reason, the role of imaging for detection of bone disease in MM is clinically important. The International Myeloma Working Group (IMWG) diagnostic criteria from 2014 states that more than one focal lesion on magnetic resonance imaging (MRI) and more

J. H. O · I. R. Yoo (✉)
Department of Nuclear Medicine, Seoul St. Mary's Hospital, The Catholic University of Korea, College of Medicine, Seoul, Republic of Korea
e-mail: ojoohyun@songeui.ac.kr; iryoo@catholic.ac.kr

S.-O. Yang et al. (eds.), *Atlas of Nuclear Medicine in Musculoskeletal System*,
https://doi.org/10.1007/978-981-19-2677-8_19

than one osteolytic lesion on computed tomography (CT) scan meet the criteria for bone damage requiring treatment; CT here means either the whole-body CT (WBCT) or the CT portion of the positron emission tomography (PET)/CT [2].

Pre-therapy imaging has traditionally included whole-body X-ray (WBXR) and WBCT. Typical finding is punched-out osteolytic lesion without sclerotic margin. WBCT is superior to the WBXR for assessing risk of fracture or lesion characterization but does have higher radiation exposure. That the osseous lytic lesions persist over time is the limitation of both modalities [9–11].

MRI is far superior for assessing the extent of bone marrow disease compared to X-ray and CT. Typical finding is hypointensity on T1-weighted image and slightly hyperintense signal on T2 sequence. Fat suppression sequence is utilized to overcome the high signal intensity of the normal bone marrow [11, 12]. For diffuse type of MM, MRI can be the superior choice of modality compared to PET, but the persistent signal change is a limitation for use in response assessment [13–15]. With the more recent use of diffusion-weighted imaging (DWI), better detection of diffuse infiltration of the bone marrow and differentiation of active and treated bone marrow lesions are feasible [16].

PET/CT utilizing ^{18}F-fluorodeoxyglucose (FDG) is suitable for detection of both intramedullary and extramedullary diseases due to the capability of the FDG PET/CT to survey the whole body and the fusion of both the functional and anatomical imaging modalities. FDG PET/CT can be valuable in the assessment of disease burden and distinguishing metabolically active and inactive lesions [4, 13] (Case 19.1). The pooled sensitivity of FDG PET/CT for detecting BM involvement in MM is reported as 61% and 91% and the pooled specificity 69% and 94% [17, 18]. The sensitivity and specificity for detecting extramedullary disease are reported to be 96% and 78%, respectively [17]. The FDG uptake in MM may be focal, multifocal, or diffuse in pattern, and abnormality needn't always be present in the corresponding CT images. The sensitivity can be lower for diffuse pattern, and differentiation from reactive BM hyperplasia can be problematic. The pitfalls of FDG PET/CT include false-positive results due to fracture, bone remodeling, BM biopsy or postoperative changes, red marrow hyperplasia/expansion, or inflammation/infection. Lesions 5 mm or less in size, especially when located in the skull, diffuse disease involvement, and non-FDG-avid plasma cell may be causes of false-negative findings [4, 19]. Mesguich et al. recommended different FDG PET/CT assessment criteria for pre-treatment and post-treatment cases [4]. The modified criteria adapted by IMWG compared focal FDG uptake to the physiologic bone marrow or liver uptake prior to treatment, but considered only lesions showing uptake higher than the liver to be significant post-treatment. Diffuse BM uptake pattern should be considered significant when the intensity is higher than the liver uptake and requires correlation with MRI findings [19] (Case 19.2). Incorporation of FDG PET/CT is recommended for routine diagnostic work-up of MM. Especially when the WBXR is negative and whole-body MRI is unavailable, FDG PET/CT is useful for distinguishing active MM from SMM.

Solitary plasmacytoma may manifest as single lytic bone lesion or soft tissue mass and can be diagnosed only when systemic BM plasma cell infiltration (<10%) and end-organ damage are absent [20] (Case 19.3). When solitary plasmacytoma is suspected, functional imaging technique is recommended for accurate assessment of tumor extent and exclusion of additional occult lesions. Particularly when whole-body MRI is unavailable, FDG PET/CT has a clear role [19, 21]. In addition, FDG PET/CT is a useful tool for predicting the prognosis, early assessment of therapeutic response, and detection of minimal residual disease.

Case 19.1

A 63-year-old man was diagnosed with relapsed MM, with multifocal hypermetabolic intramedullary and extramedullary lesions. FDG PET/CT

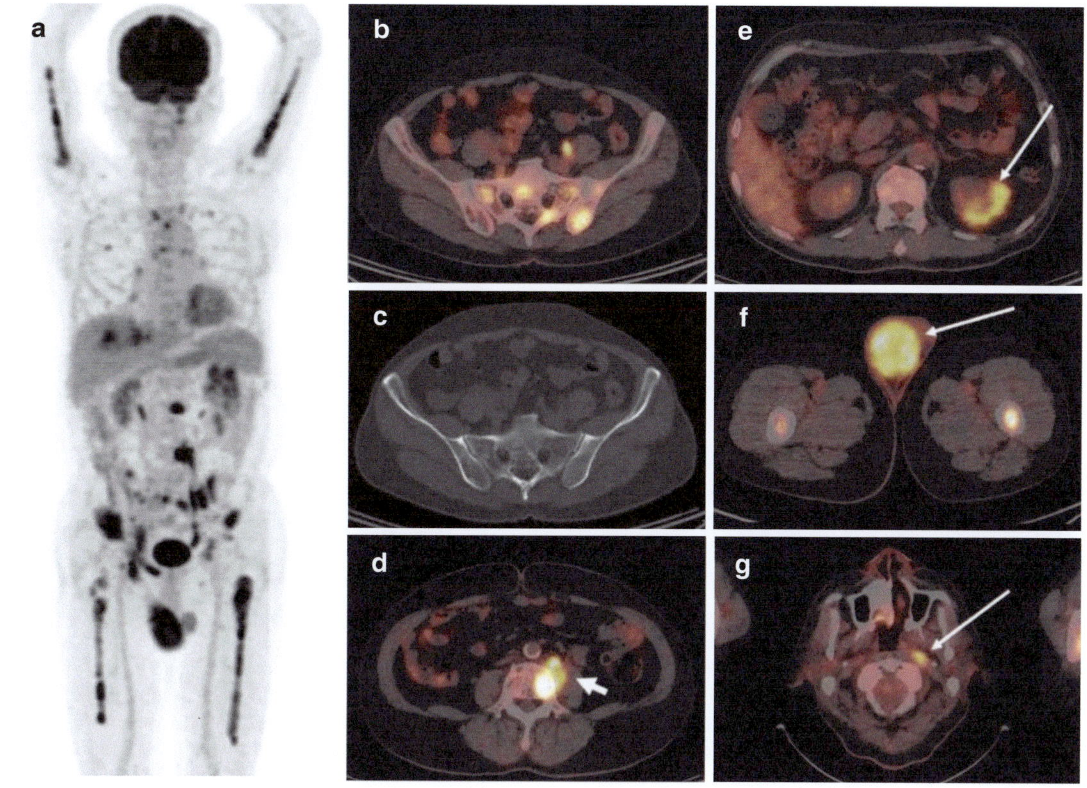

Fig. 19.1 Maximum intensity projection (MIP) image of FDG PET/CT (**a**) showed multifocal hypermetabolic intramedullary and extramedullary lesions. In axial fusion PET/CT (**b**) and CT (**c**) images, multifocal hypermetabolic lesions were noted in sacrum and pelvic bones without corresponding CT abnormality. Paramedullary extension from L4 vertebral lesion (short arrow) was seen on axial fusion PET/CT image (**d**). Axial fusion PET/CT images (**e–g**) showed multifocal extramedullary disease in left perinephric area, right scrotal sac, and LN of left retropharyngeal region (arrows)

can accurately assess the extent of intramedullary lesions as well as extramedullary lesions in unusual locations that are difficult to detect by anatomical imaging (Fig. 19.1).

Case 19.2
A 61-year-old man presented with acute renal injury and hypercalcemia. Following BM biopsy, initial work-up for MM was performed (Fig. 19.2).

Case 19.3
A 63-year-old man diagnosed with solitary plasmacytoma. Because whole-body MRI is often not available in daily practice, FDG PET/CT is used to confirm the diagnosis of solitary plasmacytoma with advantage of whole-body survey (Fig. 19.3).

19.2 Lymphoma and Leukemia

19.2.1 Clinical Findings

According to the revised World Health Organization classification of neoplasm of the hematopoietic and lymphoid tissues, lymphoma can be classified into more than 90 subtypes depending firstly on the cell origin—mature B cells, T cells, and natural killer cells [22]. The most common aggressive lymphoma worldwide is diffuse large B cell lymphoma (DLBCL), and bone marrow involvement is seen in up to 11%–25% of DLBCL cases [23, 24]. With bone involvement, the lymphoma stage becomes IV, the international prognostic index (counting toward number of involved extra-nodal sites)

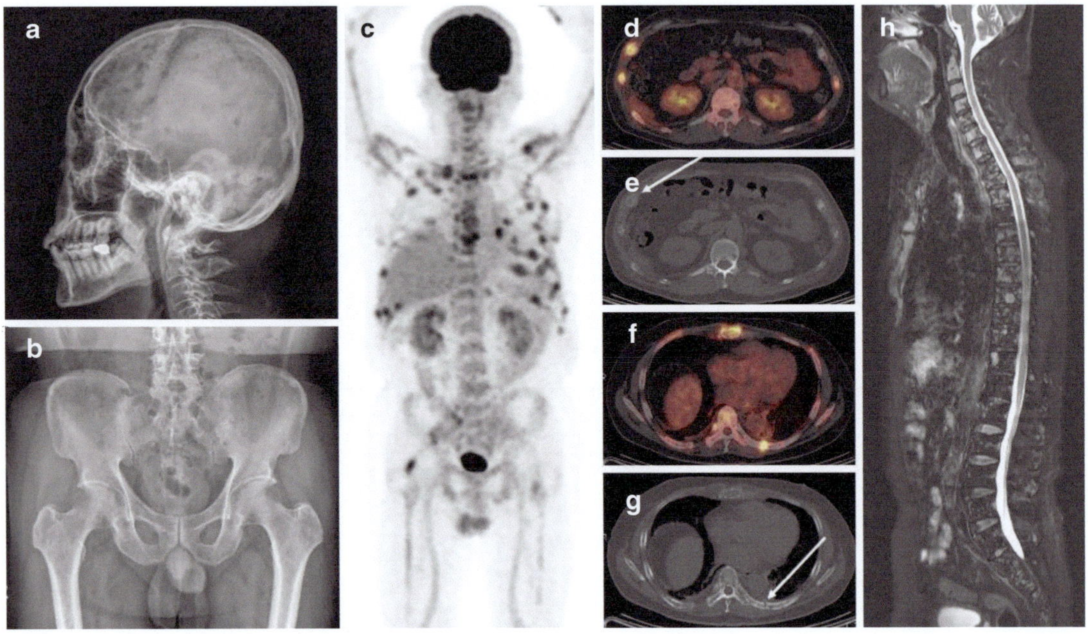

Fig. 19.2 Skull lateral (**a**) and pelvis AP (**b**) radiographs showed multiple small osteolytic lesions without sclerotic rim. FDG PET/CT MIP (**c**) image shows diffuse bone marrow activity slightly more intense than the liver uptake. Multiple focal FDG uptake lesions are present in the rib cage, sternum, and right clavicle, which are mostly accompanied by fracture findings in the CT portion (arrows) (**d–g**). There were diffuse and focal BM lesions on fat-saturated T2-weighted whole spine sagittal MRI (**h**)

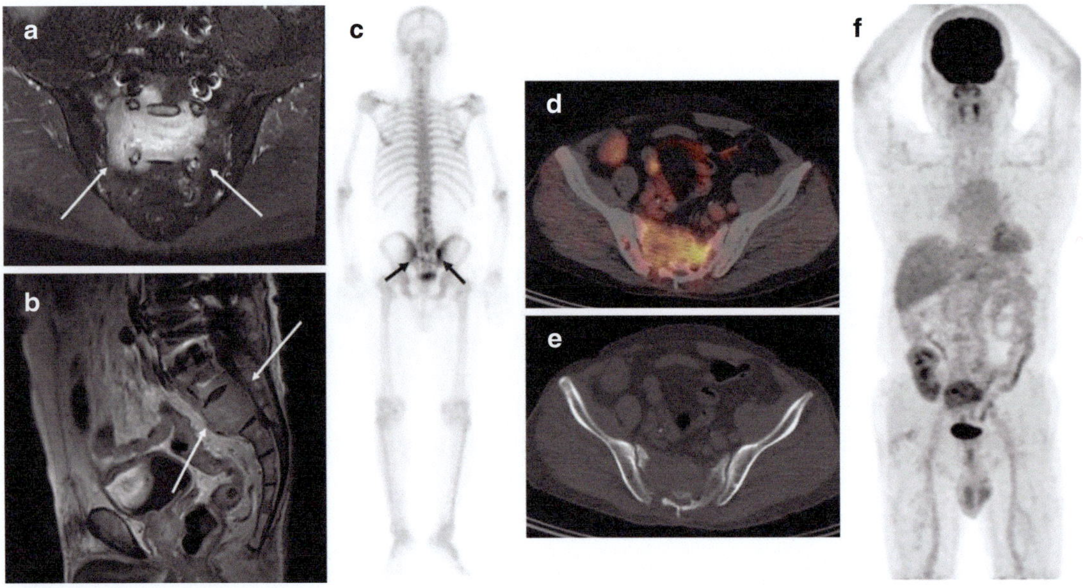

Fig. 19.3 MRI (**a**, **b**) showed large mass with T2 high and T1 intermediate signal intensity in sacrum (arrows). On posterior view of whole-body bone scintigraphy with ^{99m}Tc-HDP (**c**), photon defect area with rim activity was noted in sacrum (short arrows). Axial fusion FDG PET/CT (**d**) and CT (**e**) images showed large osteolytic lesion with intense heterogeneous FDG uptake and paramedullary extension. MIP image (**f**) of PET/CT showed no evidence of other intramedullary and extramedullary lesion nor diffusely increased marrow activity

score increases, and worse prognosis and outcome are expected. Leukemia is by definition malignancy with extensive involvement of the bone marrow, and bone marrow biopsy becomes essential for accurate diagnosis and subtype classification.

Clinically, the gold standard for diagnosis of bone marrow involvement has been biopsy obtained from posterior iliac crest. However, it is now widely known that bone marrow biopsy from iliac bone alone can present false-negative results. Conversely, FDG PET/CT can be negative for abnormal bone uptake, while the bone marrow biopsy is positive. Such discordant findings between the two tests are not uncommon, and iliac bone marrow biopsy alone cannot fully represent the wide spectrum of tumor behavior [25–27]. In cases with fibrosis of the bone marrow, aspiration biopsy may not be feasible, and bone biopsy could be required.

19.2.2 Image Findings

Depending on the subtype of lymphoma and leukemia, FDG uptake can vary from imperceptible to remarkably intense. Most of the aggressive forms demonstrate high FDG avidity. There is no objective FDG uptake threshold or imaging criteria for determining bone involvement of lymphoma or leukemia. Most readers would consider intense discrete FDG uptake in the bones to be positive for malignant involvement, in the absence of obvious signs of benign findings such as fracture or post-surgical remodeling (Case 19.4). Leukemia can often appear as diffuse intense FDG activity throughout the axial and appendicular skeleton before treatment, similar to the bone marrow uptake following growth stimulating factor, or multiple focal FDG uptake areas resembling bone metastases (Case 19.5). Lymphoma and leukemia with known bone marrow involvement can also show FDG uptake similar to the liver or even lower. After chemotherapy, it becomes difficult to distinguish regressed but viable lymphoma/leukemia involvement of the bones from benign bone marrow hyperplasia.

It should be noted that bone involvement is not limited to the axial skeleton or long bones. Lymphoma and leukemia can be present in any bone, from skull to phalanges of feet.

The radiology findings could be nonspecific and may be normal, lytic, sclerotic, or mixed in the plain X-ray and CT [28]. Though MRI is not usually performed for the purpose of detection of lymphoma or leukemia involving the bones, the high resolution of MRI images allows more accurate assessment of extent of disease involvement in structures such as spinal cord and head and neck region. Involved bone marrow may show low signal intensity on T1 and high signal on T2 [29].

Case 19.4

A young man with acute lymphocytic leukemia initially achieved complete remission following chemotherapy and allogeneic bone marrow transplant. However, 2 years after the transplant, the patient started experiencing pain in the right hip. The radiating pain without sensory change worsened over a couple of weeks, and the patient visited the emergency room due to severe sharp pain that kept him awake at night. The patient denied any recent fall or excessive exercise. The subsequent image findings were consistent with leukemic involvement in the right femur. Following therapy with anti-CD22 monoclonal antibody and radiotherapy, the patient is in remission (Fig. 19.4).

Case 19.5

A 49-year-old man who was initially diagnosed with nodal marginal zone lymphoma 2 years ago received chemotherapy and reached complete remission. During surveillance period, palpable nodes were discovered in the axillary area, and restaging work-up was performed. Biopsy from the liver revealed diffuse large B cell lymphoma, activated B-cell type (Fig. 19.5).

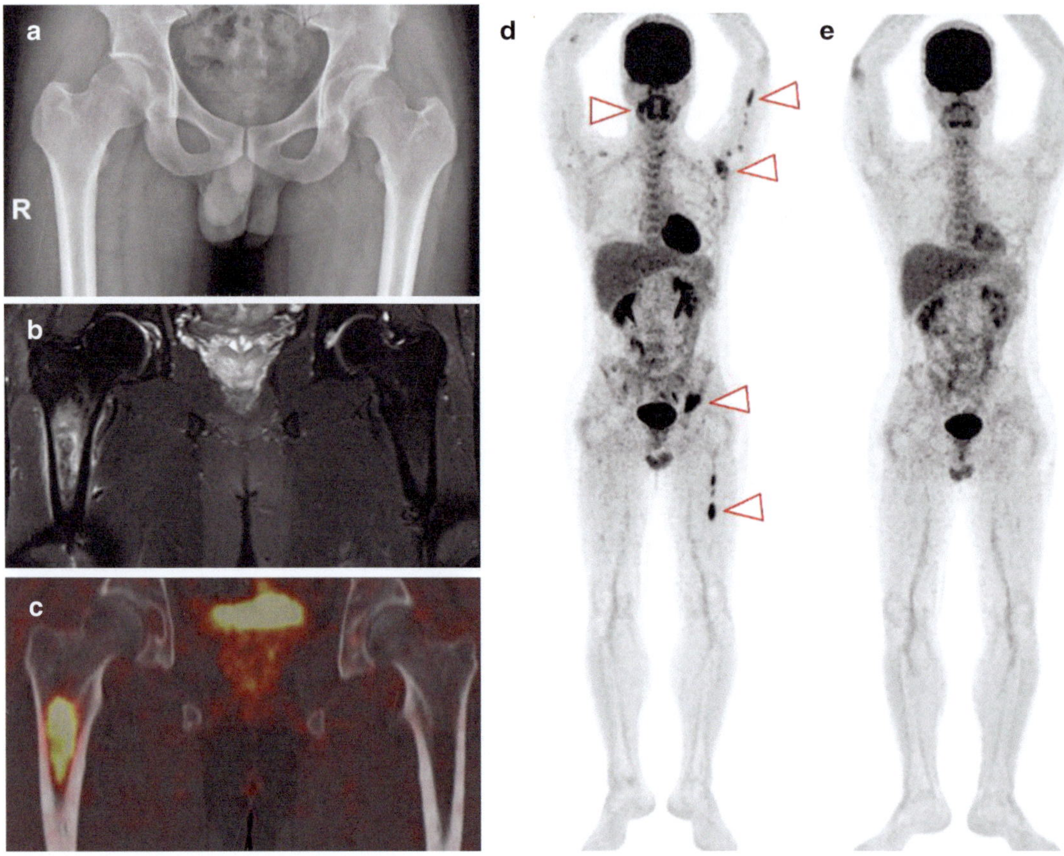

Fig. 19.4 No abnormal findings were noted to account for the pain in the X-ray of the hips (**a**). Coronal view MRI of the hips showed intramedullary bone lesion in right proximal femur with circumferential periosteal reaction consistent with leukemic infiltration (**b**). Fusion PET/CT showed intense FDG uptake in the corresponding femoral lesion (**c**). After radiotherapy the right femur lesion shows diminished FDG uptake, but focal FDG uptakes newly developed in multiple bones including right mandible, left humerus, left scapula, left iliac bone, and left femur (**d**, arrowheads). FDG PET/CT performed after inotuzumab and radiotherapy shows markedly diminished FDG uptakes in multiple bone sites (**e**)

Case 19.6

A 45-year-old patient started experiencing frequent gum bleeding and fatigue since 1 month ago. The patient also noticed black and blue marks more often throughout the body. The skin of lower leg showed swelling and redness suggestive of cellulitis. Initial MRI findings were suggestive of cellulitis and myositis with abscess. Biopsy confirmed myeloid sarcoma from underlying acute myeloid leukemia (Fig. 19.6).

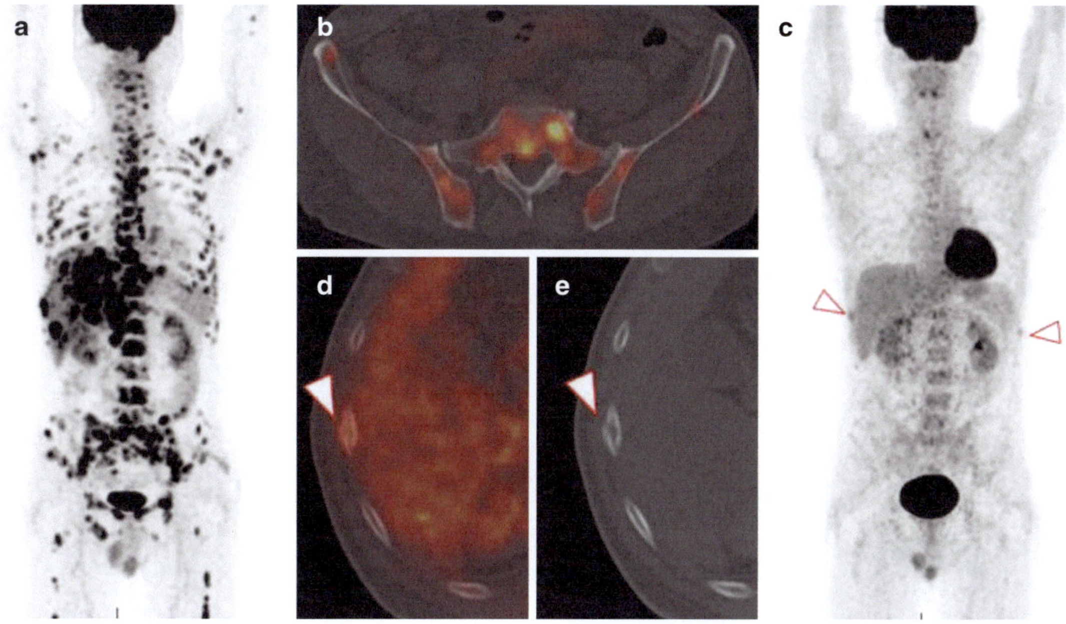

Fig. 19.5 There are multiple focal FDG uptakes throughout the axial and appendicular skeleton, as well as the liver and the nodal stations in the MIP image (**a**). The FDG uptake pattern is heterogeneous in the iliac bones (**b**), and depending on the position of the needle, the biopsy could yield false-negative result, as in this patient. Follow-up FDG PET/CT performed after chemotherapy shows good response, without discrete FDG uptake in the interim MIP image (**c**). There are mild FDG uptakes in the ribs in the interim PET/CT image (arrowheads in **c**, **d**), corresponding to fracture line in the CT portion (**e**)

Teaching Points

- The bone marrow is involved in myeloid and lymphoid neoplasms.
- CT or MRI is often used for preliminary assessment of bone lesions, but FDG PET/CT has the advantage of allowing assessment of multiple bones.
- FDG PET/CT shows high sensitivity for detection of extramedullary lesions.
- FDG PET/CT is a valuable tool for both newly diagnosed and relapsed multiple myeloma.
- FDG PET/CT is the preferred modality for monitoring response to therapy in multiple myeloma patients.
- In patients with suspected solitary plasmacytoma, FDG PET/CT is indispensable for confirming the diagnosis, if whole-body MRI is unavailable.
- FDG PET/CT has complimentary role to bone marrow biopsy and is a useful tool for staging, monitoring response to therapy, and restaging in lymphoma/leukemia.

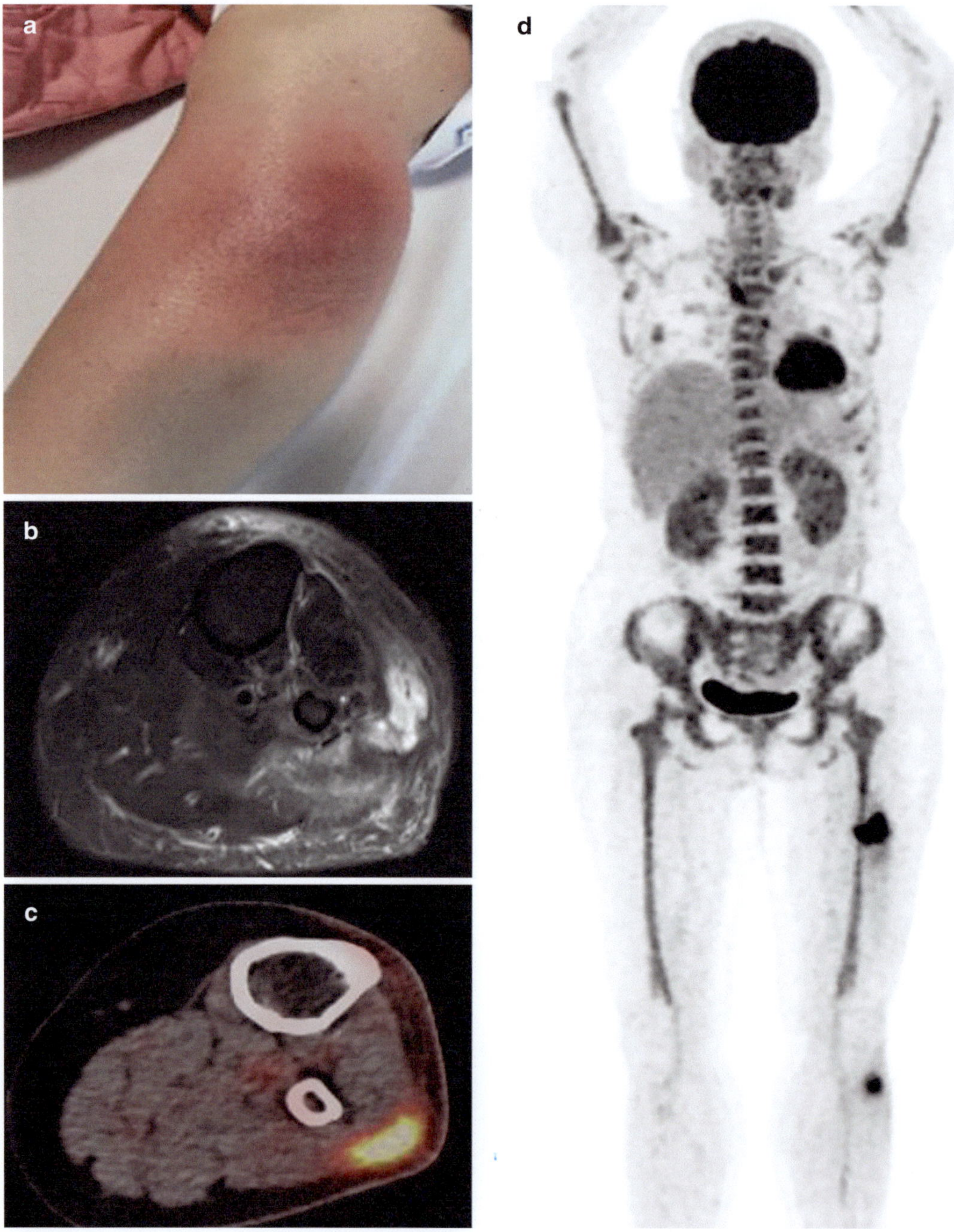

Fig. 19.6 Photograph of lower leg shows erythema and purpura at lower level (**a**). Diffuse reticular thickening with enhancement of subcutaneous layer, patchy edema with enhancement of peroneal longus and soleus muscles, and peripherally enhancing nodular lesion were suggestive of cellulitis and myositis with abscess on MRI (**b**). Biopsy confirmed myeloid sarcoma in left lower leg, which shows intense FDG uptake even after antibiotics therapy (**c**). The MIP images show additional extramedullary involvement in the muscles of left thigh and both lungs, as well as diffuse bone marrow involvement (**d**)

References

1. Palumbo A, Anderson K. Multiple myeloma. N Engl J Med. 2011;364:1046–60.
2. Rajkumar SV, Dimopoulos MA, Palumbo A, Blade J, Merlini G, Mateos MV, et al. International Myeloma Working Group updated criteria for the diagnosis of multiple myeloma. Lacet Oncol. 2014;15:e538–48.
3. Kazandjian D. Multiple myeloma epidemiology and survival, a unique malignancy. Semin Oncol. 2016;43(6):676–81.
4. Mesguich C, Fardanesh R, Tanenbaum L, Chari A, Jagannath S, Kostakoglu L. State of the art imaging of multiple myeloma: comparative review of FDG PET/CT imaging in various clinical settings. Eur J Radiol. 2014;83:2203–23.
5. Rajkumar SV, Landgren O, Mateos MV. Smoldering multiple myeloma. Blood. 2015;125:3069–75.
6. Landgren O, Kyle RA, Pfeiffer RM, Katzmann JA, Caporaso NE, Hayes RB, et al. Monoclonal gammopathy of undetermined significance (MGUS) consistently precedes multiple myeloma: a prospective study. Blood. 2009;113:5412–7.
7. Kumar S, Paiva B, Anderson KC, Durie B, Landgren B, Moreau P, et al. International Myeloma Working Group consensus criteria for response and minimal residual disease assessment in multiple myeloma. Lancet Oncol. 2016;17:e328–46.
8. Terpos E, Dimorpoulos MA. Myeloma bone disease: pathophysiology and management. Ann Oncol. 2005;16:1223–31.
9. Dimopoulos M, Terpos E, Comenzo RL, Tosi P, Beksac M, Sezer O, et al. International myeloma working group consensus statement and guidelines regarding the current role of imaging techniques in the diagnosis and monitoring of multiple myeloma. Leukemia. 2009;23(9):1545–56.
10. Baur MA, Buhmann S, Becker C, Schoenberg SO, Lang N, Barkl R, et al. Whole-body MRI versus whole-body MDCT for staging of multiple myeloma. Am J Roentgenol. 2008;190(4):1097–104.
11. Zamagni E, Tacchetti, Michele C. Imaging in multiple myeloma: how? When? Blood. 2019;133:644–51.
12. Mosebach J, Thierjung H, Schlemmer HP, Stefan D. Multiple myeloma guidelines and their recent updates: implications for imaging. Rofo. 2019;191:998–1009.
13. Van Lammeren-Venema D, Regelink JC, Riphagen II, Zweegman S, Hoekstra OS, Zijlstra JM. ^{18}F-fluorodeoxyglucose positron emission tomography in assessment of myeloma-related bone disease: a systemic review. Cancer. 2012;118:1971–1981.
14. Regelink JC, Minnema MC, Terpos E, Kamphuis MH, Raijmakers PG, Pieters-van den Bos IC, et al. Comparison of modern and conventional imaging techniques in establishing multiple myeloma-related bone disease: a systematic review. Br J Haematol. 2013;162:50–61.
15. Caers J, Withofs N, Hillengass J, Simoni P, Zamagni E, Hustinx R, et al. The role of positron emission tomography-computed tomography and magnetic resonance imaging in diagnosis and follow up of multiple myeloma. Haematologica. 2014;99:629–37.
16. Hameed M, Sandhu A, Soneji N, Amiras D, Rockall A, Messiou C, et al. Pictorial review of whole body MRI in myeloma: emphasis on diffusion-weighted imaging. Br J Radiol. 2020;93:20200312. Epub
17. Lu YY, Chen JH, Lin WY, Liang JA, Wang HY, Tsai SC, et al. FDG PET or PET/CT for detecting intramedullary and extramedullary lesions in multiple myeloma: a systematic review and meta-analysis. Clin Nucl Med. 2012;37(9):833–7.
18. Weng WW, Dong MJ, Zhang J, Yang J, Xu Q, Zhu YJ, et al. A systemic review of MRI, scintigraphy, FDG-PET and PET/CT for diagnosis of multiple myeloma related bone disease – which is best? Asian Pac J Cancer Prev. 2014;15:9879–84.
19. Cavo M, Terpos E, Nanni C, Moreau P, Lentzsch S, Zweegman S, et al. Role of ^{18}F-FDG PET/CT in the diagnosis and management of multiple myeloma and other plasma cell disorders: a consensus statement by the International Myeloma Working Group. Lancet Oncol. 2017;18:e206–17.
20. Warsame E, Gertz MA, Lacy MQ, Kyle RA, Buadi F, Dingli D, et al. Trends and outcome of modern staging of solitary plasmacytoma of bone. Am J Hematol. 2012;87:4468–74.
21. Albano D, Bosio G, Treglia G, Giubbini R, Bertagna F. ^{18}F-FDG PET/CT in solitary plasmacytoma: metabolic behavior and progression to multiple myeloma. Eur J Nucl Med Mol Imaging. 2018;45:77–84.
22. Swerdlow SH, Campo E, Pileri SA, Harris NL, Stein H, Siebert R, et al. The 2016 revision of the World Health Organization classification of lymphoid neoplasms. Blood. 2016;127:2375–90.
23. Sehn LH, Scott DW, Chhanabhai M, Berry B, Ruskova A, Berkahn L, et al. Impact of concordant and discordant bone marrow involvement on outcome in diffuse large B-cell lymphoma treated with R-CHOP. J Clin Oncol. 2011;29(11):1452–7.
24. Adams HJ, Nievelstein RA, Kwee TC. Opportunities and limitations of bone marrow biopsy and bone marrow FDG-PET in lymphoma. Blood Rev. 2015;29(6):417–25.
25. Berthet L, et al. Newly diagnosed diffuse large B-cell lymphoma, determination of bone marrow involvement with 18F-FDG PET/CT provides better diagnostic performance and prognostic stratification than does biopsy. J Nucl Med. 2013;54:1244–50.
26. Hong J, Lee Y, Park Y, Kim SG, Hwang KH, Park SH, et al. Role of FDG-PET/CT in detecting lymphomatous bone marrow involvement in patients with

newly diagnosed diffuse large B-cell lymphoma. Ann Hematol. 2012;91(5):687–95.
27. Paone G, Itti E, Haioun C, Gaulard P, Dupuis J, Lin C, et al. Bone marrow involvement in diffuse large B-cell lymphoma: correlation between FDG-PET uptake and type of cellular infiltrate. Eur J Nucl Med Mol Imaging. 2009;36(5):745–50.
28. Lim CY, Ong KO. Imaging of musculoskeletal lymphoma. Cancer Imaging. 2013;13(4):448–57.
29. Krishnan A, Shirkhoda A, Tehranzadeh J. et-al. Primary bone lymphoma: radiographic-MR imaging correlation. Radiographics. 2003;23(6):1371–83.

Part VI

Miscellaneous Features in Musculoskeletal Nuclear Imaging

Soft Tissue Uptake of Bone Scan Agents

20

Yun Young Choi and Soo Jin Lee

Abstract

Unexpected soft tissue uptake of bone scan agents is often a source of uncertainty and doubt to inexperienced physicians, but sometimes provides information that enhances the diagnostic value of the study. This chapter reviews several remarkable cases showing soft tissue uptake associated with extraosseous heterotopic new bone formation, soft tissue calcification, abnormal intracellular flux of ionic calcium after damage to cell membrane integrity, and expansion of the interstitial fluid component.

Keywords

Heterotopic ossification · Dystrophic calcification · Metastatic calcification · Tumoral calcinosis · Rhabdomyolysis · Bone scan · Bone SPECT/CT

Y. Y. Choi (✉)
Department of Nuclear Medicine, Hanyang University College of Medicine, Seoul, Republic of Korea
e-mail: yychoi@hanyang.ac.kr

S. J. Lee
Department of Nuclear Medicine, Hanyang University College of Medicine, Seoul, Republic of Korea

20.1 Heterotopic Ossification

Heterotopic new bone formation is the presence of bone in soft tissue, where it does not normally exist. Vast majority of conditions are acquired following trauma, and rarely it can be congenital (e.g., myositis ossificans progressiva). The pathogenetic mechanism is believed to be due to transformation of certain primitive cells of mesenchymal origin in the connective tissue septa within muscles into bone-forming cells [1]. Bone scan is more sensitive than plain film in detecting heterotopic ossification. Three-phase bone scan can be used for determining the optimum time for surgical removal. As heterotopic bone formation progresses from immature to mature, all the three phases of bone scan typically show progressive decreased uptake, leading to steady state over a period of 2–3 months. Then, it could minimize the risk of recurrence after excision [2].

Case 20.1
Evolution of heterotopic ossification after trauma (Fig. 20.1).

20.2 Soft Tissue Calcification

Besides heterotopic ossification, major types of extraosseous calcification include dystrophic calcification and metastatic calcification.

S.-O. Yang et al. (eds.), *Atlas of Nuclear Medicine in Musculoskeletal System*,
https://doi.org/10.1007/978-981-19-2677-8_20

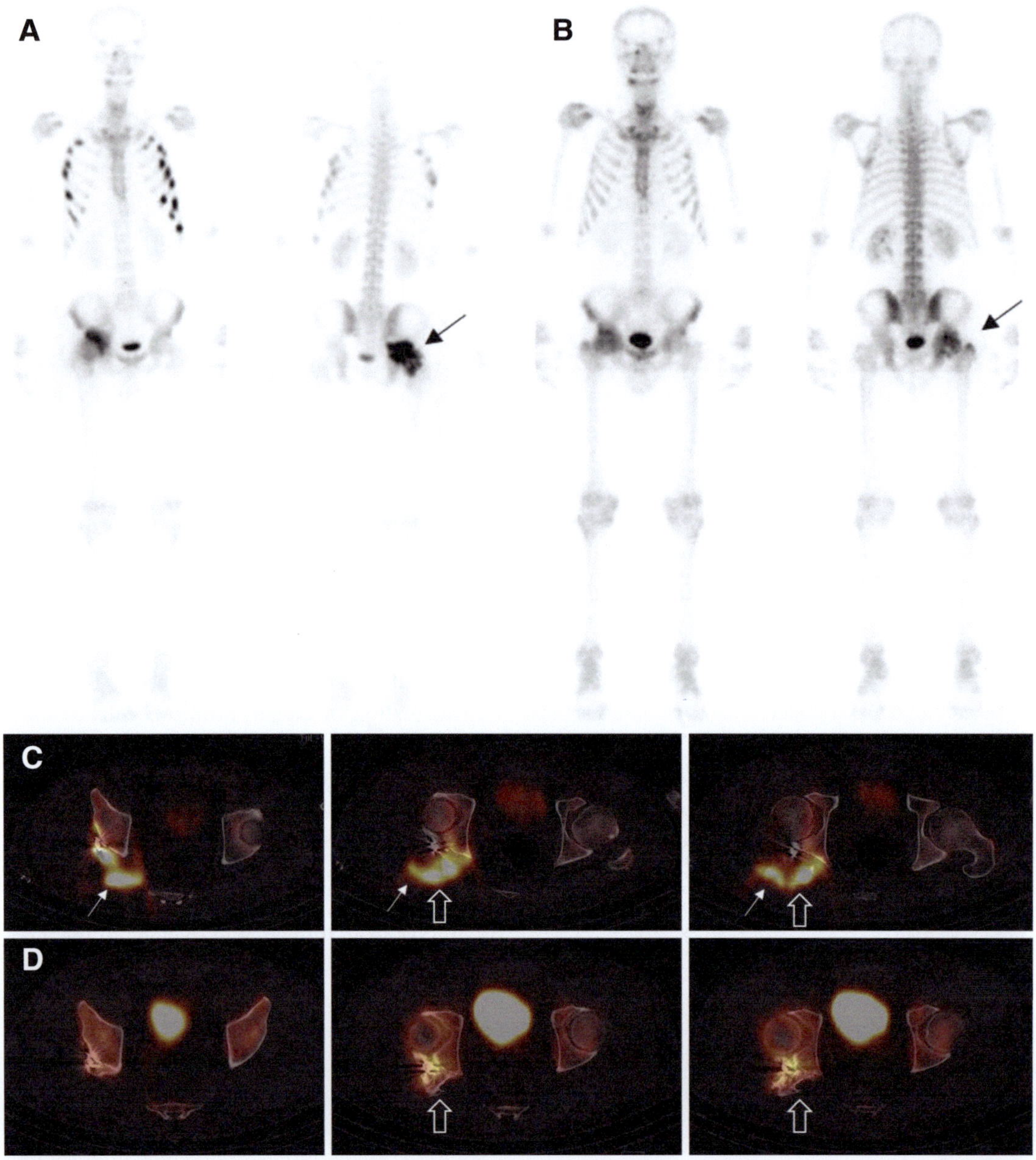

Fig. 20.1 A 33-year-old man with the right acetabular fracture. Bone scan taken 2 weeks after trauma shows focal intense uptake mainly in the posterior aspect of right acetabulum (**A**), which is markedly decreased after 1 year (**B**). Serial SPECT/CT images show the evolution of the focal intense uptake lesions detected immediately after trauma (**C**, upper row) and 1 year later (**D**, lower row): majority of the uptake lesion became mature heterotopic bone (open arrows), and part of the lesion has been resolved (arrow)

20.2.1 Dystrophic Calcification

Dystrophic calcification involves the calcification of damaged tissue and occurs in the setting of normal serum calcium and phosphate level. Tissue damage might be from inflammation, neoplasm, or necrosis. Increased calcium-binding capacity of the exposed denatured proteins of the injured cells which preferentially bind with phosphate ions, in turn react with calcium and form calcium deposits. Examples include calcification in infarcted myocardium, atheromas, amyloid tissue, and the center of tumors [3].

Case 20.2
Tumor uptake: dystrophic calcification (Fig. 20.2).

Case 20.3
Foreign body uptake: dystrophic calcification of paraffinoma (Fig. 20.3).

Oblong soft tissue uptake in subcutaneous areas around both knees and calfs on SPECT/CT images (arrows in B-a & B-a′) are matched with soft tissue masses with spotty calcifications on CT images (arrows in B-b & B-b′), proven to be paraffinoma. The patient had a history of paraffin injection decades ago.

20.2.2 Metastatic Calcification

Metastatic calcification is the calcification of viable, undamaged, normal tissue as a result of hypercalcemia and/or hyperphosphatemia associated with increased calcium phosphate product, locally or systemically. This can be due to (1) metabolic abnormalities as renal failure, hypervitaminosis D, and hyperparathyroidism and (2) increased bone demineralization from bone tumors or disseminated metastasis.

Tumoral calcinosis is a form of metastatic calcification, which shows large, calcified, periarticular soft tissue masses of calcium phosphate near the large joints such as hip, shoulder, and elbow, outside the joint capsule. This can be observed in the primary form (idiopathic, con-

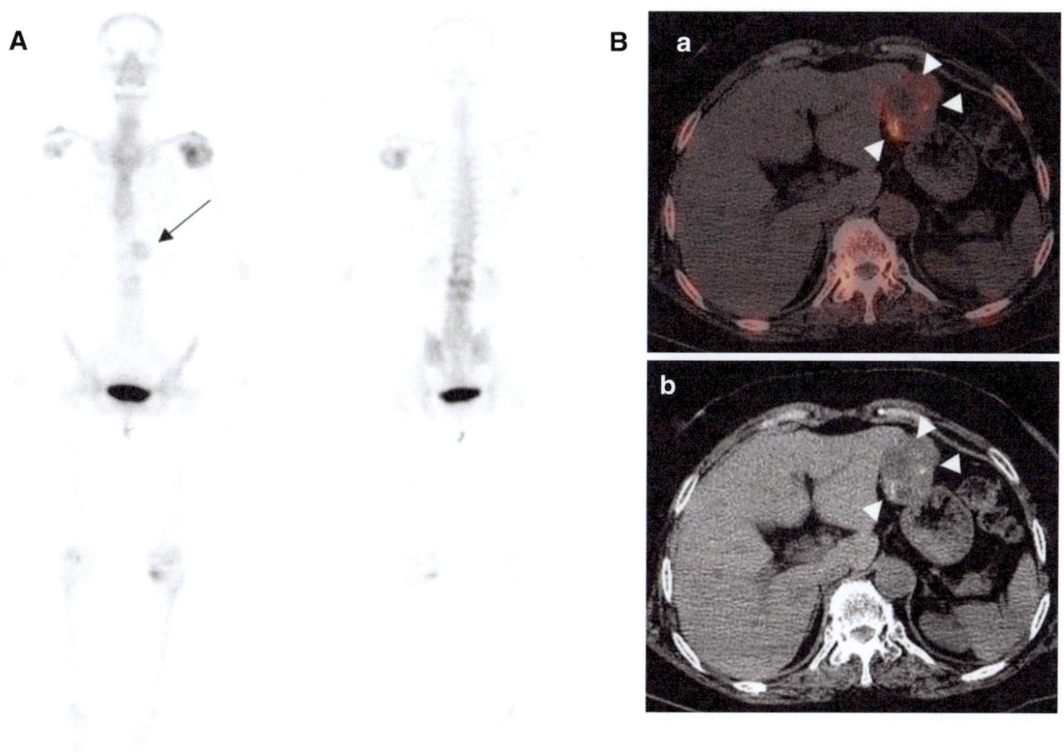

Fig. 20.2 A 72-year-old woman with left shoulder pain. Doughnut-shaped focal uptake is incidentally detected in the left upper abdomen (arrow) on whole-body bone scan (**A**). Abdominal CT taken on the next day shows gastric submucosal tumor. Curvilinear increased MDP uptake is noted at the margin of gastric submucosal tumor on SPECT/CT images (**B-a**, white arrowheads), matched with dystrophic calcification on non-enhanced CT image (**B-b**, white arrowheads). The mass was surgically removed and proven to be malignant GIST. Careful evaluation of soft tissue uptake made a contribution to early diagnosis of malignant tumor

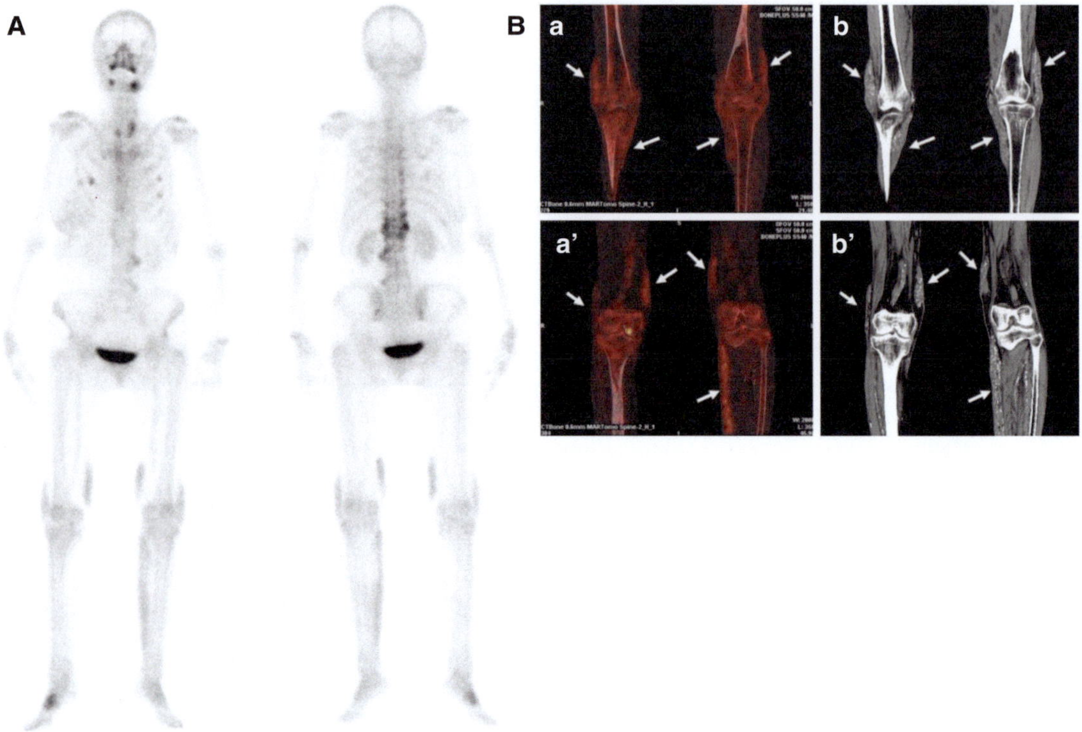

Fig. 20.3 An 88-year-old woman with right breast cancer shows incidentally detected soft tissue uptake along bilateral lower extremities on whole-body bone scan (**A**). Oblong soft tissue uptake in subcutaneous areas around both knees and proximal legs on SPECT/CT images (arrows in **a** & **a′**) are soft tissue masses with spotty calcifications on CT images (arrows in **b** & **b′**), proven to be paraffinoma (**B**). The patient had a history of paraffin injection decades ago

genital) but also be found in various conditions including primary or secondary hyperparathyroidism, scleroderma, hypervitaminosis D, chronic renal failure on dialysis, etc [4].

Case 20.4
Metastatic calcification: tumoral calcinosis in secondary hyperparathyroidism due to end-stage renal disease undergoing dialysis (Fig. 20.4).

20.3 Causes of Soft Tissue Uptake Other than Calcification

20.3.1 Rhabdomyolysis

Rhabdomyolysis is a condition that follows muscle damage due to various causes including viral or bacterial infection, certain drugs, alcohol abuse, trauma, and excessive physical activity, characterized by excess myoglobin in urine, since intracellular muscle protein is released and excreted by dark-colored urine. Variable degrees of muscle death cause abnormal influx of calcium ions into muscle cells after damage to cell membrane integrity, which allows bone scan agents to form stable complexes inside muscle cells and results in variable degree of abnormally increased uptake in damaged muscles shown on bone scan. Rhabdomyolysis can lead to serious complications such as renal failure [5].

Case 20.5
Various features of rhabdomyolysis are associated with causative factors: excessive physical activity, chronic use of clutch, lying unconscious on a hard surface under the influence of alcohol, and drug induce, etc. (Fig. 20.5).

Case 20.6
Focal uptake in resolving hematoma after contusion of abdominal wall (Fig. 20.6).

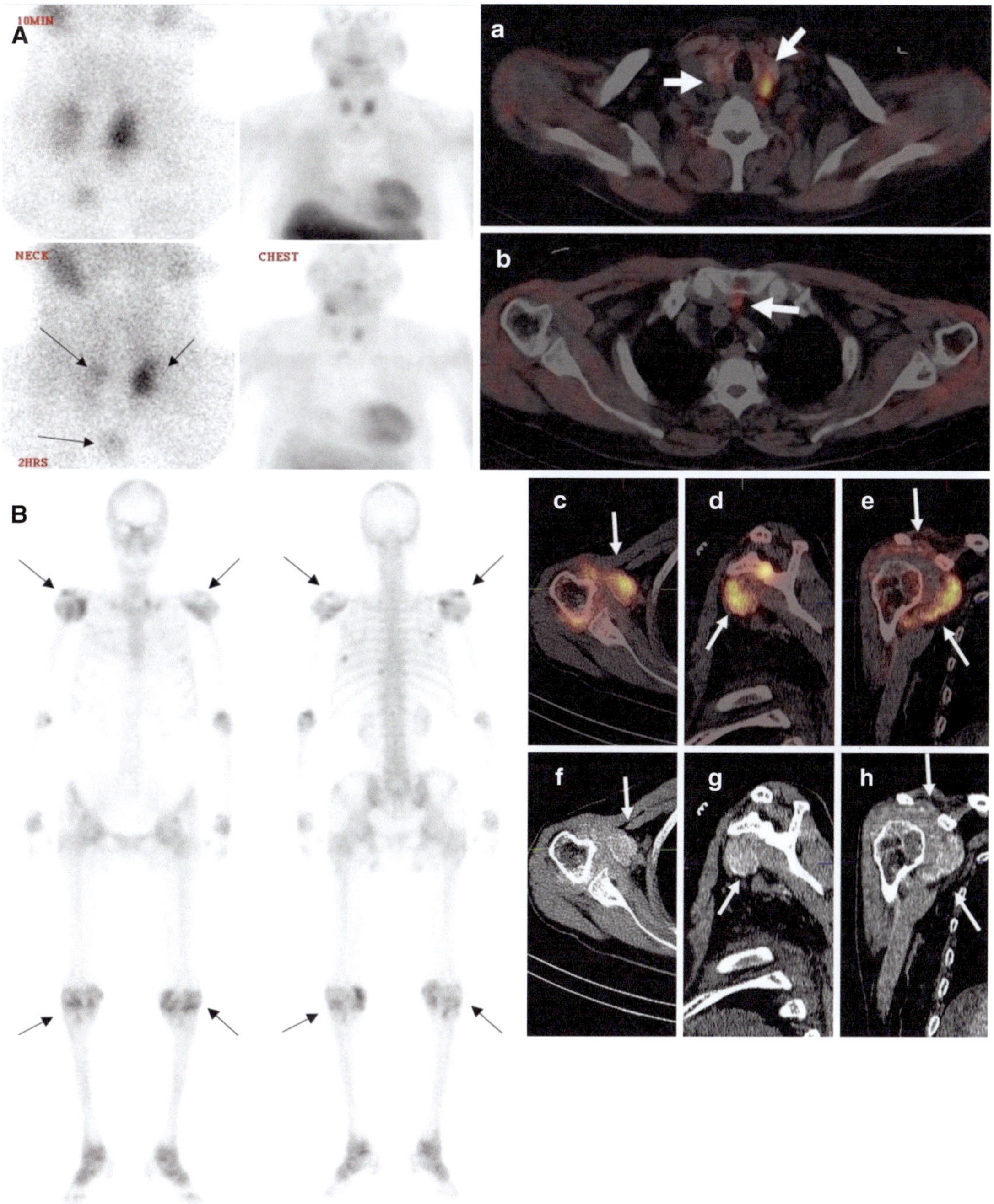

Fig. 20.4 A 66-year-old woman with hypercalcemia and hyperphosphatemia. She had end-stage renal disease and underwent peritoneal dialysis for 13 years. Serum-intact PTH was elevated as high as 987.1 pg/ml (normal, 14–64 pg/ml), and secondary hyperparathyroidism was suspected clinically. Parathyroid scan (**A**) shows multifocal nodular lesions revealing delayed washout on the regional image of neck taken 2 h after Tc-99m MIBI injection (arrows). SPECT/CT images show three hot nodules: two are posterior to thyroid upper pole (**a**, white arrows) and one is inferior to thyroid gland (**b**, white arrow), suggestive of parathyroid hyperplasia. Multiple periarticular uptake lesions are noted, especially involving both shoulders and knees (arrows) on whole-body bone scan (**B**). Shoulder SPECT/CT images show focal intense uptake lesions around the right shoulder (**c**–**e**), which are proven to be mass-like calcifications outside the joint capsule (**f**–**h**) on CT images

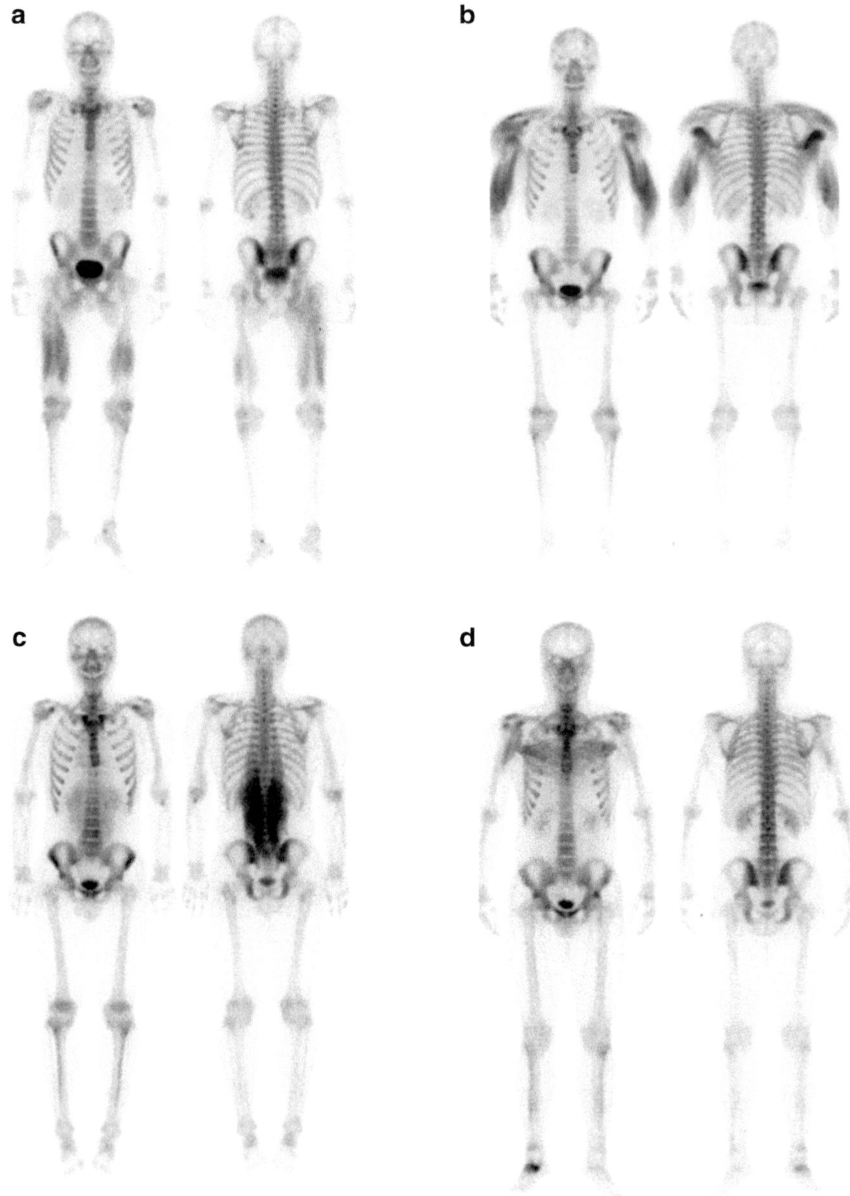

Fig. 20.5 (**a**)–(**c**) Cases with severe exercise-induced rhabdomyolysis with exercise-related muscle pain and dark-colored urine and elevated muscle enzyme and urine myoglobin. Areas of rhabdomyolysis shows focal increased uptake lesions on whole-body bone scan images (arrows). (**a**) A 24-year-old man with anterior thigh pain after squat exercise 2 days ago, serum-creatine kinase (s-CK) > 20,000, urine-myoglobin 9478 (normal, 0–21). (**b**) A 25-year-old man with both upper arm pain 2 h after exercise, s-CK > 20,000, urine myoglobin >3000. (**c**) A 21-year-old man with back pain after kettlebell exercise 2 days ago, s-CK > 20,000 urine myoglobin >1200. (**d**) A 31-year-old man with clutch-induced rhabdomyolysis, due to a fracture of right foot 18 months ago. (**e**) A 42-year-old man with weakness, especially right side, on the next day of heavy drinking and over-night sleep outdoors on a mountain rock (s-CK > 20,000; CK-MB, 42.8; u-myoglobin, 759.2). (**f**) A 35-year-old man, who is a severe alcoholic with uremic encephalopathy and methicillin-sensitive *S. aureus* bacteremia, shows multifocal rhabdomyolysis. Multiple factors could be concerned for causatives of rhabdomyolysis, but neuropsychiatric medication was concerned for the causative factor clinically (s-CK, 53728; CK-MB, 233.4). (**g**) A 77-year-old man with diabetes nephropathy on hemodialysis for 3 years had drug-induced rhabdomyolysis. He had general weakness 3 weeks after administration of statin

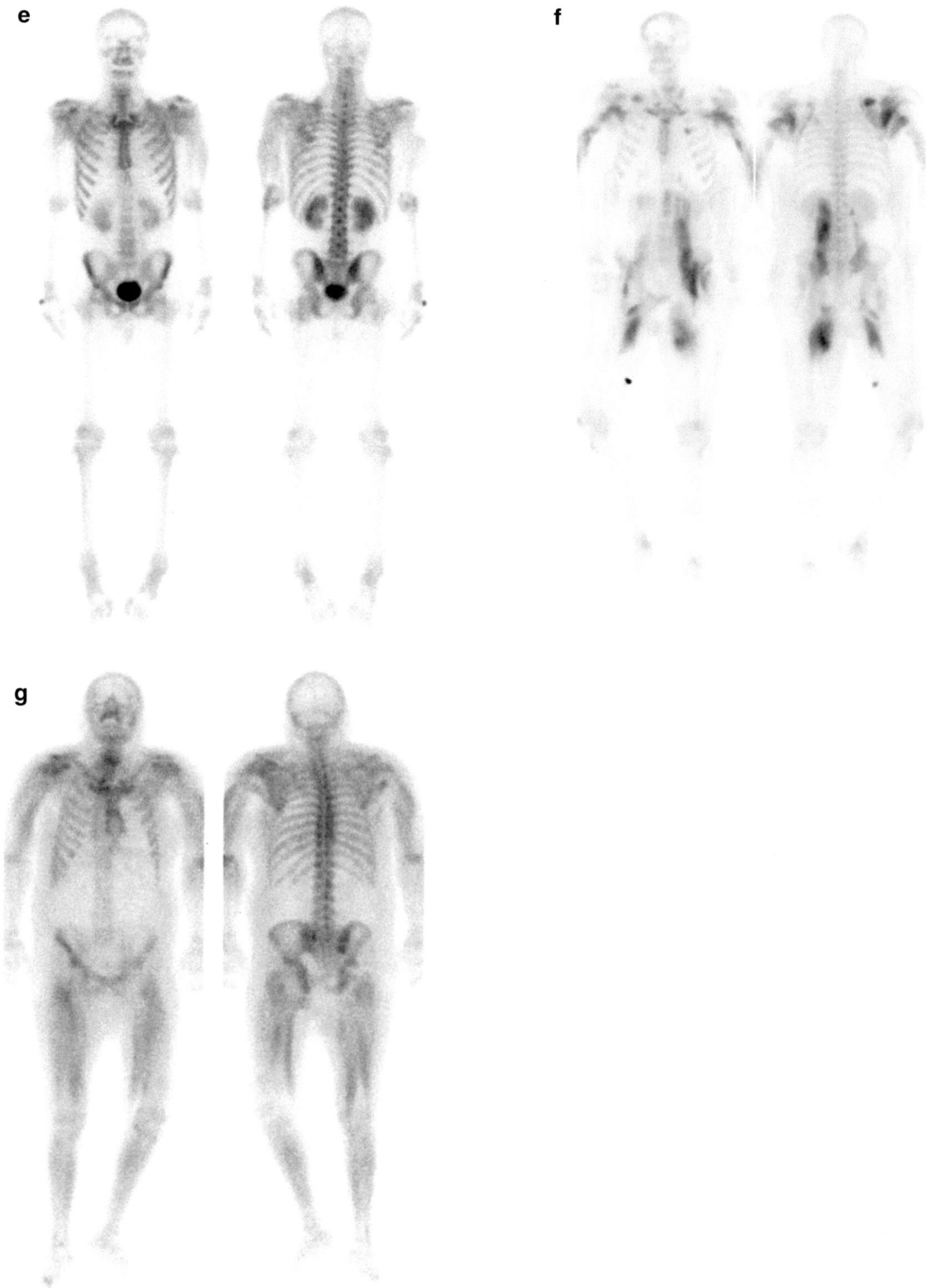

Fig. 20.5 (continued)

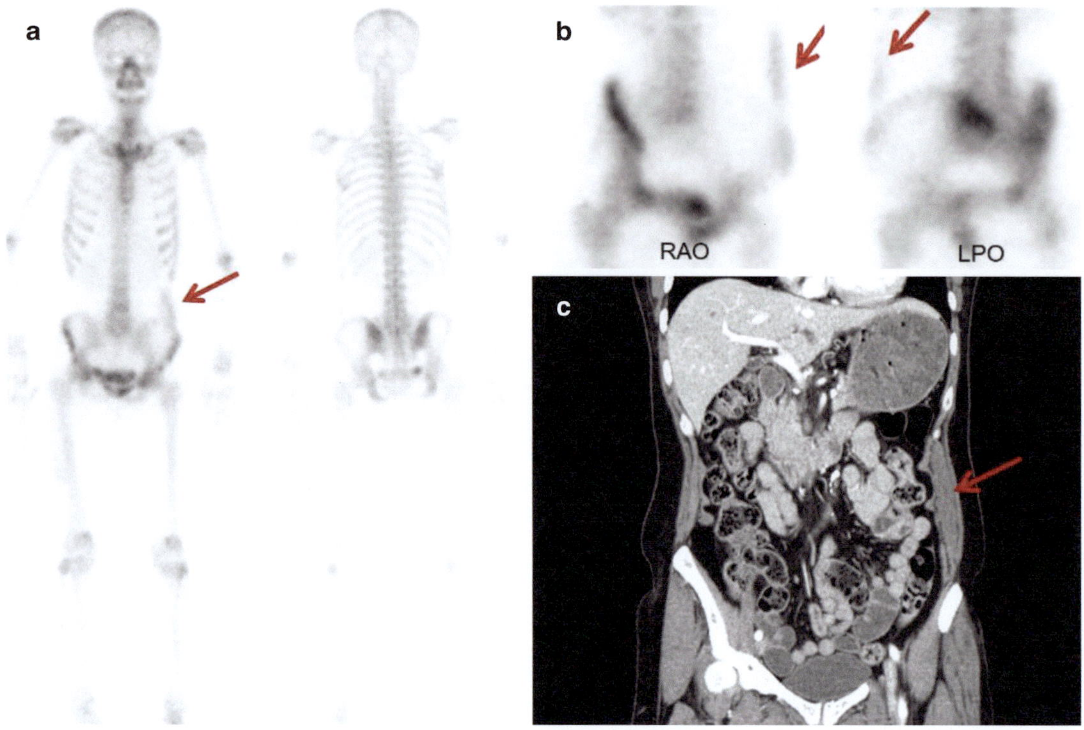

Fig. 20.6 A 57-year-old woman was hit by a motorcycle a day before. She complained about left hip and elbow pain. Linear increased soft tissue uptake is noted along the left lower anterior abdominal wall on whole-body (**a**) and regional (**b**) images of bone scan, which is proven to be resolving hematoma on abdominal CT image (**c**)

20.3.2 Expansion of the Interstitial Fluid Compartment

Another common mechanism of soft tissue localization bone scan agents is associated with expansion of interstitial fluid compartment (e.g., lymphedema, ascites, pleural effusion).

Case 20.7
Expansion of the interstitial fluid compartment: lymphedema (Figs. 20.7 and 20.8) [5].

Case 20.8
Expansion of the interstitial fluid compartment: ascites (Fig. 20.9).

20.3.3 Primary or Metastatic Tumor Uptake Associated with Tumor Hypervascularity

Malignant tumors show various spectra of uptake ranges from ill-defined and barely detectable to intense and sharply marginated. Multiple factors may play the role in localization of bone scan agents. Histologic evidence of calcium correlates most strongly with avid tracer uptake, but tumor vascularity also plays a secondary but important role [3, 6].

Case 20.9
Tumor uptake: neovascularization of hypervascular tumor (Fig. 20.10).

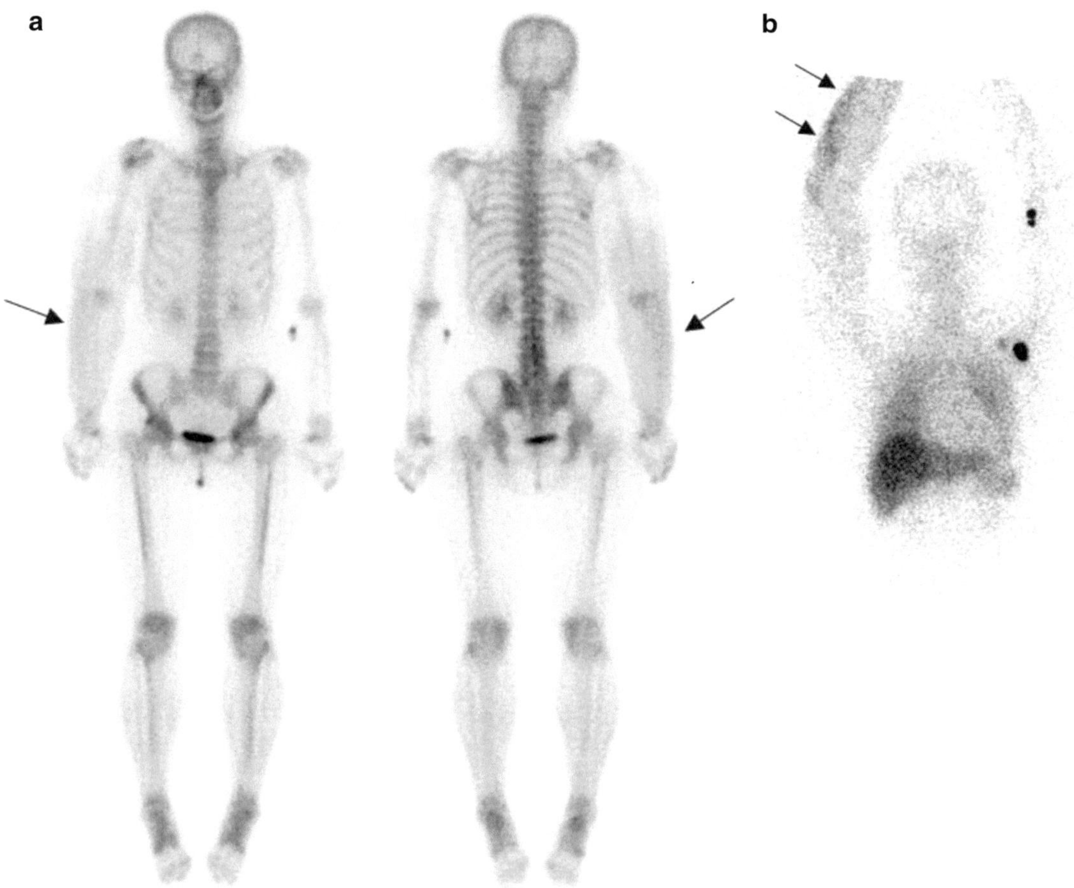

Fig. 20.7 Lymphedema of upper extremity in breast cancer. A 51-year-old woman complained of swelling in her right upper extremity. She had a history of right breast cancer and underwent radiation therapy 4 years ago. Diffuse soft tissue uptake of swollen right upper extremity (**a**, arrow) is noted on whole-body bone scan. On lymphoscitigraphy, non-visualization of normal lymphatic flow and skin backflow in right upper extremity (**b**, arrows), suggestive of secondary lymphedema

Case 20.10
Tumor uptake: hypervascular tumor with internal necrosis (Fig. 20.11).

20.4 Artificial Uptake of Bone Scan Agents

Urinary activity and bowel activity are most frequently shown artifactual soft tissue uptake [7].

Case 20.11
Unusual bowel uptake (Fig. 20.12).

Case 20.12
Incidental uptake in bladder diverticulum (Fig. 20.13).

Case 20.13
Urinoma due to urine leakage from percutaneous nephrectomy (PCN) catheter (Fig. 20.14).

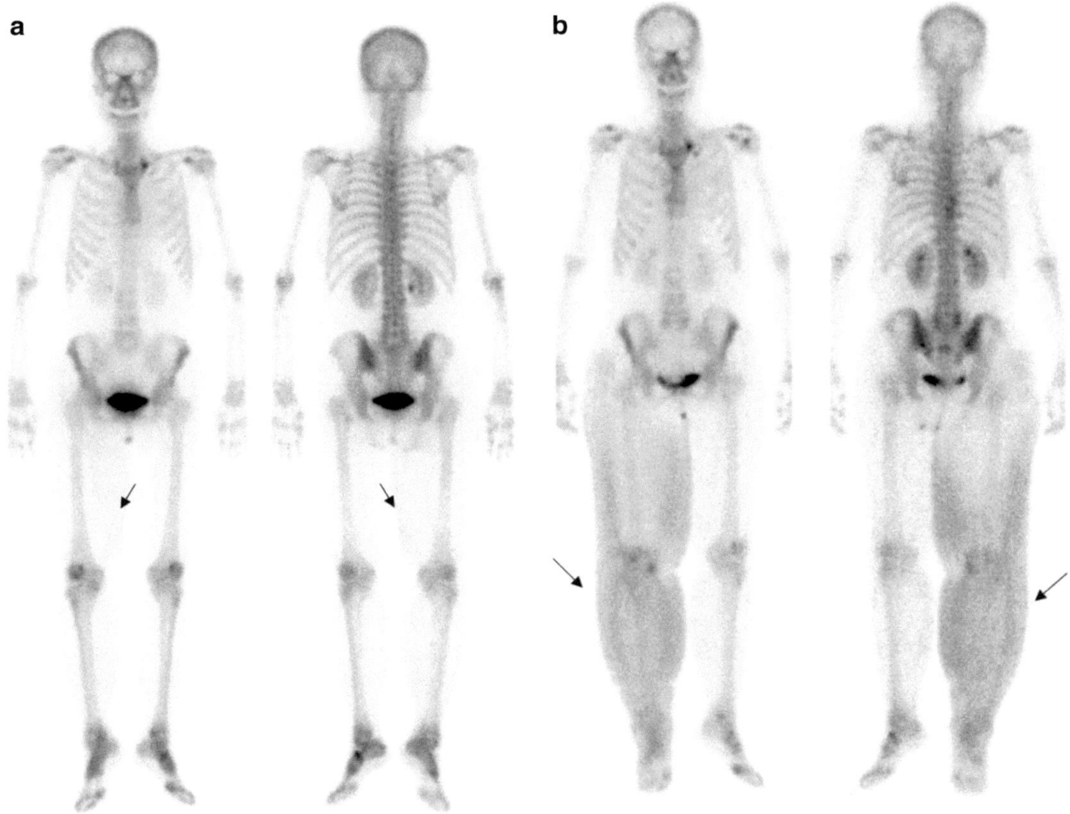

Fig. 20.8 Lymphedema of lower extremity in cervix cancer. A 59-year-old woman presented progressive right lower extremity swelling over several years. She had a history of radical hysterectomy and pelvic lymph node dissection due to cervix cancer 10 years ago. She complained of heaviness of the right lower extremity, which occured suddenly, 10 years after operation. There is subtle soft tissue uptake in the right medial thigh on bone scan (**a**), which is aggravated to diffuse, intense soft tissue uptake of right lower extremity 2 years later (**b**), suggestive of secondary lymphedema

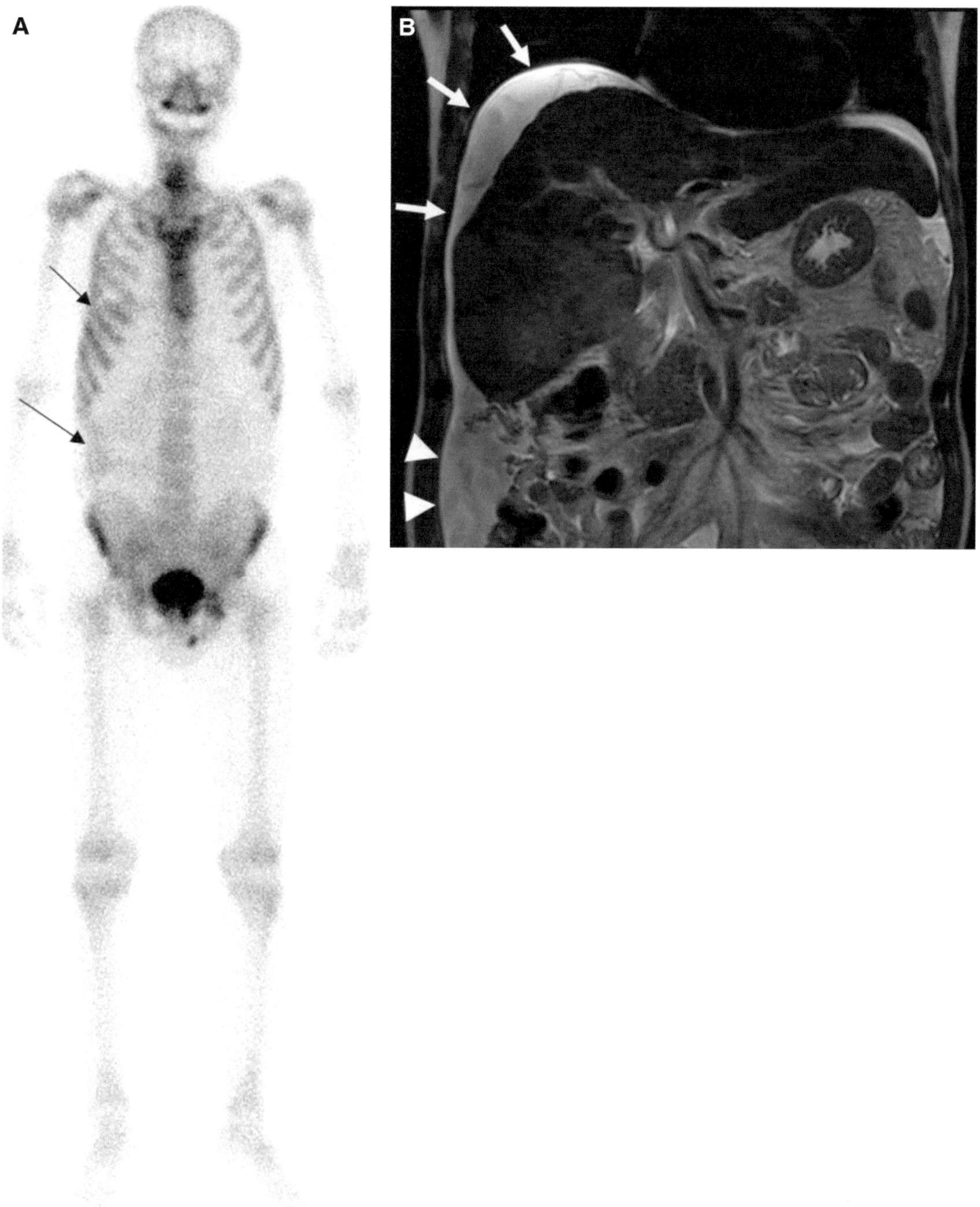

Fig. 20.9 A 53-year-old man with hepatocellular carcinoma shows increased soft tissue uptake in abdomen (black arrows) on bone scan (**A**), which matched with ascites in perihepatic subdiaphragmatic space (white arrows) and right paracolic gutter (arrow heads) on MRI (**B**)

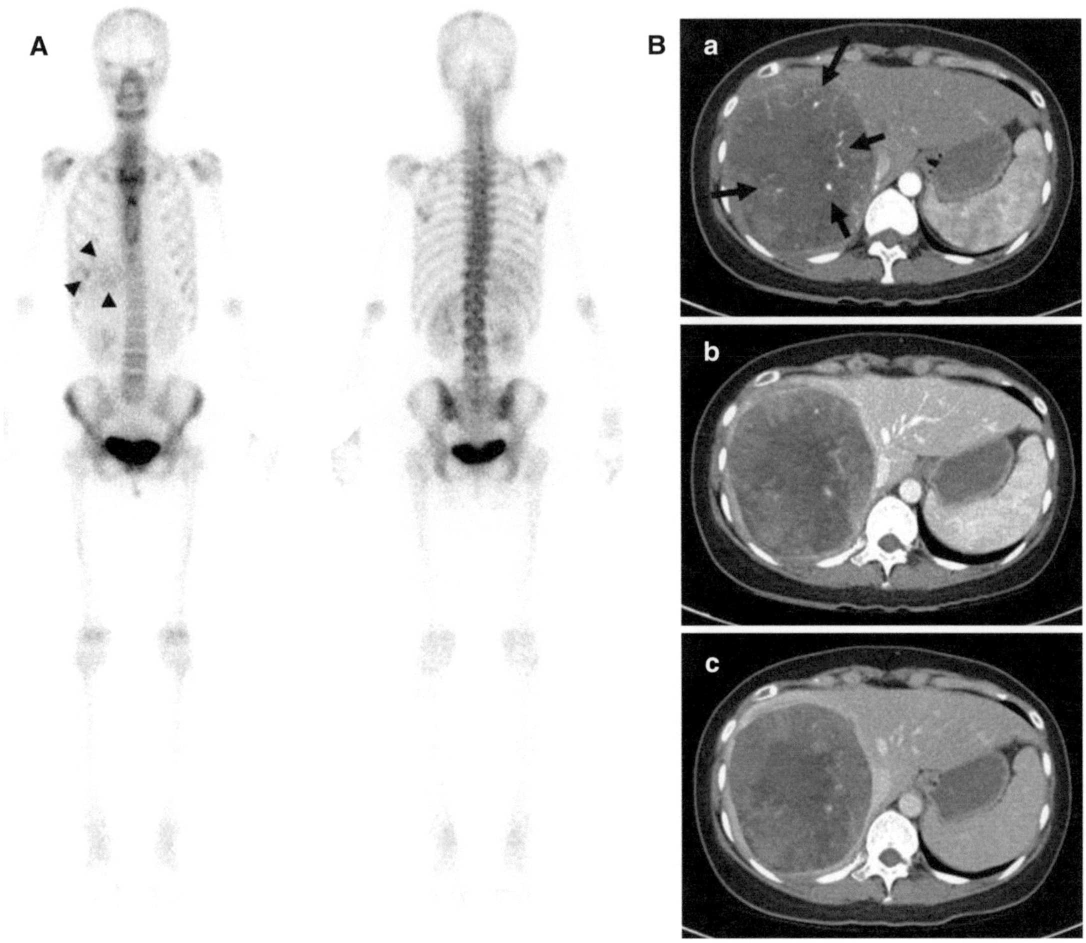

Fig. 20.10 A 37-year-old woman with hepatocellular carcinoma. Focal soft tissue uptake in right upper abdomen (arrow heads) presenting uptake of huge hepatocellular carcinoma on whole-body bone image (**A**). Abdominal CT images show neovascularization of hypervascular hepatocellular carcinoma on arterial (**B**-**a**, arrows) and portal phase (**B**-**b**) and peripheral enhancement on delayed phase (**B**-**c**), suspected to be associated with increased soft tissue uptake on bone scan

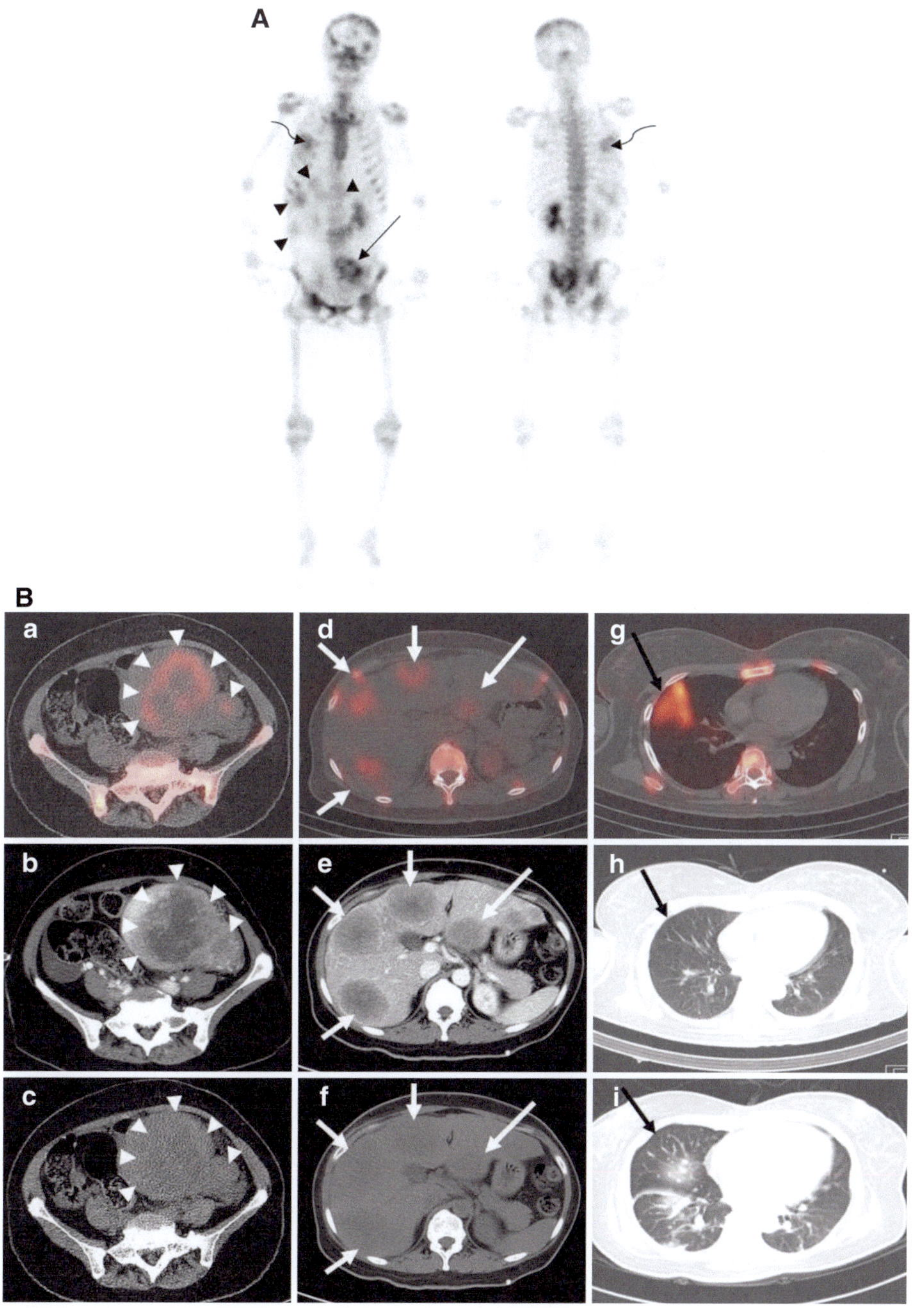

Fig. 20.11 A 34-year-old woman with azotemia due to post-renal AKI presented huge endometrial cancer in abdomen. Uneven soft tissue uptake in left pelvic cavity (arrow), left upper abdomen (arrow heads), and right thorax (curved arrow) on whole body bone scan (**A**). SPECT/CT of abdomen shows increased MDP uptake along the margin of necrosis in the hypervascular endometrial cancer (**B**-**a**, white arrowheads) and well-enhancing hepatic metastatic nodules (**B**-**d**, white arrows) on enhanced CT images (**B**-**b** & **B**-**e**). The tumors do not show definite calcific densities on non-contrast CT images (**B**-**c** & **B**-**f**). Incidentally detected lung uptake in RML lateral segment (**B**-**g**, arrows), without definite anatomic abnormality on lung window CT image (**B**-**h**), but progress to multiple lung and pleural metastasis, revealing multiple small lung nodules with pleural effusion in right hemithorax on lung window CT image taken 2 weeks later (**B**-**i**)

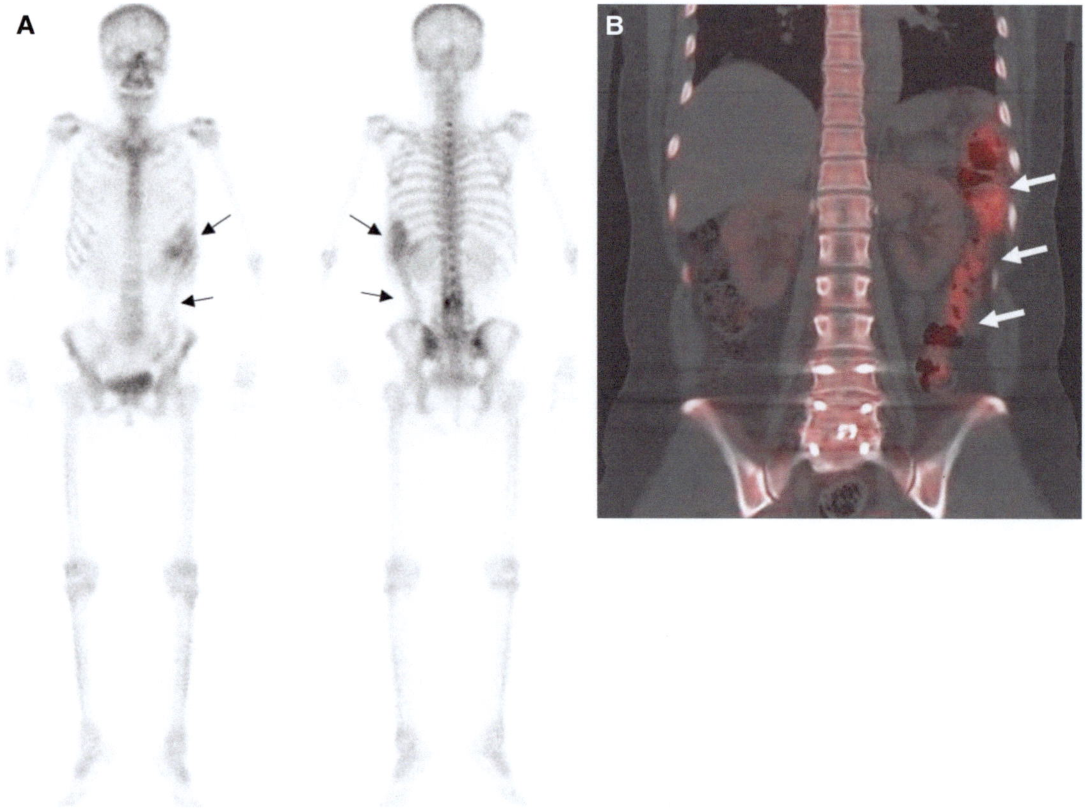

Fig. 20.12 A 55-year-old woman shows abnormal bowel uptake in left abdomen on bone scan (**A**, arrows), which is in the colonic loops on coronal SPECT/CT image (**B**, white arrows). Diffuse colonic uptake can be seen normally after intravenous CT contrast injection or other pathologic conditions including primary intestinal lymphangiectasia, protein-losing enteropathy, and systemic amyloidosis

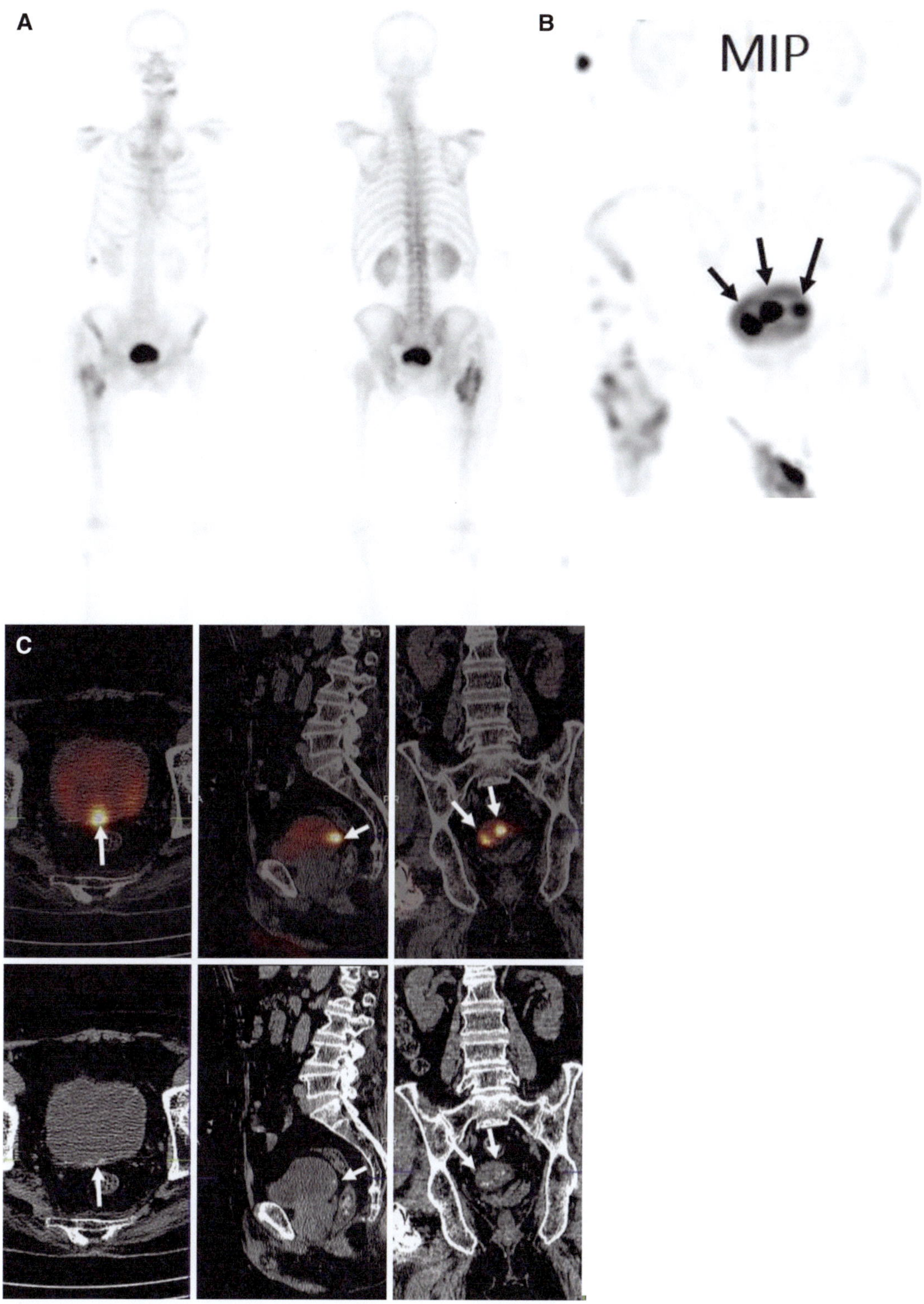

Fig. 20.13 A 79-year-old man with a right femur neck fracture. There are three hot spots in the bladder on the MIP image of SPECT/CT (**B**, arrows), which were not evident on the whole-body image (**A**). On the SPECT-CT image, tiny calcific densities are scattered in the dependent portion of the bladder, and focal radioactivity retention is seen between the calcifications (**C**, white arrows). Bladder diverticulums were detected by the cystoscopic examination

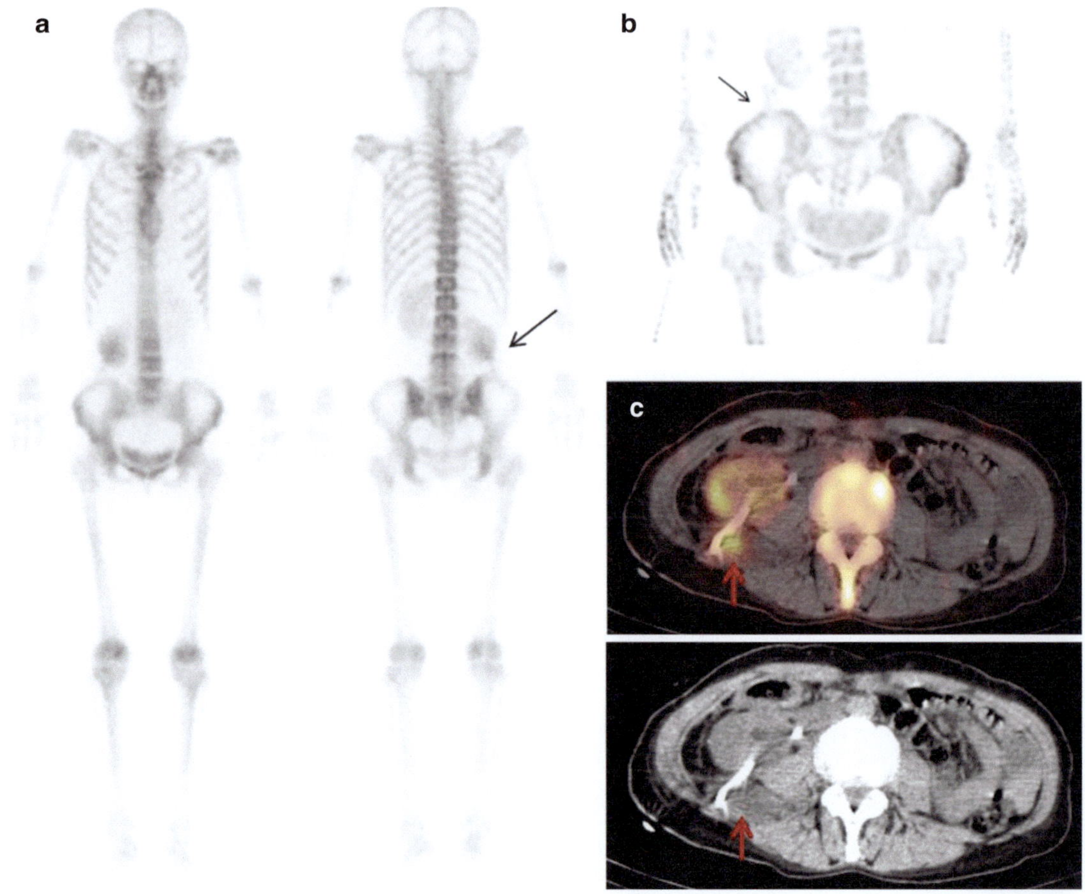

Fig. 20.14 A 50-year-old woman complained of right pelvic pain for 1 week. She had a total gastrectomy due to stomach cancer 8 years ago. Right PCN catheter was inserted 3 weeks before, because of right hydronephrosis resulting from peri-ureteral metastasis. Asymmetric radioactivity retention is noted in the right kidney, with linear increased uptake in soft tissue, which was suspected to be PCN catheter activity (**a**). Pelvic SPECT/CT was taken for evaluation of pelvic pain (**b**, **c**). There is focal radioactivity retention in the right back muscle adjacent to the catheter route, which is swollen compared to the contralateral side, due to intramuscular urinoma

Teaching Points

- In this section, we reviewed various clinical cases of non-osseous soft tissue uptake of bone scan agents including heterotopic ossification, dystrophic calcification of tumor and foreign body, metastatic calcifcation in tumoral calcinosis, rhabdomyolysis, third space leakage including lymphedema and ascites, hypervascular tumor uptake, and artifical activity in bowel and of urine.
- The mechanisms of non-osseous uptake of bone scan agents including soft tissue calcification, abnormal intracellular flux of ionic calcium, expansion of the interstitial fluid component, hypervascularity of tumor, and artificial uptake were presented.
- Some of the questionable lesions on planar bone scan were correctly identified on additional SPECT/CT.

References

1. Urist MR, Nakagawa M, Nakata N, Nogami H. Experimental myositis ossificans: cartilage and bone formation in muscle in response to diffusible bone matrix-derived morphogen. Arch Pathol Lab Med. 1978;102:312–6.
2. Shehab D, Elgazzar AH, Colllier BD. Heterotopic ossification. J Nucl Med. 2002;43:346–53.
3. Peller PJ, Ho VB, Krasdorf MJ. Extraosseous Tc-99m MDP uptake: a pathophysiologic approach. Radiographics. 1993;13:715–34.
4. Steinbach LS, Johnston JO, Tepper EF, Honda GD, Martel W. Tumoral calcinosis: radiologic-pathologic correlation. Skelet Radiol. 1995;24:573–8.
5. Gray HW, Krasnow AZ. Soft tissue uptake of bone agents. In: Collier BD, Fogelman I, Rosenthall L, editors. Skeletal nuclear medicine. St. Louis, Missouri: Mosby-Year book; 1996. p. 374–99.
6. Silberstein EB. Nonosseous localization of bone seeking radiopharmaceuticals. In: Silberstein EB, editor. Bone scintigraphy. Mount Kisco, NY: Futura; 1985. p. 347–70.
7. Loutfi I, Collier BD, Mohammed A. Nonosseous abnormalities on bone scans. J Nucl Med Technol. 2003;31:149–53.

Musculoskeletal Nuclear Imaging Pitfalls

21

Yun Young Choi, Ji Young Kim, and Seoung-Oh Yang

Abstract

Factors related to clinical history and physical examination (previous trauma or recent radionuclide studies), related to patient's condition (age, body habitus, underlying diseases, medications, hydration status, lack of cooperation during scanning), related to radiopharmaceuticals (radiochemical impurities, introduction of air into vial during preparation), related to technique (intra-arterial injection, extravasation, suboptimal image due to inadequate count collection, full bladder), and related to interpretation (normal and abnormal pattern recognition) are well-known possible sources of diagnostic errors [1].

Recently, SPECT/CT has been introduced, and the additional role of SPECT/CT has been stressed: enabling accurate diagnosis through enhanced sensitivity of SPECT and additional anatomic information from CT.

In this section, clinical cases of some classical artifacts associated with technical and patient-related factors and clinical cases of whole-body bone scan with equivocal diagnosis at presentation, which were correctly diagnosed with additional SPECT/CT, will be presented.

Keywords

Pitfall · Artifact · Bone scan · Bone SPECT/CT

21.1 Instrument-Related

21.1.1 Improper Photopeak Window Setting

Gamma cameras are equipped with pulse height analyzer which allows the operator to select an optimal range of energies for accepting photons for the bone scan images, which are centered at photopeak energy of Tc-99m. The typical energy window for Tc-99m bone scan agents is 10–20% window centered at 140 keV [2].

Co-57 flood sources are used for daily quality control of field homogeneity, which has an energy peak (122 keV) similar to that of Tc-99m. The energy peak of the gamma camera should be reset after the daily QC before imaging bone scan. If it is not done, subsequent scanning using Tc-99m

Y. Y. Choi (✉)
Department of Nuclear Medicine, Hanyang University College of Medicine, Seoul, Republic of Korea
e-mail: yychoi@hanyang.ac.kr

J. Y. Kim
Department of Nuclear Medicine, Hanyang University College of Medicine, Seoul, Republic of Korea

S.-O. Yang
Department of Nuclear Medicine, Dongnam Institute of Radiological and Medical Sciences, Busan, Republic of Korea

S.-O. Yang et al. (eds.), *Atlas of Nuclear Medicine in Musculoskeletal System*,
https://doi.org/10.1007/978-981-19-2677-8_21

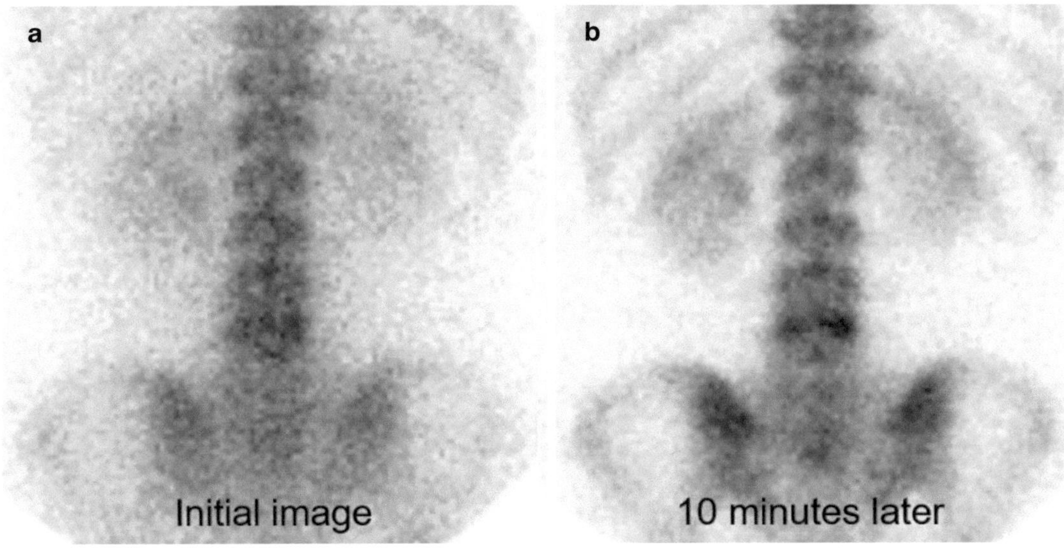

Fig. 21.1 What happened between two images (**a**, **b**) taken 10 min apart? On initial image (**a**), diffusely increased soft tissue activity with poor visualization of the bones is noted. A technical problem was concerned, and the photopeak energy window was found to be centered erroneously lower at 122 keV, the energy of Co-57, instead of that of Tc-99m

bone scan agents will show low-resolution images, resulting from loss of photopeak count and increased lower energy scatter counts [3, 4].

Case 21.1 Off-photopeak energy window (Fig. 21.1)

21.2 Technique-Related

21.2.1 Intra-arterial Injection

The uptake mechanism of bone-seeking agent is influenced not only by osteoblastic activity but also by other factors including blood flow, sympathetic tone, and bone surface area. Intra-arterial injection may cause increased delivery of bone-seeking agent to the area distal to injection site and results in increased bone uptake. "Glove phenomenon" was previously described in cases with increased uptake in distal forearm bone and soft tissue after intra-arterial injection on the antecubital region. "Sock" pattern was also introduced as an intra-arterial injection artifact of lower limb [5]. The explanation for hyperfixation mechanism could be secondary to the increased arterial blood flow at the first step of the radiotracers binding mechanism. Intra-arterial injection should be considered when exaggerated diffuse increased bone uptake is seen in an extremity distal to injection site, especially with no demonstrable history and radiographic findings. Differential diagnosis includes reflex sympathetic dystrophy [6], frostbite injury, and tourniquet effect [7].

Case 21.2 Intra-arterial injection (Fig. 21.2)

21.2.2 Injection into Central Venous Catheter

Injection into the central venous catheter results in residual radioactivity within the plastic tubing or reservoir. Therefore, sufficient saline flushing into the venous catheter is required in those cases.

Case 21.3 Radiotracer retention along chemoport catheter (Fig. 21.3)

21.2.3 Tourniquet Effect

It has been known that release of tourniquet results in increase of blood flow and radiotracer

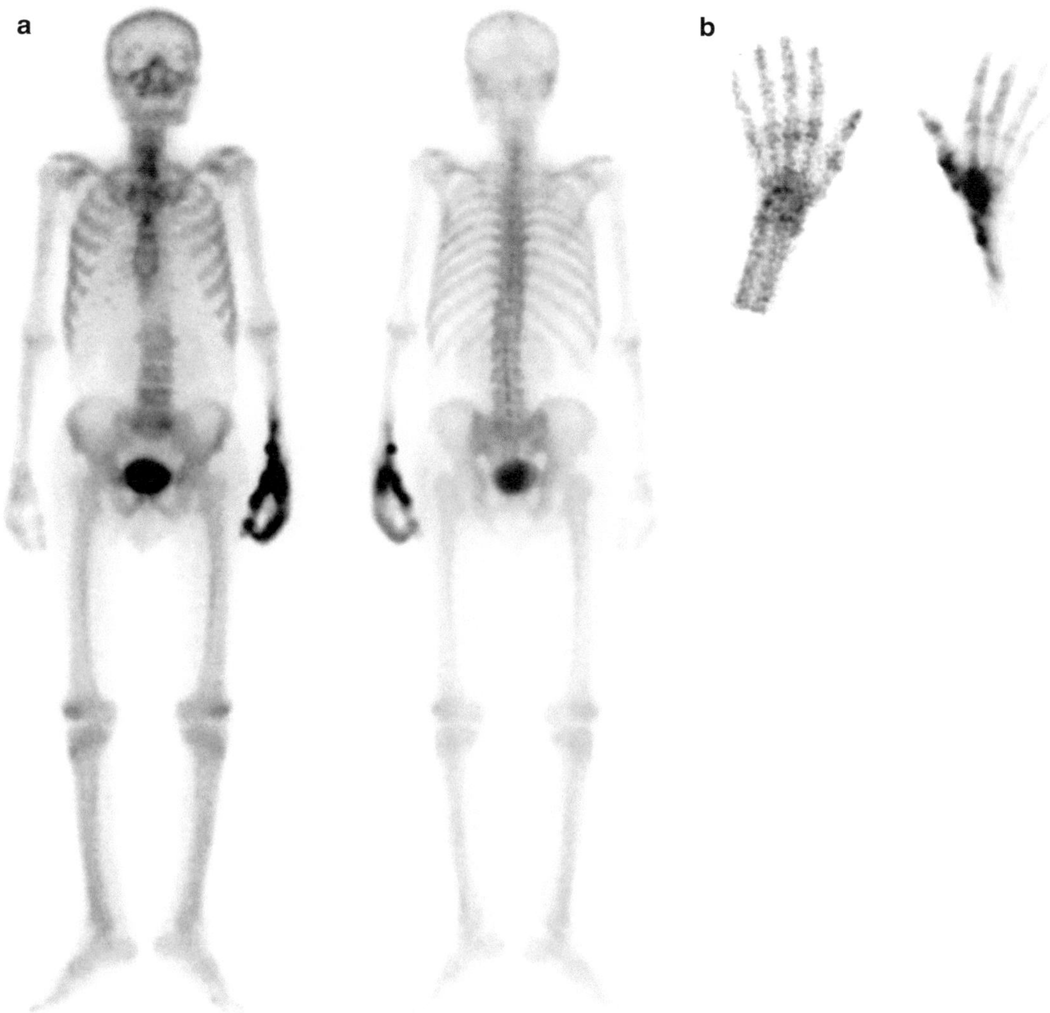

Fig. 21.2 A 75-year-old man performed a bone scan for evaluation of back pain. Intense uptake in left hand distal to IV site in left wrist is noted (**a**). On regional image (**b**), increased uptake of the radiopharmaceutical is more prominent in radial side, where the radial artery supplies dominantly. The above finding is due to injection of bone-seeking agent into the left radial artery, instead of vein

uptake in distal parts of injection site. The phenomenon is associated with reactive hyperemia induced by transient ischemia during perfusion and blood pool phases of three-phase bone scan, due to prolonged compression [8, 9]. On delayed bone scan, diffusely increased uptake in the extremity distal to injection site can be shown in cases with maintaining the tourniquet in place during injection [10–12].

The opposite finding of decreased localization of radionuclide in an extremity can also occur due to tight elastic stockings or elastic bandage wrappings, representing ischemic condition [12].

Case 21.4 Tourniquet effect (Fig. 21.4)

Case 21.5 Elastic bandage wrapping (Fig. 21.5)

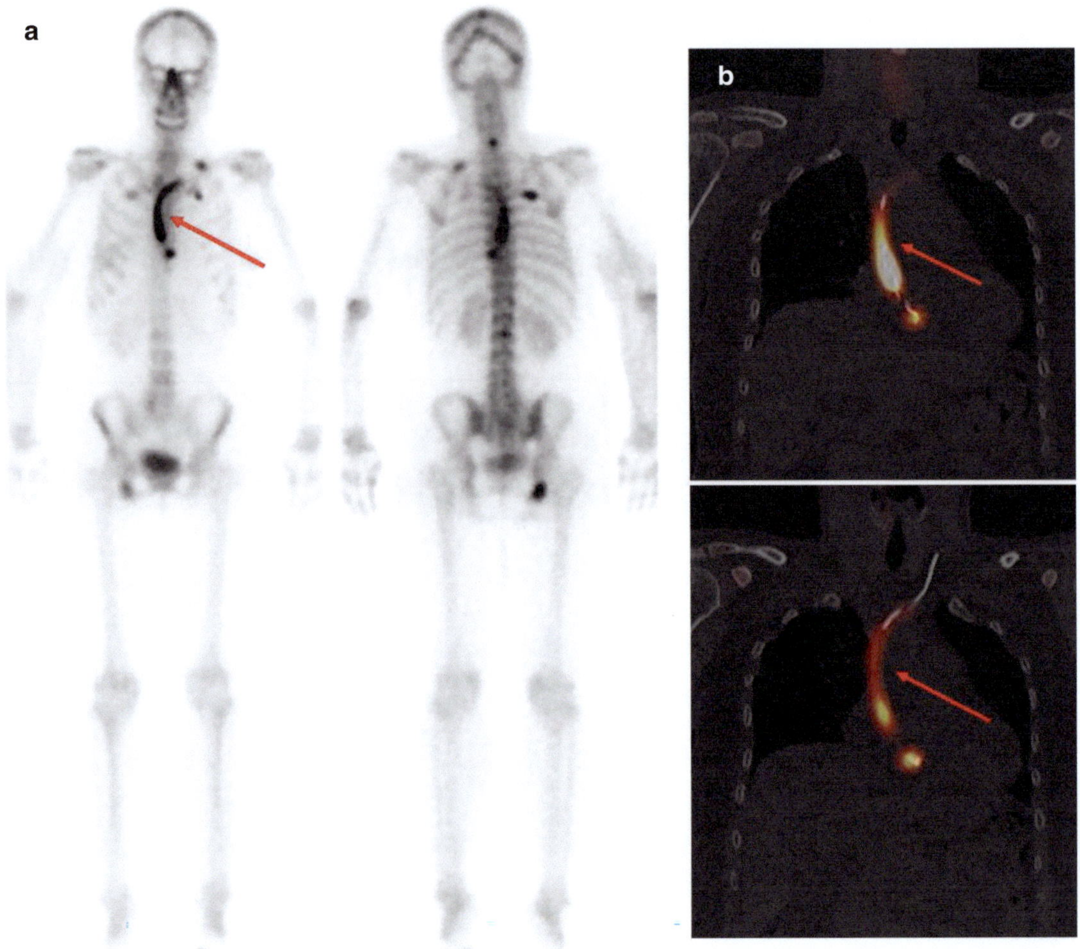

Fig. 21.3 A 43-year-old woman undergoing chemotherapy for breast cancer with multiple bone metastasis. Whole-body bone scan shows multiple focal increased uptake at lower C-spine, left first rib, right fifth rib, L2, and right ischial tuberosity suggested as bone metastasis. Also unusual curvilinear increased tracer retention was noted overlapped with sternum and manubrium (arrow) (**a**), which was proven as radiotracer retention along chemoport catheter on regional SPECT/CT image (**b**)

21.2.4 Extravasation of Radiopharmaceutical

Extravasation and subcutaneous infiltration of radiopharmaceutical into surrounding soft tissues induce increased activity at the site of injection, which can make star artifacts on bone scan if large amounts have been leaked [13]. Incidental visualization of the ipsilateral axillary or elbow lymph node has been reported [14, 15]. The lymphatic system is an accessory route for drainage of interstitial fluid. Large molecular weight substances, which cannot be directly absorbed into capillaries, are readily accommodated by lymphatics and incorporated into the chylous network draining into regional nodes. Tc-99m MDP is a large molecular weight substance and therefore is preferentially captured by the lymphatic

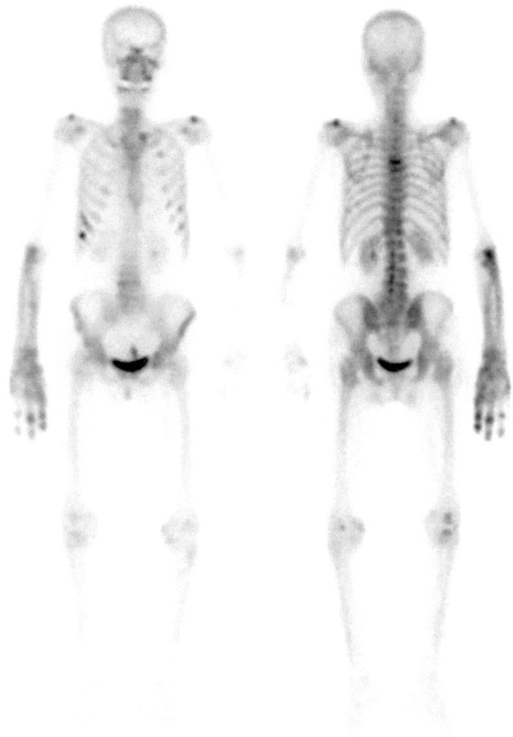

Fig. 21.4 An 82-year-old woman complained of pain in chest wall and upper back after sitting on a massage machine several times. She was injected in her right antecubital vein after binding tightly with rubber tourniquet. Diffusely increased uptake in right arm distal to right elbow injection site is incidentally detected. This finding is associated with tight binding of tourniquet. Focal uptake lesions detected on the right and left anterior thoracic cage were confirmed as acute fractures, and another focal uptake in T5–6 level was revealed as acute compression fracture

system. Axillary lymph node uptake should be differentiated from superimposed bony structure by adding oblique spot views, and not be misinterpreted as a pathologic focus [15, 16].

Case 21.6 Axillary lymph node uptake of extravasated radiopharmaceutical (Fig. 21.6)

21.2.5 Improper Preparation of Radiopharmaceuticals

Case 21.7 Free pertechnetate in stomach and small bowel loops (Fig. 21.7)

21.3 Patient-Related

21.3.1 Influence of Recent Nuclear Medicine Study

Unexpected abnormal uptake lesions can be noted by the influence of recent nuclear medicine study. Prior administration of a higher-energy radionuclide or of a preceding examination with another Tc-99m radiopharmaceutical that accumulates in an organ could obscure or confound skeletal activity [17]. Therefore, relevant information that may assist in interpretation of imaging findings including the history of recent nuclear medicine studies should be checked with the patient before injection of radiopharmaceutical [17, 18].

Case 21.8 Influence of recent nuclear medicine study (Fig. 21.8)

In lymphoscintigraphy using a very small dose, compared to bone scan, most of injected colloid material remains at the intradermal or subdermal injection site and could be seen as focal uptake even 48 h after injection. This could be postulated that intradermal injection of a small dose of Tc-99m colloid has not been cleared via tthe kidney or liver.

21.3.2 Attenuation Artifact

Photon-deficient areas detected on the bone scan are commonly attenuation artifacts caused by metallic objects external to the patients, such as jewelry, pacemakers, coins in pockets, metallic belt buckles, snaps, zippers, and external breast prosthesis. Therefore, patients should be asked to remove metallic objects wherever possible before performing the scan [19]. Photon-deficient areas due to avascular change may be differentiated in some cases.

Case 21.9 Attenuation artifact (Fig. 21.9)

Case 21.10 Differential diagnosis of photon-deficient lesions (Fig. 21.10)

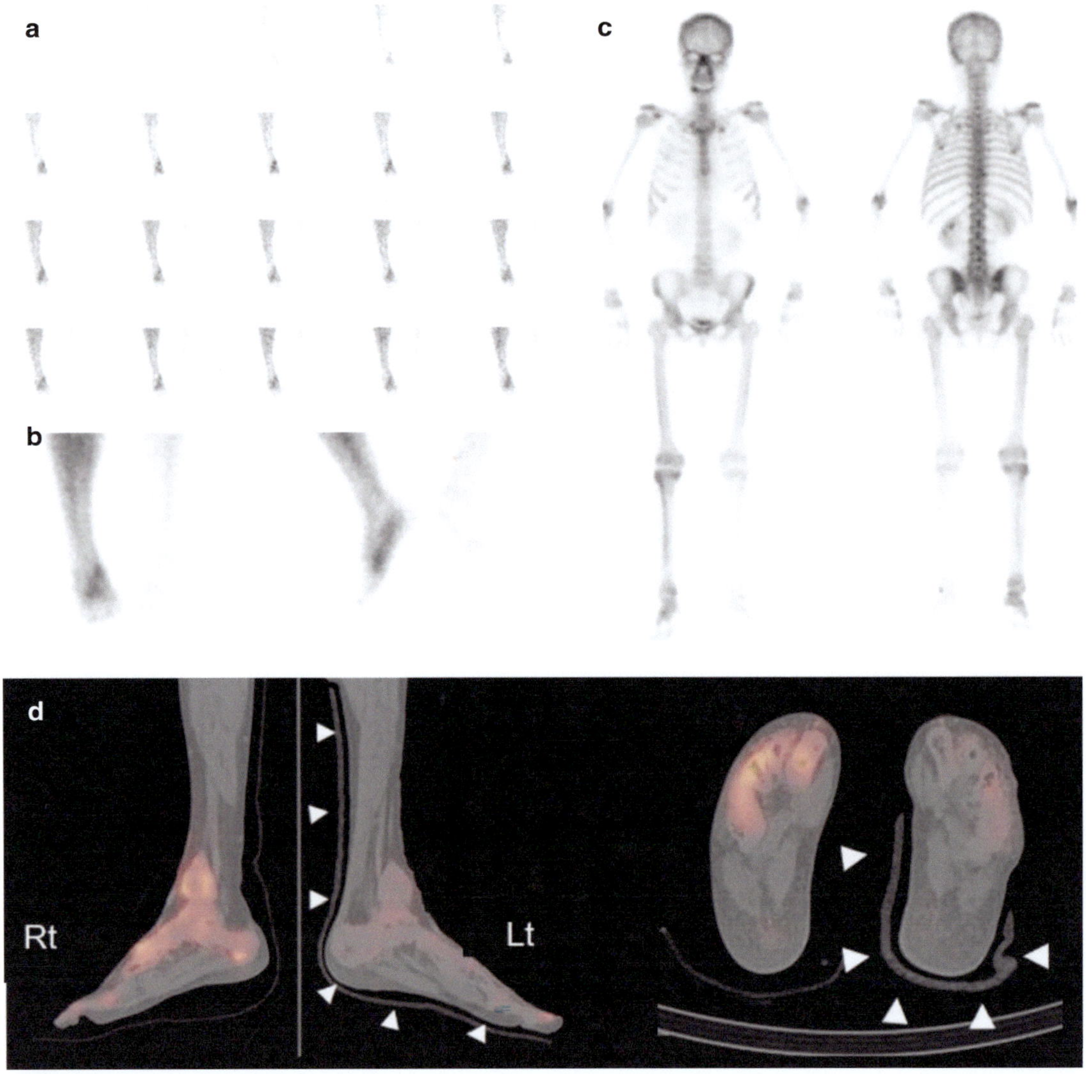

Fig. 21.5 A 52-year-old woman had pain and tenderness in the lateral malleolar area of left ankle after slipping down. Eleven days after trauma, she underwent a three-phase bone scan. Asymmetric diffusely decreased perfusion (**a**), blood pool activity (**b**), and bone uptake (**c**). Above findings could be noted in the chronic phase of complex regional pain syndrome. But the patient's secret was revealed on SPECT/CT image (**d**). She had applied elastic bandage and short leg cast (arrow heads) during three-phase bone scan, which is proved on SPECT/CT image

21.3.3 Optimum Timing of Bone Scan After Trauma

The whole-body bone scan is a highly sensitive modality in the evaluation of fractures, and the majority of fractures will manifest a positive three-phase bone scan immediately, but potential false-negative result is concerned, because it may take up to a week for the scan to become positive in a small percentage of the elderly patients [20, 21].

Case 21.11 Optimum time of bone scan after trauma (Fig. 21.11)

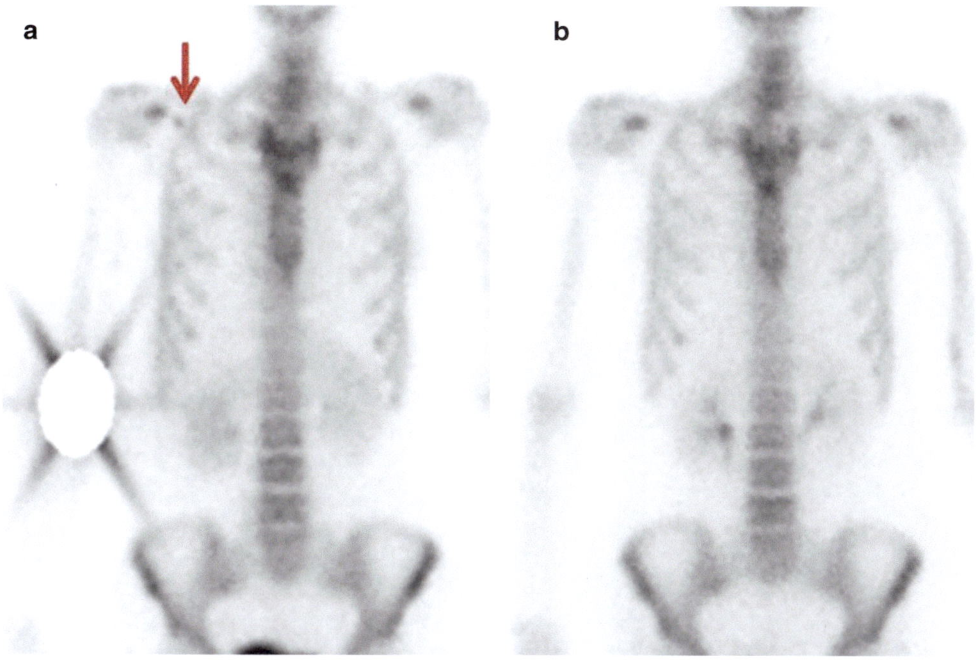

Fig. 21.6 A 36-year-old woman complained of polyarthralgia. Star artifact in right elbow, which resulted from leakage of radiopharmaceutical at the IV site, was masked. There is a focal uptake lesion in the right axillary area (**a**, arrow), axillary lymph node activity, which was newly visualized compared to prior bone scan taken 3 months before (**b**)

Fig. 21.7 A 44-year-old woman with breast cancer and liver metastasis underwent bone scan for evaluation of metastasis. Incidentally detected stomach and small bowel activity in initial bone scan (**a**) but disappeared on followed bone scan after 6 months (**b**). Incidentally detected bowel uptake including stomach could be from free pertechnetate and metastatic calcification. The patient didn't show any clinical condition for metastatic calcification and presents disappearance of bowel uptake on the following image; it was concerned for free pertechnetate activity due to improper preparation

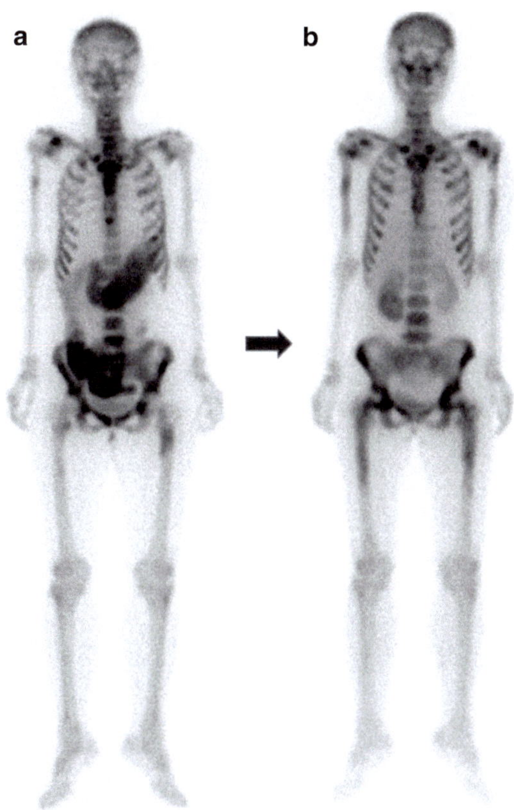

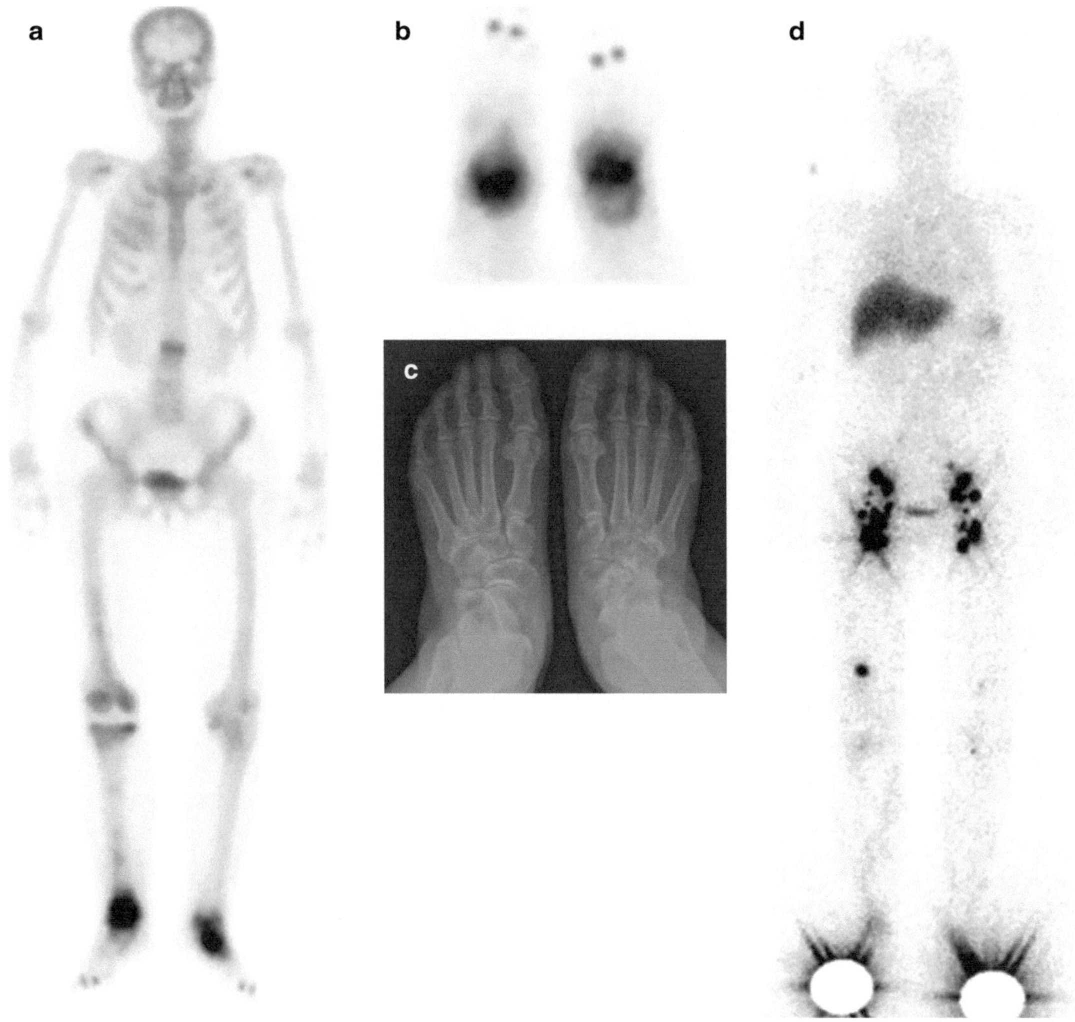

Fig. 21.8 A 65-year-old woman complained with both legs swelling for 3 weeks. She had a 4-year history of rheumatoid arthritis and underwent right total knee replacement 3 months before. On the whole-body bone scan (**a**) and regional images (**b**), there are increased uptake lesions in both ankles and left hind-foot. Unexpectedly, focal spotty uptake lesions are noted in second and third MTP joint area of both feet. There is no demonstrable joint lesion on plain radiograph of both feet (**c**). The definition of lesions is too clear; therefore artificial conditions could be considered. Past history of the patient was reviewed, and it was found that she had lymphoscintigraphy (**d**) 2 days before the whole-body bone scan. Tc-99m phytate (1 mCi syringe was prepared for each site; residual activity in each syringe was about 0.25 mCi, so net injected dose was 0.75 mCi) was given. Intradermal injection of such a small dose of Tc-99m colloid could be remained after 2 days, because it has not been excreted via the kidney or liver

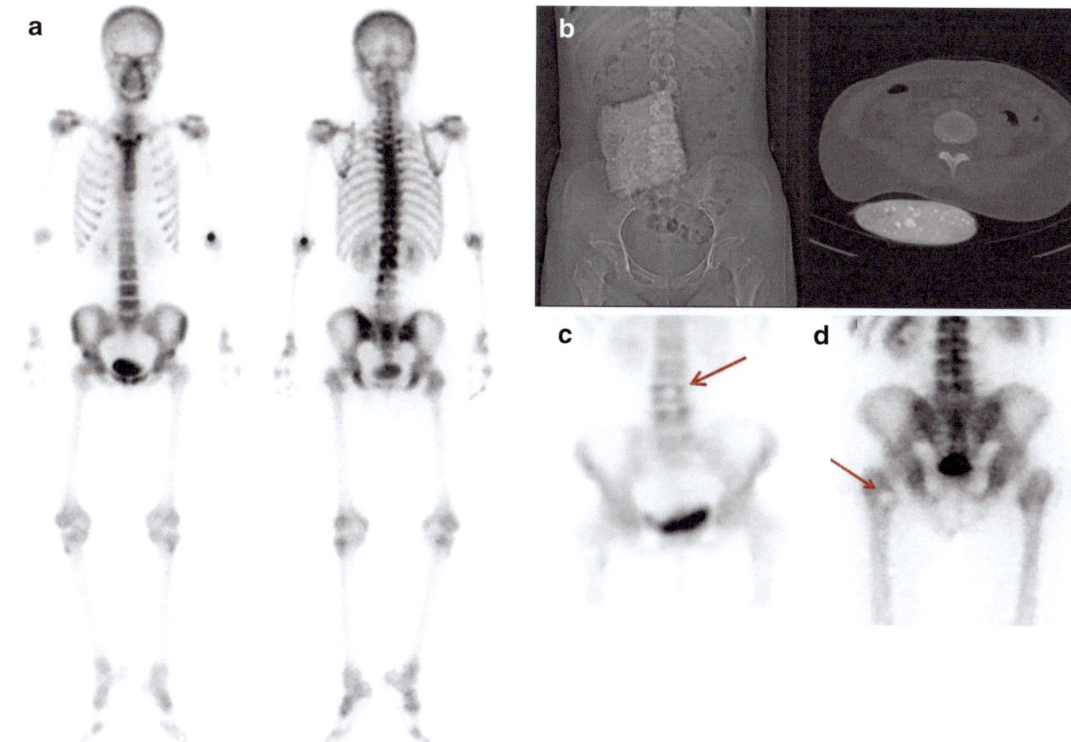

Fig. 21.9 Whole-body bone scan of an 18-year-old girl with intestinal lymphoma shows diffusely decreased uptake in L3–5 level on posterior image (**a**), which has proven to be attenuation artifact due to sandbag applied after bone marrow aspiration biopsy (**b**). Focal decreased uptake associated with attenuation artifacts due to metallic button (**c**) and coin (**d**) is noted

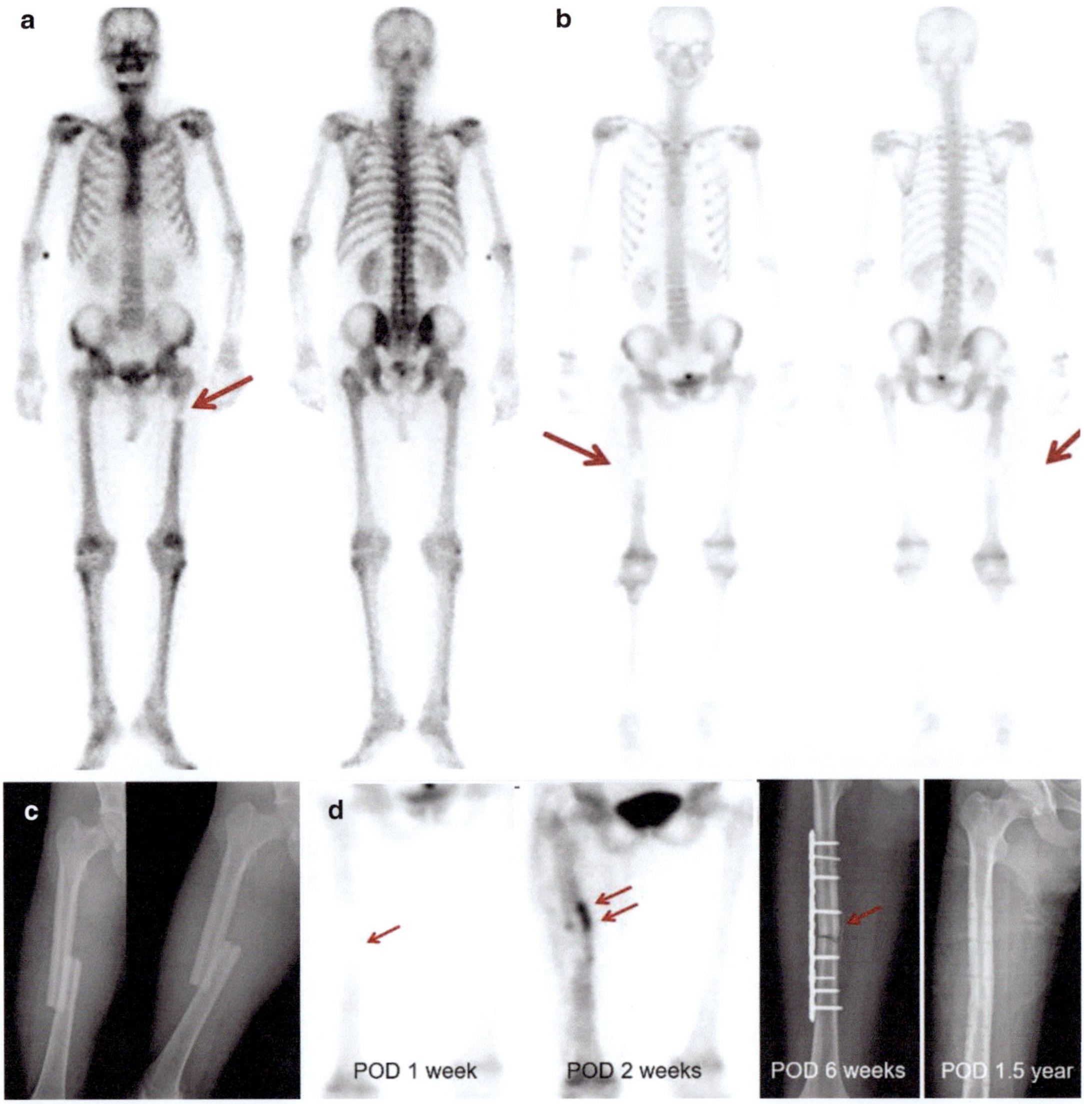

Fig. 21.10 A 75-year-old man with lung cancer shows focal defect in left proximal femoral shaft (**a**), while a 16-year-old boy shows cold defect in right femur mid shaft (**b**). These two patients have similar whole-body bone anterior images, showing cold defects in femur. One is an attenuation artifact, and the other is a true lesion. Guess what? The tip is looking carefully at the posterior images. There is no defect in the left proximal femur on posterior image in (**a**), while there is still noted cold defect in (**b**). The 16-year-old boy has left femur shaft fracture and dislocation (**c**); therefore the cold defect is thought to be avascular change. On followed bone scan and radiographic images (**d**), cortical bone uptake is seen in medial femur, matched with periosteal bone formation, but still noted is cold defect in lateral cortex, suggestive of avascular state. After 1 year, healed fracture with minimal lateral angulation is noted

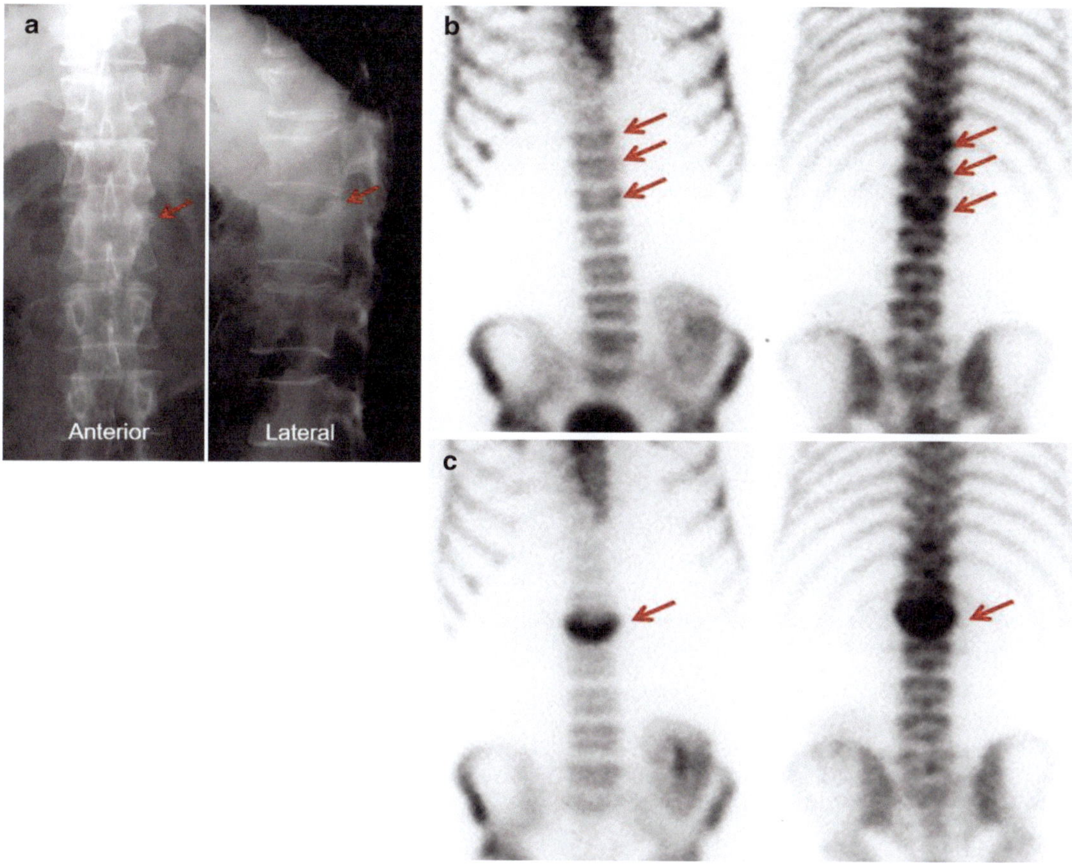

Fig. 21.11 A 58-year-old man had back pain after slipping down. Plain radiograph shows multiple compression fractures in lower T- and upper L-spine (**a**). Bone scans taken after 2 days show subtle uptake in T11-L1 level (**b**). The patient was concerned of acute compression fracture, and bone scan was repeated after 1 week (**c**). L1 showed intense uptake, and T11 and T12 did not show increased activity compared to initial study. Those findings are suggestive of acute compression fracture of L1 and old compression fractures of T11 and T12 level

Teaching Points

- In this section, we reviewed some clinical cases of instrument-related, technique-related, and patient-related pitfalls and artifacts on bone scintigraphy.
- Some of these pitfalls and artifacts were correctly diagnosed with additional SPECT/CT.
- The factors for best possible quality and interpretation include (1) obtaining the relevant clinical information, (2) proper preparation of patients, (3) meticulous positioning of patients and adequate acquisition, (4) familiarity of the normal appearance of different age groups and normal variants, (5) awareness of technical pitfalls, and (6) knowledge of strengths and limitations of each modality.

References

1. Naddaf SY, Collier BD, Elgazzar AH, Magdy MK. Technical errors in planar bone scanning. J Nucl Med Technol. 2004;32:148–53.
2. Wyngaert T, Strobel K, Kampen WU, et al. The EANM practice guidelines for bone scintigraphy. Eur J Nucl Med Mol Imaging. 2016;43:1723–38.
3. Sokole EB, Plachcinski A, Britten A, Georgakopoulou ML, Tindale W, Klett R. Routine quality control recommendations for nuclear medicine instrumentation. Eur J Nucl Med Mol Imaging. 2010;37:662–71.
4. Giammarile F, Mognetti T, Paycha F. Injection artefact displaying "sock" pattern on bone scan: "glove" sign equivalent resulting from bisphosphonate-(99mTc) injection in the foot venous system. Eur J Nucl Med Mol Imaging. 2014;41: 1644–5.
5. Bozkurt MF, Uğur O. Intra-arterial Tc-99m MDP injection mimicking reflex sympathetic dystrophy. Clin Nucl Med. 2001;26:154–6.
6. Gunay EC, Erdogan A. Asymmetrically increased uptake in upper extremities on 99mTc-MDP bone scintigraphy caused by intra-arterial injection: DIFFERENT uptake patterns in three cases. Rev Esp Med Nucl. 2011;30:372–5.
7. Lecklitner ML, Douglas KP. Increased extremity uptake on three-phase bone scans caused by peripherally induced ischemia prior to injection. J Nucl Med. 1987;28:108–11.
8. Kirsh JC, Tepperman PS. Assessment of hand blood flow: a modified technique. Am J Roentgenol. 1985;144:781–3.
9. Orzel JA, Rosenbaum DM, Weinberger E. "Tourniquet effect" can alter delayed static bone scan. Am J Roentgenol. 1989;152:896.
10. Sohn MH, Lim ST, Jeong YJ, Kim DW, Jeong HJ, Yim CY. Abnormally increased uptake on bone scintigraphy in the long bone proximal to a tourniquet: an injection artifact. Clin Nucl Med. 2010;35:349–50.
11. Weiss SC, Conway JJ. An injection technique artifact. J Nuc Med Technol. 1984;12:10–2.
12. Andrich MP, Chen CC. Bone scan injection artifacts. Clin Nucl Med. 1996;21:260–2.
13. Shih WJ, Collins J, Kiefer V. Visualization in the ipsilateral lymph nodes secondary to extravasation of a bone-imaging agent in the left hand: a case report. J Nucl Med Technol. 2001;29:154–5.
14. Ongseng F, Goldfarb R, Finestone H. Axillary lymph node uptake of technetium-99m-MDP. J Nucl Med. 1995;36:1797–9.
15. Wallis JW, Fisher S, Wahl RL. 99Tcm-MDP uptake by lymph nodes following tracer infiltration: clinical and laboratory evaluation. Nucl Med Commun. 1987;8:357–63.
16. Wyngaert T, Strobel K, Kampen WU, et al. The EANM practice guideline for bone scintigraphy. Eur J Nucl Med Mol Imaging. 2016;43:1723–38.
17. Donohoe KJ, Henkin RE, Royal HD, et al. Procedure guideline for bone scintigraphy:1.0. J Nucl Med. 1996;37:1903–6.
18. Gnanasegaran G, Cook G, Adamson K, Fogelman I. Patterns, variants, artifacts, and pitfalls in conventional radionuclide bone imaging and SPECT/CT. Semin Nucl Med. 2009;39:380–95.
19. Martin P. The appearance of bone scans following fractures, including immediate and long-term studies. J Nucl Med. 1979;20:1227–31.
20. The skeletal system. In: Taylor A, Schuster DM, Alazraki N. A clinician's guide to nuclear medicine. 2nd ed. Reston (VA): Society of Nuclear Medicine; 2000, p. 209–229.
21. Weiner GM, Jenicke L, Muller V, Bohuslavizki KH. Artifacts and non-osseous uptake in bone scintigraphy. Imaging reports of 20 cases. Radiol Oncol. 2001;35:185–91.

Index

S.-O. Yang et al. (eds.), *Atlas of Nuclear Medicine in Musculoskeletal System*, https://doi.org/10.1007/978-981-19-2677-8

MIX
Papier aus verantwortungsvollen Quellen
Paper from responsible sources
FSC® C105338
FSC
www.fsc.org

If you have any concerns about our products,
you can contact us on
ProductSafety@springernature.com

In case Publisher is established outside the EU,
the EU authorized representative is:
Springer Nature Customer Service Center GmbH
Europaplatz 3, 69115 Heidelberg, Germany

Printed by Libri Plureos GmbH
in Hamburg, Germany